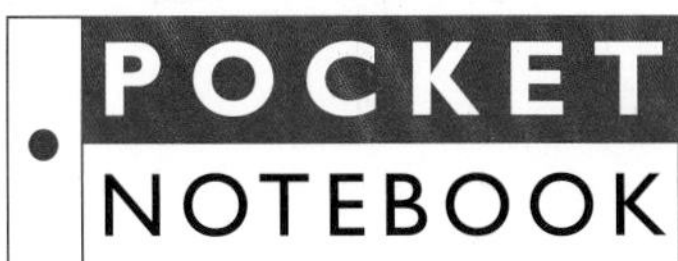

Pocket RADIATION ONCOLOGY

The MD Anderson Cancer Center Handbook of Radiation Oncology

Edited by

CHAD TANG, MD

AHSAN FAROOQI, MD, PhD

Advisors

STEPHEN HAHN, MD

PRAJNAN DAS, MD, MPH

THE UNIVERSITY OF TEXAS
MD Anderson Cancer Center
Making Cancer History®

Wolters Kluwer

Philadelphia • Baltimore • New York • London
Buenos Aires • Hong Kong • Sydney • Tokyo

Acquisitions Editor: Ryan Shaw
Development Editor: Sean McGuire
Editorial Coordinator: Jeremiah Kiely
Editorial Assistant: Kathryn Sherrer
Marketing Manager: Rachel Mante-Leung
Production Project Manager: Sadie Buckallew
Design Coordinator: Elaine Kasmer
Artist/Illustrator: Jen Clements
Manufacturing Coordinator: Beth Welsh
Prepress Vendor: SPi Global

9 8 7 6 5 4 3 2

Printed in China

Library of Congress Cataloging-in-Publication Data
Names: Tang, Chad, editor. | Farooqi, Ahsan, editor. | University of Texas M.D. Anderson Cancer Center, sponsoring body.
Title: Pocket radiation oncology : the MD Anderson Cancer Center handbook of radiation oncology / [edited by] Chad Tang, Ahsan Farooqi.
Other titles: MD Anderson Cancer Center handbook of radiation oncology | Pocket notebook.
Description: Philadelphia : Wolters Kluwer, 2019. | Series: Pocket notebook series | Includes index.
Identifiers: LCCN 2019005774 | ISBN 9781496398574 (loose-leaf)
Subjects: | MESH: Neoplasms—radiotherapy | Handbook
Classification: LCC RC270.3.T65 | NLM QZ 39 | DDC 616.99/407572—dc23 LC record available at https://lccn.loc.gov/2019005774

CCS0220

shop.lww.com

DEDICATION

We dedicate this book in memory of Dr. James D. Cox, MD, who dedicated much of his life to MDACC, RTOG, ABR, and the Red Journal. He was and will always be a lifelong mentor to all past, current, and future trainees in radiation oncology.

CONTRIBUTORS

Mitchell S. Anscher, MD
Professor and Genitourinary Section Chief
Department of Radiation Oncology
University of Texas MD Anderson Cancer Center
Houston, Texas

Alexander Augustyn, MD, PhD
Resident Physician
Department of Radiation Oncology
University of Texas MD Anderson Cancer Center
Houston, Texas

Zeina Ayoub, MD
Clinical Instructor
Department of Radiation Oncology
American University of Beirut Cancer Center
Beirut, Lebanon

Alexander F. Bagley, MD, PhD
Resident Physician
Department of Radiation Oncology
University of Texas MD Anderson Cancer Center
Houston, Texas

Houda Bahig, MD
Staff Radiation Oncologist
Centre hospitalier de l'Université de Montréal
Montréal, Quebec, Canada

Peter Balter, PhD
Professor, Department of Radiation Physics
Division of Radiation Oncology
University of Texas MD Anderson Cancer Center
Houston, Texas

Vincent Bernard, PhD
Postdoctoral Fellow
Translational Molecular Pathology
University of Texas MD Anderson Cancer Center
Houston, Texas

Michael Bernstein, MD
Assistant Attending
Department of Radiation Oncology
Memorial Sloan Kettering Cancer Center
New York City, New York

Andrew J. Bishop, MD
Assistant Professor
Department of Radiation Oncology
University of Texas MD Anderson Cancer Center
Houston, Texas

Eric D. Brooks, MD, MHS
Resident Physician
Department of Radiation Oncology
University of Texas MD Anderson Cancer Center
Houston, Texas

Samantha M. Buszek, MD
Resident Physician
Department of Radiation Oncology
University of Texas MD Anderson Cancer Center
Houston, Texas

Joe Y. Chang, MD, PhD, FASTRO
Professor
Department of Radiation Oncology
University of Texas MD Anderson Cancer Center
Houston, Texas

Bhavana S. Vangara Chapman, MD
Resident Physician
Department of Radiation Oncology
University of Texas MD Anderson Cancer Center
Houston, Texas

Seungtaek Choi, MD
Associate Professor
Department of Radiation Oncology
University of Texas MD Anderson Cancer Center
Houston, Texas

Kaitlin Christopherson, MD
Resident Physician
Department of Radiation Oncology
University of Texas MD Anderson Cancer Center
Houston, Texas

Caroline Chung, MD, MSc
Associate Professor
Department of Radiation Oncology
University of Texas MD Anderson Cancer Center
Houston, Texas

Lauren Elizabeth Colbert, MD, MSCR
Resident Physician
Department of Radiation Oncology
University of Texas MD Anderson Cancer Center
Houston, Texas

Bouthaina Dabaja, MD
Professor and Lymphoma Section Chief
Department of Radiation Oncology
University of Texas MD Anderson cancer center
Houston, Texas

Prajnan Das, MD, MPH
Professor and GI Section Chief
Department of Radiation Oncology
Deputy Department Chair for Education
Residency and Fellowship Program Director
University of Texas MD Anderson Cancer Center
Houston, Texas

Brian J. Deegan, MD, PhD
Radiation Oncologist
Department of Radiation Oncology
Cancer Specialists of North Florida
Jacksonville, Florida

Patricia J. Eifel, MD
Professor
Department of Radiation Oncology
University of Texas MD Anderson Cancer Center
Houston, Texas

Adnan Elhammali, MD, PhD
Resident Physician
Department of Radiation Oncology
University of Texas MD Anderson Cancer Center
Houston, Texas

Penny Fang, MD, MBA
Resident Physician
Department of Radiation Oncology
University of Texas MD Anderson Cancer Center
Houston, Texas

Ahsan Farooqi, MD, PhD
Resident Physician
Department of Radiation Oncology
University of Texas MD Anderson Cancer Center
Houston, Texas

Steven J. Frank, MD
Professor and Deputy Division Head
Department of Radiation Oncology
University of Texas MD Anderson Cancer Center
Houston, Texas

Clifton David Fuller, MD, PhD
Associate Professor
Department of Radiation Oncology
University of Texas MD Anderson Cancer Center
Houston, Texas

Adam Seth Garden, MD
Professor
Department of Radiation Oncology
University of Texas MD Anderson Cancer Center
Houston, Texas

Amol Jitendra Ghia, MD
Associate Professor
Department of Radiation Oncology
University of Texas MD Anderson Cancer Center
Houston, Texas

Daniel Gomez, MD
Associate Professor and Thoracic Section Chief
University of Texas MD Anderson Cancer Center
Houston, Texas

Stephen Grant, MD
Resident Physician
Department of Radiation Oncology
University of Texas MD Anderson Cancer Center
Houston, Texas

Aaron Joseph Grossberg, MD, PhD
Assistant Professor
Department of Radiation Medicine
Cancer Early Detection Advanced Research Center
Brenden-Colson Center for Pancreatic Care
Oregon Health and Science University
Portland, Oregon

David Grosshans, MD, PhD
Associate Professor
Department of Radiation Oncology
University of Texas MD Anderson Cancer Center
Houston, Texas

B. Ashleigh Guadagnolo, MD, MPH
Professor and Sarcoma Section Chief
Department of Radiation Oncology
University of Texas MD Anderson Cancer Center
Houston, TX

Jillian Gunther, MD, PhD
Assistant Professor
Department of Radiation Oncology
University of Texas MD Anderson Cancer Center
Houston, Texas

Stephen Hahn, MD
Professor
Department of Radiation Oncology
University of Texas MD Anderson Cancer Center
Chief Medical Executive
Houston, Texas

Jennifer C. Ho, MD
Resident Physician
Department of Radiation Oncology
University of Texas MD Anderson Cancer Center
Houston, Texas

Karen Elizabeth Hoffman, MD, MPH
Associate Professor
Department of Radiation Oncology
University of Texas MD Anderson Cancer Center
Houston, Texas

Emma B. Holliday, MD
Assistant Professor
Department of Radiation Oncology
University of Texas MD Anderson Cancer Center
Houston, Texas

Anuja Jhingran, MD
Professor
Department of Radiation Oncology
University of Texas MD Anderson Cancer Center
Houston, Texas

Ann H. Klopp, MD
Associate Professor and Gynecology Section Chief
Department of Radiation Oncology
University of Texas MD Anderson Cancer Center
Houston, Texas

Albert C. Koong, MD, PhD
Professor and Chair
Department of Radiation Oncology
University of Texas MD Anderson Cancer Center
Houston, Texas

Rachit Kumar, MD
Adjunct Assistant Professor
Division of Radiation Oncology
Banner MD Anderson Cancer Center
Gilbert, Arizona

Jing Li, MD, PhD
Associate Professor and CNS/Pediatric Section co-Chief
Department of Radiation Oncology
University of Texas MD Anderson Cancer Center
Houston, Texas

Anna Likhacheva, MD, MPH
Adjunct Assistant Professor
Department of Radiation Oncology
Banner MD Anderson Cancer Center
Gilbert, Arizona

Lilie L. Lin, MD
Associate Professor
Department of Radiation Oncology
University of Texas MD Anderson Cancer Center
Houston, Texas

Jennifer Logan, MD
Resident Physician
Department of Radiation Oncology
University of Texas MD Anderson Cancer Center
Houston, Texas

Ethan Bernard Ludmir, MD
Resident Physician
Department of Radiation Oncology
University of Texas MD Anderson Cancer Center
Houston, Texas

Geoffrey V. Martin, MD
Resident Physician
Department of Radiation Oncology
University of Texas MD Anderson Cancer Center
Houston, Texas

Mary Frances McAleer, MD, PhD
Associate Professor
Department of Radiation Oncology
University of Texas MD Anderson Cancer Center
Houston, Texas

Shane Mesko, MD, MBA
Resident Physician
Department of Radiation Oncology
University of Texas MD Anderson Cancer Center
Houston, Texas

Sarah Milgrom, MD
Assistant Professor
Department of Radiation Oncology
University of Colorado
Denver Colorado

Bruce Minsky, MD
Professor and Frank T. McGraw Memorial Chair
Department of Radiation Oncology
University of Texas MD Anderson Cancer Center
Houston, Texas

Shalini Moningi, MD
Resident Physician
Department of Radiation Oncology
University of Texas MD Anderson Cancer Center
Houston, Texas

Amy C. Moreno, MD
Resident Physician
Department of Radiation Oncology
University of Texas MD Anderson Cancer Center
Houston, Texas

Quynh-Nhu Nguyen, MD
Associate Professor
Department of Radiation Oncology
University of Texas MD Anderson Cancer Center
Houston, Texas

Hubert Young Pan, MD
Resident Physician
Department of Radiation Oncology
University of Texas MD Anderson Cancer Center
Houston, Texas

Dario Pasalic, MD
Resident Physician
Department of Radiation Oncology
University of Texas MD Anderson Cancer Center
Houston, Texas

Arnold C. Paulino, MD
Professor and CNS/Pediatric Section co-Chief
Department of Radiation Oncology
University of Texas MD Anderson Cancer Center
Houston, Texas

Curtis A. Pettaway, MD
Professor
Department of Urology
University of Texas MD Anderson Cancer Center
Houston, Texas

Jack Phan, MD, PhD
Associate Professor
Department of Radiation Oncology
University of Texas MD Anderson Cancer Center
Houston, Texas

Chelsea C. Pinnix, MD, PhD
Associate Professor
Department of Radiation Oncology
University of Texas MD Anderson Cancer Center
Houston, Texas

Courtney Pollard III, MD, PhD
Resident Physician
Department of Radiation Oncology
University of Texas MD Anderson Cancer Center
Houston, Texas

Jay Paul Reddy, MD, PhD
Assistant Professor
Department of Radiation Oncology
University of Texas MD Anderson Cancer Center
Houston, Texas

Mohammed Salehpour, PhD
Professor and Director of Education
Department of Radiation Physics
University of Texas MD Anderson Cancer Center
Houston, Texas

Tommy Sheu, MD, MPH
Resident Physician
Department of Radiation Oncology
University of Texas MD Anderson Cancer Center
Houston, Texas

Shervin 'Sean' Shirvani, MD, MPH
Adjunct Assistant Professor
Department of Radiation Oncology
Banner MD Anderson Cancer Center
Gilbert, Arizona

Lisa Singer, MD, PhD
Instructor
Department of Radiation Oncology
Dana-Farber Cancer Institute and Brigham and Women's Hospital
Boston, Massachusetts

Shane R. Stecklein, MD, PhD
Resident Physician
Department of Radiation Oncology
University of Texas MD Anderson Cancer Center
Houston, Texas

Erik P. Sulman, MD, PhD
Professor and Vice-Chair of Research
Department of Radiation Oncology
Co-Director, Brain Tumor Center
Laura and Isaac Perlmutter Cancer Center
New York City, New York

Chad Tang, MD
Assistant Professor
Department of Radiation Oncology
University of Texas MD Anderson Cancer Center
Houston, Texas

Cullen Taniguchi, MD, PhD
Assistant Professor
Department of Radiation Oncology
University of Texas MD Anderson Cancer Center
Houston, Texas

Nikhil G. Thaker, MD
Radiation Oncologist
Division of Radiation Oncology
Arizona Oncology/The US Oncology Network
Tucson, Arizona

Jeena Varghese, MD
Assistant Professor
Department of Endocrine Neoplasia and Hormonal Disorders
University of Texas MD Anderson Cancer Center
Houston, Texas

Gary Walker, MD, MPH
Staff Physician
Department of Radiation Oncology
Banner MD Anderson Cancer Center
Gilbert, Arizona

Christopher Wilke, MD, PhD
Assistant Professor
Department of Radiation Oncology
University of Minnesota
Minneapolis, Minnesota

Wendy Woodward, MD, PhD
Associate Professor and Breast Section Chief
Department of Radiation Oncology
University of Texas MD Anderson Cancer Center
Houston, Texas

Debra Nana Yeboa, MD
Assistant Professor
Department of Radiation Oncology
University of Texas MD Anderson Cancer Center
Houston, Texas

FOREWORD

In the fast-paced world we live in today, it can be challenging to find time to keep abreast of the current standards of care and the constantly evolving technologic and practical innovations. National guidelines are often too vague when it comes to how we deliver radiation therapy for specific disease sites, and textbooks are either too broad or too lengthy for practitioners to interpret key concepts necessary to deliver care. While we recognize that there are other pocket books available, we have intentionally narrowed our focus and scope of this pocket handbook to include the best practices that we have determined are necessary to deliver safe, multidisciplinary evidence-based care to our patients. This was accomplished through capturing years of experience and expertise of senior radiation oncologists at MD Anderson, many of which created the cutting edge technologies discussed in this handbook. The MD Anderson residents and fellows both past and current played a major part in the creation of this pocket handbook and reviewed each of the chapters.

The goal of this pocket handbook is to provide a snapshot in a user-friendly presentation that can be used to guide the active management and review of specific cases. While we acknowledge that it is not a comprehensive resource, the handbook provides the basic fundamentals that can guide the practitioner with the necessary tools and information to dig deeper into specific cases.

In this handbook, we have covered all of the major stages of commonly treated diseases and included treatment techniques for both common and rare malignancies. Unlike most pocket references, we have a section that is dedicated to treatment planning and dose constraints. This section also includes specific figures which are helpful in determining how blocks should be drawn and which areas should be avoided during radiation therapy. We also provide insight into emerging technologies and identify clinical pearls related to these technologies as well as areas of concern that could lead to catastrophic complications.

Recognizing the limited time that physicians and trainees have, we included only those specific references that drive the current clinical standards. We hope that this handbook will serve as a valuable resource for you and your peers as we endeavor to provide appropriate, safe, and quality care to our patients.

ALBERT C. KOONG, MD, PHD
Professor and Department Chair, Radiation Oncology

JOSEPH M. HERMAN, MD
Professor and Division Head, Radiation Oncology

PREFACE

We are delighted to introduce the first edition of *Pocket Radiation Oncology: The MD Anderson Cancer Center Handbook of Radiation Oncology*. While there are many excellent textbooks on radiation oncology, in an era of constantly evolving evidence and rapidly changing technology, there appears to be great need for an easily accessible handbook with clinically relevant and evidence-based information, presented in a concise and easily accessible format. We feel that this handbook will appeal to the learning styles of today's generation of adult learners.

We are grateful to all the contributors at the University of Texas MD Anderson Cancer Center who made *Pocket Radiation Oncology* possible. All chapters were created by current or past members of the MD Anderson Cancer Center, Department of Radiation Oncology. The chapters were created by resident and attending pairs, and all chapters were reviewed by a senior attending who specialized in that disease site. We are also grateful to the past and present faculty at the University of Texas MD Anderson Cancer Center, whose clinical experience and knowledge is reflected in this handbook.

STEPHEN HAHN AND PRAJNAN DAS, ADVISORS

CONTENTS

THORACIC

Section Editors: Eric D. Brooks, Daniel Gomez

GASTROINTESTINAL

Section Editors: Lauren Elizabeth Colbert, Prajnan Das

BREAST

Section Editors: Jennifer Logan, Amy C. Moreno, Wendy Woodward

GENITOURINARY

Section Editors: Geoffrey V. Martin, Shalini Moningi, Mitchell S. Anscher

GYNECOLOGIC

Section Editors: Shane R. Stecklein, Ann H. Klopp

SKIN/SARCOMA

Section Editors: Kaitlin Christopherson, B. Ashleigh Guadagnolo

LYMPHOMA

Section Editors: Tommy Sheu, Bouthaina Dabaja

RADIATION EMERGENCIES, BENIGN DISEASE, AND PALLIATION

Section Editors: Adnan Elhammali, Amol Jitendra Ghia

RADIATION BIOLOGY

AARON JOSEPH GROSSBERG • AHSAN FAROOQI • CULLEN TANIGUCHI

4 Rs of Radiobiology

- **Repair**
  Lethal and sublethal ***damage repair*** *increases cell survival after fractionated radiation*
- **Reoxygenation**
  Hypoxic cells *are radioresistant; hypoxic fraction ↑ with treatment.*
- **Redistribution**
  Lethality increases as cells redistribute to more radiosensitive stages of ***cell cycle****.*
- **Repopulation**
  Repopulation increases cell survival over ***long treatment time****; accelerated in some cancers.*

Molecular Signaling and Pathways

- **Oncogene:** Normal function is to positively regulate cellular growth, that is *RAS, MYC, ABL, ERBB2.*
- **Tumor suppressor gene:** Normal function is to negatively regulate cellular growth, that is *TP53, RB, VHL, PTEN.*
- **Cellular signaling pathways**
  - EGFR-MAPK: Pro-survival pathway involving the EGFR family of tyrosine kinases
    - EGFR (ErbB-1): Targeting by cetuximab
    - HER2/neu (ErbB-2): Targeted by trastuzumab
    - Her3 and Her4: Not as commonly mutated in cancer
  - Ras: G protein bound to cellular membrane that transmits signals from activated tyrosine kinases
    - K-RAS: Mutated in colon and lung cancer
    - N-RAS: Mutated in neuroblastoma
    - H-RAS: Bladder cancer
- VEGFR: Leads to angiogenesis, also involves tyrosine kinase pathways. Targeted by bevacizumab
- PI3K-Akt-mTOR pathway: PI3K is a membrane-bound protein that is negatively regulated by PTEN, and whose downstream targets include Akt and mTOR, which activate cellular survival, proliferation, and angiogenesis. Targeted by rapamycin, temsirolimus, and everolimus (immune-suppressive drugs), which can also inhibit various cancers that activate this pathway (ie, renal cell carcinoma)
- BCR-ABL: Tyrosine kinase pathway activated in chronic myelogenous leukemia (via classic 9:22 translocation) that is targeted by imatinib
- ALK: Tyrosine kinase that is pro-survival and found mutated in NSCLC and hereditary neuroblastoma. Targeted by ALK inhibitor crizotinib

Telomeres, Telomerase and Cancer

- Due to the end-replication problem, a cell loses between 50 and 200 bp per cell division.
- Telomeres are repetitive elements consisting of the (TTAGGG)n repeats found at the ends of our chromosomes that serve as a buffer to our coding DNA.
- After ~40-50 population doublings, most cell lines in culture reach critically short telomere lengths, which triggers senescence/apoptosis (Hayflick limit).
- Cancer cells counteract telomere shortening by activating telomere maintenance mechanisms.
  - Telomerase: Activated in ~85% of all cancers. Increased telomerase activity has been associated with mutations in the *TERT* promoter gene (which encodes the catalytic component of telomerase) seen in tumors of neural or mesenchymal origin (*Killela PNAS* 2013).
  - Alternative lengthening of telomeres: Activated in 10%-15% of cancers. Poorly understood mechanism but thought to utilize homologous recombination machinery to maintain telomere length

DNA Damage and Repair

- **DNA damage:** Defined as any covalent modifications of the nucleotide backbone (exception being cytosine methylation)
  - Occurs at a high frequency from both endogenous and exogenous sources

- Approximately 1 Gy of ionizing radiation leads to ~40 double-strand breaks (DSBs), >1000 base damages, and ~1000 single-strand breaks (SSBs)
- DNA repair pathways
  - Base excision repair (*APE1, PCNA, FEN1, XRCC1*): Functions to repair base damage utilizing DNA glycosylase and endonucleases
  - Nucleotide excision repair: Can be initiated by either the global genomic pathway (*ERCC1, XPF, XPG*) or transcription coupled (stalled RNA polymerase complexes). Defects in this pathway lead to hereditary xeroderma pigmentosum.
  - Mismatch repair: *MLH1 MSH2, MSH4, MSH6*. Functions to excise the incorrect nucleotide and replace with the correct one. Mutations in genes involved in this pathway lead to microsatellite instability (MSI) and hereditary nonpolyposis colorectal cancer (HNPCC).
  - Nonhomologous end joining (NHEJ): Immediate response of a cell to correct a DNA double-strand break. Compared to homologous recombination, this process is rapid but is more prone to errors. First there is end recognition by binding of Ku proteins → recruitment of DNA-dependent protein kinases (DNA-PKcs) → end-processing, bridging, and ligation. Typically active in the G1 phase of the cell cycle, where there is no sister chromatid
  - Homologous recombination: High-fidelity mechanism compared to NHEJ for repair of DNA DSBs. Requires sequence homology to rejoin the broken DNA ends; hence this repair process is active in the S and G2 phases of the cell cycle. Following ATM-mediated DNA DSB recognition, the Mre11/Rad50/NBS1 complex is recruited for 3′ end resection. RAD51/RAD52 then mediate strand invasion of the homologous strand on the sister chromatid in conjunction with BRCA1 and BRCA2 proteins. Inactivation of HRR genes greatly increase radiosensitivity in *in vitro* models.

Mechanisms of Cell Death

- DNA is the target of radiation-induced cell lethality.
- Apoptosis: Programmed cell death mechanism that is common in embryonic development. Primary mode of cell death in hemopoietic and lymphoid cells following radiation. Importantly, this is a p53-mediated cellular death pathway (which is mutated in numerous cancers). BCL-2 counteracts the initiation of apoptosis. Can be initiated by the extrinsic pathway (via FAS-L and TRAILR) or intrinsic pathway (as a result of DNA damage, hypoxia, and metabolic stress). Both pathways lead to activation of caspases that disrupt mitochondrial outer membrane permeabilization leading to cytochrome c release and subsequent chromatin condensation → DNA fragmentation → cell death.
- Mitotic catastrophe: Results from aberrated mitosis due to radiation-induced lethal DNA DSBs. Primary mode of death following radiation in nonhematopoietic cells. Many tumors have deficient p53 and abrogated cell-cycle checkpoints that allow cells to progress into G2/M despite sustaining DNA DSBs as a result of radiation. **The three major lethal chromosomal aberrations induced from radiation are formation of dicentric chromosomes, rings, and anaphase bridges.**
- Radiation-induced senescence: Has been reported in in vitro models following extensive stress due to DNA damage induced from radiation. Classically, senescence (or permanent cellular arrest) occurs as a result of telomere shortening due to aging. However, DNA damage that results from low doses of radiation can induce accelerated senescence due to a persistently up-regulated DNA damage response proteins. There is some clinical evidence of radiation-induced senescence in slow growing tumors following radiation (ie, prostate cancer).

Acute Effects of Total Body Irradiation

- **LD_{50}**
  - **3.25-4 Gy** (without treatment)
  - **~7 Gy** (with antibiotics, supportive care)
  - **~10 Gy** (with BMT)
  - *No survivors >10 Gy exposure*
- **Prodromal syndrome**
  - <50% lethal dose: Easy fatigability, anorexia, vomiting
  - Supralethal dose: Fever, hypotension, immediate diarrhea

Vomiting Onset	Est. Dose
<10 min	>8 Gy
10-30 min	6-8 Gy
30 min to 1 h	4-6 Gy
1-2 h	2-4 Gy
>2 h	<2 Gy

- **REAC/TS triage based on vomiting onset time**
  - Vomit <4 hours → immediate hospital evaluation (median dose 3.6 Gy)
  - Vomit >4 hours → delayed (1-3 days) hospital evaluation (median dose 0.9 Gy)

- **Hematopoietic syndrome**
  - Dose: 2.5-5 Gy
  - Time: Death within 4-8 weeks
  - Symptoms: (1) Prodromal syndrome; (2) latent period; (3) ~3 weeks → chills, fatigue, petechial hemorrhages, loss of hair, infections (usually anemia not seen)
- **GI syndrome**
  - Dose: 5-12 Gy
  - Time: Death in 9-10 days, due to loss of intestinal lining
  - Symptoms: (1) Prodromal syndrome; (2) prolonged diarrhea (indicates *dose >10 Gy*)
- **Cerebrovascular syndrome**
  - Dose: >100 Gy
  - Time: Death in hours, due to capillary leakage in brain
  - Symptoms: (1) Nausea/vomiting *in minutes*; (2) disorientation, loss of coordination of muscular movement, respiratory distress, diarrhea, convulsive seizures, coma
- **Treatment**
  - <2 Gy: No treatment
  - 2-5 Gy: Expectant management (eg, antibiotics, transfusions)
  - 5-7 Gy: Prophylactic antibiotics, transfusions
  - 8-10 Gy: Bone marrow transplant
  - >10 Gy: GI death; supportive care
  - Colony-stimulating factors given for >2-3 Gy within 24-72 hours

Normal Tissue Toxicity

- **Early effects** <60 days; rapid cell turnover, due to acute cell killing; repaired within 2 months
  - High α/β; less sensitive to fraction size; toxicity based on total Gy and Gy/week
  - Prolonging radiation allows for repopulation (↓ acute effects)
  - **Latency period** = lifespan of functional cell
- **Late effects** >60 days; tissues without rapid turnover; **never completely repaired**
  - Low α/β; more sensitive to *fraction size*; toxicity based on *total Gy* and *Gy/fx*
  - *Fractionation decreases late effects, but not over a clinically relevant time.*
- **Serial organ:** Loss of function in one part causes whole organ dysfunction (CNS; GI tract).
  - No threshold volume; probability of damage proportional to volume irradiated
  - Risk dominated by D_{max}
- **Parallel organ:** Loss of function in one part only impacts that part (kidney; lung; liver).
  - Threshold volume effect
  - Risk dominated by **average dose** or **volume receiving threshold dose**
- **Skin tolerance:** ~60 Gy (depending on volume irradiated and fractionation)
  - Acute effects occur in epidermis: Erythema (rapid); desquamation (~14 days); epilation (~2-3 weeks, takes ~3 months to regrow)
  - Late effects occur in dermis: Telangiectasias and fibrosis

Oxygen Effects

- **Most potent modifying factor of cell kill by ionizing radiation**
- **Must be present within microseconds of IR**
  - **"Oxygen fixation"**: Formation of peroxyl radical permanently changes DNA structure.
  - Hydroxyl radical (·OH) most important radical for indirect damage to DNA
- **Oxygen enhancement ratio** $\frac{d_{hypoxic}}{d_{oxic}}$
  - OER range 2.5-3.0 (typically 2.8)
  - Requires very little O_2 (3 mm Hg or ~0.5% O_2)
  - Higher LET reduces OER.
  - Optimal LET: 100 keV/μM (width of double helix)
- **Tumor hypoxia**
  - Hypoxic cells thought to be "treatment resistant"
  - Diffusional capacity of O_2 **~**180 μM from capillary
  - Typical hypoxic fraction ~10%-15% with standard fractionation
  - Hypoxic fraction ↑ as tumor size ↑
  - Hypoxic fraction ↑ as dose/fx ↑

- **Therapeutic approaches to hypoxia**
  - Raising tumor oxygenation: 100% O_2, hyperbaric, carbogen, transfusion, nicotinamide
  - Hypoxic cell sensitization
  - Nimorazole was tested as a hypoxic radiosensitizer in supraglottic laryngeal and pharyngeal cancer by the Danish HNC. It was found to improve LRC (49% vs 33%) and DSS (52% vs 41%) w/ minor side effects *(Overgaard et al. Radiother Oncol 1998)*
  - Hypoxic cell cytotoxins: Mitomycin C, doxorubicin, metronidazole, tirapazamine (no clear hypoxia-modulating clinical benefit shown)

Radioprotectors

Goal: Enhance therapeutic ratio

- Reoxygenation: Vasoconstriction or free radical scavenging
  - **Sulfhydryl compounds (amifostine)**, SOD, DMSO, CO, NaCN, epinephrine
- Repair: H donation to facilitate repair
  - **Sulfhydryl compounds (amifostine)**, glutathione, cysteine
- Reassortment: Induce senescence via p53; cell-cycle arrest
- Repopulation: Enhance stem cell growth
  - For example R-spondin for intestinal stem cells

Amifostine is the only FDA-approved radioprotector

- Administer 30 minutes prior to RT; reduces mucositis and xerostomia (head and neck ca); pneumonitis and esophagitis (lung ca)
  - More effective if given in *morning*
- Selective for normal tissue because
  - Requires alk phos to activate (low in tumor tissue)
  - Hypovascularity and hypoxia of tumor limits amifostine penetration
  - Acidic environment of tumor prevents activation
- Side effects: Nausea and hypotension (~60% of pts; BP reverts w/in 15 minutes)

Carcinogenesis and Heritable Effects

Effective dose-Sievert (Sv) weighted for both radiation type and volume of tissue irradiated

$$\text{Effective dose (Sv)} = \text{dose (Gy)} \times \text{WF} \times \text{fraction of tissue irradiated}$$

- Photon/e^- *WF = 1*; proton *WF = 2*; neutron *WF up to 20*; heavy ion *WF = 20*
- Can be calculated per *tissue* or per *whole body*

Average annual human exposure to ionizing radiation

- World: 3 mSv/y
- USA: 6 mSv/y
- **Deterministic:** Effect occurs after exceeding threshold dose and severity correlates with dose.
  - For example skin erythema, epilation, sterility, cataracts, lethality, fetal abnormality
- **Stochastic:** Effect occurs randomly with probability proportional to dose (no safe threshold).
  - For example secondary malignancies and heritable effects

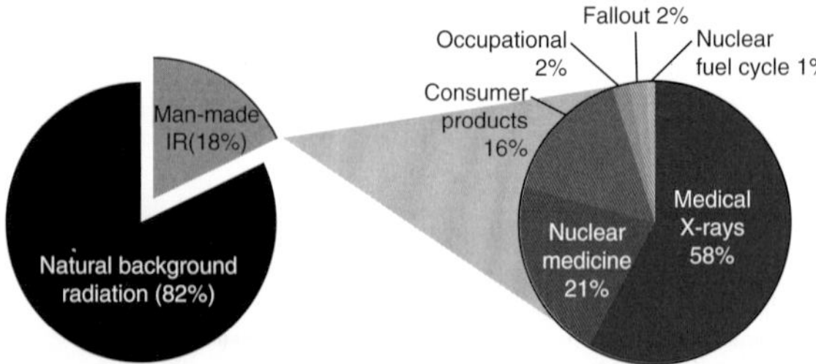

Data from the National Council on Radiation Protection and Measurements (NCRP). Report No. 93, Ionizing Radiation Exposure of the Population of the United States, 1987.

Radiation carcinogenesis

- **Solid tumors**
  - Within radiation field receiving >50 cGy
  - latency ≥5 years
  - Usually different tumor type than original
- **Leukemia**
  - latency ≥5 years
  - bone marrow >50 cGy
  - non-CLL
- Cancer induction: *Carcinogen dominant*
  - ↑ incidence of uncommon cancers assoc. w/ ↑ carcinogen exposure
  - Exposure stigmata (long-standing changes in affected tissues)
    - Radium-bone, aniline dye-bladder, uranium-lung, chimney sweep-scrotal, ALL
- Cancer enhancement: Predominant mechanism—*carcinogen participant*
  - ↑ incidence of common cancers assoc. w/ ↓ carcinogen exposure
  - Normal-appearing affected tissue
    - Thyroid (well-diff), breast, skin (SCC/BCC ≫ sarcoma), ovary, lung, colon
    - RT for Hodgkin's ↑ breast ca risk (RR = 3.2 at 4 Gy; RR = 8 at 40 Gy)
    - RT for prostate ↑ secondary ca (rectal, bladder, sarcoma) RR = 1.34 at 10 years

Risk estimate for malignancy

- **10%/Sv** for entire population and high dose (>0.2 Gy) or dose rate (>0.1 Gy/h)
- **8%/Sv** for working population and high dose or dose rate
- **5%/Sv** for entire population and low dose or dose rate
- **4%/Sv** for working population and low dose or dose rate

Hereditary effects: Radiation effects that can be transferred from parent to progeny

- Radiation-caused changes in the genetic material of sex cells (germ-line mutations)
- Radiation does not produce new, unique mutations but *increases the incidence* of the same mutations that occur spontaneously.
- Doubling dose (increase spontaneous mutation rate two-fold) = 1 Gy

Fertility effects

- **Male: >0.15 Gy** causes temporary infertility.
  - **3.5-6 Gy** causes permanent sterility.
  - 10-week delay for onset of infertility after exposure
  - can take up to 6 months for fertility to return
- **Female: 2.6-6 Gy** causes permanent infertility
  - sensitivity ↑ with age

ICRP risk estimate for hereditary effects (calculated using gonad dose)

0.41%-0.64%/Sv/child of an irradiated individual

Total population **0.2%/Sv/individual;** working population **0.1%/Sv/individual**

Not more than 1%-6% of spontaneous mutations ascribed to background radiation

Individual dose limits

- General public: 5 mSv total body, 15 mSv lens, 50 mSv other single organ
  - Continuous exposure: 1 mSv total body
- Radiation worker: 50 mSv total body, 150 mSv lens, 500 mSv other single organ
- Monthly limit of *declared pregnant woman* is **0.5 mSv/mo**

Area dose limits

- Uncontrolled area: ≤0.02 mSv/h and ≤0.1 mSv/wk
- Controlled area: ≤1 mSv/wk

Imaging	mSv	mrem	cGy
CXR	0.05	5	0.005
KUB	1	100	0.1
PET	4	400	0.4
Whole body CT	~10	1000	1

Effects on the Embryo and Fetus

- **Sensitive period: 10 days to 26 weeks of gestation**
- **Preimplantation (0-9 days)**
  - Very low dose (0.05-0.15 Gy) leads to *prenatal death*; all or nothing effect

- **Organogenesis (10 days to 6 weeks)**
  - Structural malformation and IUGR most common; growth restriction resolves over time
  - Threshold dose >0.2 Gy
- **Fetal stage (>6 weeks)**
  - LD_{50} approaches that of adults (~3.5 Gy)
  - *Permanent* growth disturbances *without* malformation
- **Dose**
  - Microcephaly >10-19 cGy
  - Cognitive decline as low as 10 cGy; <5 cGy *probably* acceptable risk
  - Discussion of birth defects and possible actions at doses >0.1 cGy
  - Therapeutic abortion considered above 10 cGy to embryo during 10 days to 26 weeks
  - Max permissible dose to fetus is 5 mSv (0.5 rem); 0.5 mSv/mo (0.05 rem)
- **Teratogenesis**
  - Exposure of 1 cGy ↑ relative risk of cancer by 40%
  - Absolute excess risk is ~6%/Gy.

Equivalent Dose

- $\text{BED}_{\alpha/\beta} = n \times d \times \left(1 + \frac{d}{\alpha/\beta}\right)$
- $\text{EQD}_{2Gy} = n \times d \times \left(\frac{\alpha/\beta + d}{\alpha/\beta + 2}\right)$
- $\text{EQD}_{\alpha/\beta} = n \times d_2 \times \left(\frac{\alpha/\beta + d_2}{\alpha/\beta + d_1}\right)$

n = no. of fractions
d = dose/fraction

Linear Energy Transfer

Radiation	LET (keV/μm)
kV x-ray, γ	2-4
MV x-ray, γ, e^-	0.2-0.5
Fast protons	0.5
Slow protons	~5
Fast neutrons	~100
α-Particles	~100
Heavy ions	200-1000
Optimal RBE	100

Alpha/Beta Ratios

Normal Tissue	Late Reaction	α/β
Spinal cord	Cervical	1.5-3.0
	Lumbar	2.3-4.9
Lung	Pneumonitis	4.0
	Fibrosis	3.1
Bladder	Frequency	5-10
Skin	Telangiectasia	2.6-2.8
	Fibrosis	1.7
Optic nerve	Neuropathy	1.6
Brachial plexus	Plexopathy	2-3.5
Small bowel		3.5-4.0
Supraglottic larynx		3.8
OC/OPX		0.8

Normal Tumor	α/β
Larynx	15-50
Nasopharynx	15-20
Oropharynx	13-19
Tonsil	7-10
Oral cavity	6.6
Skin	8.5
Esophagus	4-5
Breast	3-5
Rhabdomyosarcoma	2.8
Prostate	1-1.5
Melanoma	0.6
Liposarcoma	0.4

Normal Tissue	Early Reaction	α/β
Skin	Desquamation	9-12.5
Jejunum	Clones	6-10.7
Colon	Weight loss	13-19
	Clones	8-9
Testis	Clones	12-13
OC/OPX	Mucositis	8-15

RADIATION PHYSICS

AARON JOSEPH GROSSBERG • MOHAMMED SALEHPOUR

Photon Dosimetry

Hand calcs *(make sure to include appropriate corrections for extended SSD/SAD)*

- **SAD**

$$MU = \frac{\text{Rx dose} \times \text{beam weight}}{OF \times \left(\frac{SCD}{SPD}\right)^2 \times S_c \times S_p \times TMR \times TF \times WF \times OAR}$$

Dose to a different depth (SAD)

$$Dose_B = Dose_A \times \frac{TMR_B}{TMR_A} \times \left(\frac{SPD_A}{SPD_B}\right)^2$$

- **SSD**

$$MU = \frac{\text{Rx dose} \times \text{beam weight}}{OF \times \left(\frac{SCD}{SSD + d_{max}}\right)^2 \times S_c \times S_p \times PDD \times TF \times WF \times OAR}$$

Mayneord *F* factor (at distance *d*)

$$F = \left[\frac{SSD + d_{max}}{100 + d_{max}} \times \frac{100 + d}{SSD + d}\right]^2$$

Dose to a different depth (SSD)

$$Dose_B = Dose_A \times \frac{PDD_B}{PDD_A}$$

OF = output factor calibrated at SCD
SCD = source to calibration distance

- Typically SCD = 100 cm for SAD and 100 cm + d_{max} for SSD

SPD = source to point distance
S_c = collimator scatter factor
S_p = phantom scatter factor
TMR = tissue maximum ratio
PDD = percent depth dose = dose at depth/d_{max}

- if SSD ≠ 100, then: **PDD_{new} = Mayneord *F* factor × $PDD_{(SSD = 100)}$**

Equivalent square: $ES = \frac{2WL}{W + L}$

Photon d_{max} (cm)	Photon attenuation *in tissue*	PDD
• ^{60}Co—0.5 • 4 MV—1.0 • 6 MV—1.5 • 10 MV—2.5 • 15 MV—3.0 • 18 MV—3.3 • 20 MV—3.5 • 25 MV—4.0	• ^{60}Co ~4.0%/cm • 6 MV ~3.3%/cm • 18 MV ~2.0%/cm 1 cm of air (e. g., lung tissue) is equivalent to 0.3 cm of soft tissue/fluid	($SSD_{100\ cm}$, $ES_{10\ cm}$, d = 10 cm) • ^{60}Co—56% • 4 MV—61% • 6 MV—67% • 10 MV—73% • 20 MV—80% • 25 MV—83%

[a]1 cm lung ~ 0.3 cm tissue

ELECTRON DOSIMETRY

Factors that affect PDD

- ↑ energy → ↑ PDD
- ↑ field size → ↑ PDD
- ↑ SSD → ↑ PDD
- ↑ depth → ↓ PDD

Factors that affect skin dose

- ↑ energy → ↓ skin dose
- ↑ field size → ↑ skin dose
- ↑ SSD → ↓ skin dose
- ↑obliquity → ↑ skin dose
- beam spoiler → ↑ skin dose
- bolus → ↑ skin dose
- underwedging → ↑ skin dose

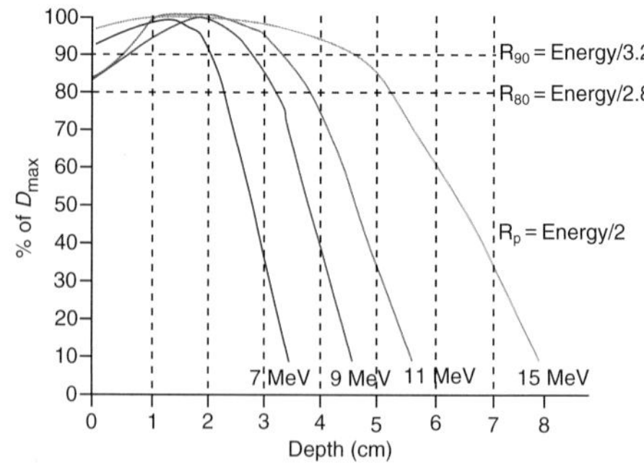

e⁻ Energy	R_{90}	R_{80}	R_p
7 MeV	2.1 cm	2.2 cm	3.5 cm
9 MeV	2.8 cm	3.2 cm	4.5 cm
11 MeV	3.4 cm	3.9 cm	5.5 cm
15 MeV	4.7 cm	5.4 cm	7.5 cm

Hand Calculations

$$MU = \frac{\text{Rx dose}}{OF \times AF \times ISF \times \text{Rx isodose}}$$

OF = output factor (typically 1 MU = 1 cGy for 10 × 10 applicator at d_{max}, 100 cm SSD)
AF = applicator factor

$$ISF = \left(\frac{\text{virtual SSD} + d_{max}}{\text{virtual SSD} + d_{max} + g}\right)^2; \quad g = SSD - 100$$

Electron shielding: Lead block thickness to attenuate 95% (mm)

Lead: t_{Pb}(mm) = (0.5 × e^- energy (MeV)) + 1
Cerrobend: t_{Cerr}(mm) = t_{Pb}(mm) × 1.2

Treatment Techniques

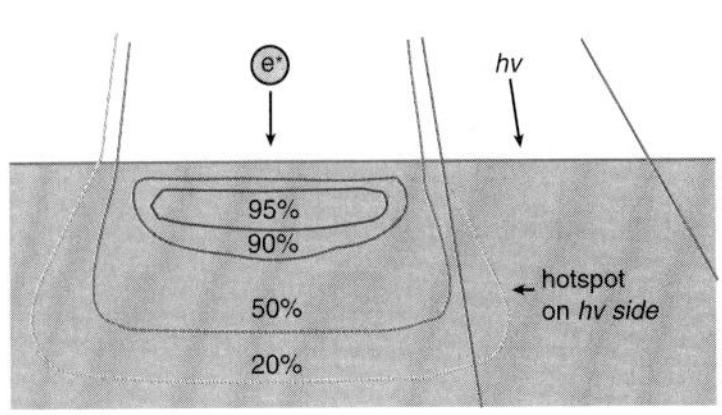

Matched photon/electron

- High electron isodose lines pull in
- Low electron isodose lines bow out
- Hotspot always on photon side
- Cold triangle on e^- side

Wedges

Underwedged

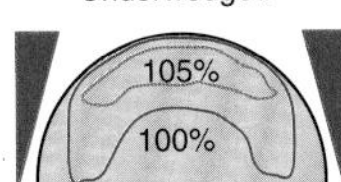

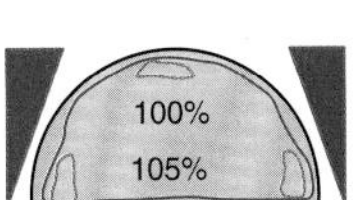

Overwedged

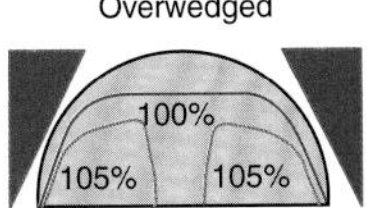

Wedge pair

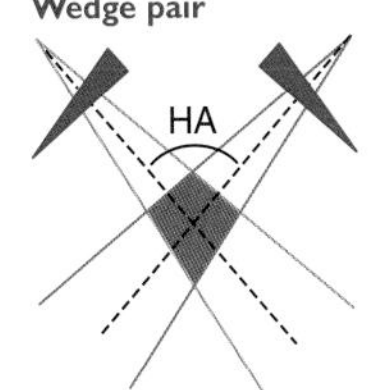

- Wedge angle (WA): Angle between wedged isodose line and a straight line at 10 cm depth
- Hinge angle (HA): Angle between central axes of incident beams
- WA = 90 – HA / 2

Craniospinal irradiation

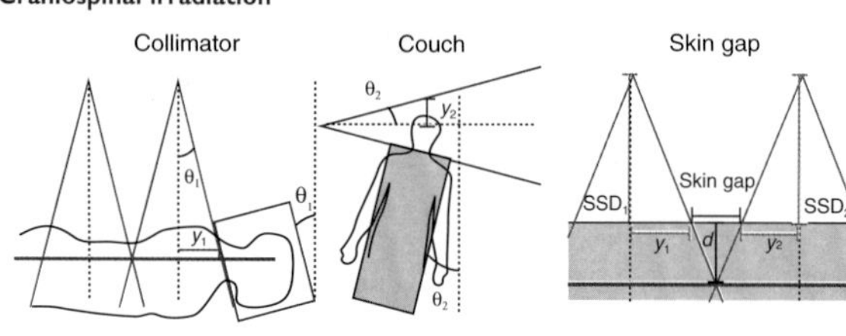

Collimator rot $\Theta_1 = \arctan\left(\frac{\text{spine}\, y_1}{\text{SAD}}\right)$	Skin gap $= d \times \frac{y_1}{\text{SSD}_1} + d \times \frac{y_2}{\text{SSD}_2}$
Couch kick $\Theta_2 = \arctan\left(\frac{\text{brain}\, y_2}{\text{SAD}}\right)$	

Brachytherapy

- 1 Becquerel (Bq) = 1 disintegration/second
- 1 curie (Ci) = 3.7×10^{10} Bq
- Source strength = air kerma rate at distance of 1 m. 1 U = 1 μGy/h/m²

Exponential decay: $A(t) = A_0\, e^{-\lambda t}$	Half-life: $t_{1/2} = \frac{\ln 2}{\lambda} = \frac{0.693}{\lambda}$
Mean life: $t_{avg} = 1.44 \times t_{1/2}$	Total dose $= \dot{D}_0 \times 1.44 \times t_{1/2}$ (permanent implant) $\dot{D}_0$ = initial dose rate
Effective half-life: $\frac{1}{t_{eff}} = \frac{1}{t_b} + \frac{1}{t_p}$ t_p = physical $t_{1/2}$; t_b = biological $t_{1/2}$	
Radium equivalent (mCi) = $\frac{\Gamma A \times \text{mgRaEq}}{8.25\,\text{R/cm}^2\text{/h}}$ for source of activity A and gamma constant Γ	

Hand calcs

$$\dot{D}(r,\Theta) = S_k \times \Lambda \times \frac{G(r,\Theta)}{D(1,\pi/2)} \times F(r,\Theta) \times g(r,\Theta)$$

- S_k: Air kerma rate
- Λ: Lambda (dose rate) constant. Converts kerma in air to dose in water
- $G(r, \Theta)$: Geometry Factor. Inverse square equation
  - Point source, $G(r) = 1/r^2$
  - Line source, $G(r, \Theta) = (\Theta_2 - \Theta_1)/Ly$
    - If $r \gg$ source length, $G(r, \Theta) \approx 1/r^2$
- $F(r, \Theta)$: Anisotropy factor
  - At perpendicular angles ($\Theta = \pi/2$), $F(r, \Theta) = 1$
  - Value changes as you move off axis
- $g(r)$: Radial dose function
  - High-energy γ sources (^{192}Ir), scatter ≈ attenuation ($r < 5$ cm)
    - $g(r) \approx 1$
  - Low-energy sources (^{125}I), attenuation ≫ scatter
    - $g(r) \ll 1$

Brachytherapy loading

- **Uniform loading:** More dose at center
- **Peripheral loading:** Uniform dose achieved by increasing source strength at ends

Brachytherapy systems

- **Fletcher-Suit:** Intracavitary tandem and ovoids; classically prescribed to *point A*
- **Patterson-Parker:** *Interstitial* crossed needles, peripheral loaded for uniform dose

- **Quimby:** *Interstitial* crossed needles, uniform loading, hot in center
- **Paris:** *Interstitial* parallel needles, hot in center
- **Modified peripheral loading**: Prostate interstitial implants

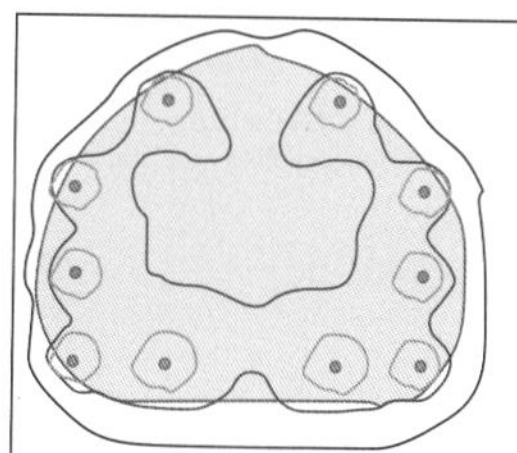	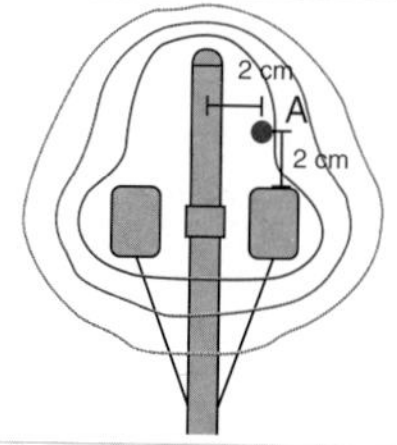
• Prostate interstitial brachytherapy using modified peripheral loading for uniform dose	• Fletcher-Suit applicator • Dose classically prescribed to point A • Start with 15/10/10 mgRaEq in tandem and 6-12 mgRaEq in each ovoid, and then optimize per GEC-ESTRO guidelines.

Common Radioisotopes

	$t_{1/2}$	Decay	Avg Energy	Use
^{60}Co	5.26 y	$\beta+\rightarrow\gamma$ emis	1.25 MeV	EBRT, SRS
^{192}Ir	73.83 d	$\beta-\rightarrow\gamma$ emis	0.38 MeV	brachy
^{125}I	60 d	e^- cap$\rightarrow\gamma$	28 keV	brachy
^{103}Pd	17 d	e^- cap	21 keV	brachy
^{131}Cs	9.7 d	e^- cap	30 keV	brachy
^{137}Cs	30.17 y	$\beta-\rightarrow\gamma$ emis	662 keV	brachy
^{223}Ra	11.4 d	α	5-7.5 MeV	bone mets
^{89}Sr	50 d	$\beta-$	1.46 MeV	bone mets
^{131}I	8 d	$\beta-$	190 keV	thyroid
^{32}P	14.3 d	$\beta-$	695 keV	craniopharyngeal
^{90}Y	64 h	$\beta-$	940 keV	liver
^{18}F	110 min	$\beta+$	640 keV	PET
^{99m}Tc	6 h	γ emis/IC	140 keV	Nuc med

Dose Specification

ICRU 50

- **GTV:** gross tumor volume—visually, palpably or radiographically apparent disease
- **CTV:** clinical target volume—GTV + volume *suspected to harbor microscopic disease*
- **PTV:** planning target volume—CTV + margin for setup error and target motion
- **TV:** treated volume—volume receiving prescribed dose
- **IV:** irradiated volume—volume receiving dose appropriate for normal tissue toxicity
- **Dose reported to ICRU reference point** (PTV within 95%-107% of Rx dose)
  - Relevant and representative of PTV dose
  - Easy to unambiguously define
  - Located where dose can be accurately calculated
  - Away from penumbra/steep dose gradients

ICRU 62

- **IM:** internal margin—physiologic variation in *shape* and *position*
- **ITV:** internal target volume—GTV + IM
- **SM:** setup margin—uncertainty in dose calc, machine alignment, and pt setup
- **PRV:** planning risk volume—organs at risk (OARs) + IM and SM

- **CI:** conformity index = TV/PTV
- *ICRU reference point not valid for IMRT*
  - Report DVHs for target volumes and OARs instead

Shielding

Half-value layer: HVL = $\ln 2/\mu$; **Tenth-value layer:** TVL = HVL × 3.3
μ = linear attenuation coefficient; dependent on material, energy, field size, and depth
Attenuation: $N = N_0 \times \left(\frac{1}{2}\right)^n$, where n is number of HVLs

Primary barrier: $P = \frac{WUT}{d^2} \times B$

Secondary barrier: $P = \frac{WUT}{d^2} \times B$

P = permissible dose-equivalent:
Controlled area: 0.1 cGy/wk
Uncontrolled area: 0.01 cGy/wk (infrequent exposure)
W = workload (# patients/wk × dose/pt = cGy/wk)
U = use factor (floor = 1, ceiling = ¼–½, walls = ¼, secondary barrier = 1)
T = occupancy factor (fraction of working day occupied; work areas/office/nurse station = 1, corridors/restrooms = ¼, waiting rooms/stairways/elevators = 1/16–1/8
d = distance (m)
B = transmission factor (HVLs or TVLs)
Neutron shielding: Wax, concrete, or borated polyethylene

Basics of Radiation Physics

Radioactive decay

- *α-decay*: Releases a helium nucleus. Very heavy nuclei ($Z > 52$), monoenergetic, 2-8 MeV
$$^{A}_{Z}X \rightarrow {}^{(A-4)}_{(Z-2)}Y + {}^{4}_{2}\alpha + E$$
- *β-decay*: Releases either b– (negatron) or b+ (positron). No change in *A*. Polyenergetic, energy shared between β and neutrino/antineutrino. Typical energy is 1/3 of maximum.
$$\beta\text{-minus: } {}^{A}_{Z}X \rightarrow {}^{A}_{(Z+1)}Y + {}^{0}_{-1}\beta + \hat{\nu} + E$$
$$\beta\text{-plus: } {}^{A}_{Z}X \rightarrow {}^{A}_{(Z-1)}Y + {}^{0}_{+1}\beta + \nu + E$$
- *Gamma emission*: Photon emitted by excited nucleus, typically after α- or β-decay
- *Electron capture*: Proton-rich nuclei; converts P→N and releases gamma ray/internal conversion electrons and characteristic x-rays or Auger e^-

Photon interactions

- *Rayleigh scatter*: Dominant <10 keV. Probability (P) ∝ Z. Photon "bounces off" e^-. **No dose contribution**
- *Photoelectric effect*: Dominant at 10-26 keV. $P \propto Z^3/E^3$. Photon ejects e^- and characteristic x-ray/Auger e^-. **Responsible for high-contrast imaging**
- *Compton scatter*: Dominant at 26 keV to 24 MeV. Photon hits e^- and sends it at angle ≤90 degrees. P ∝ electron density (Z-independent). **Underlies radiotherapy dose delivery**. Poor for imaging
- *Pair production*: Dominant at >10 MeV. $P \propto Z^2$ and dramatically increases with E. Photon splits energy of 1.02 MeV into electron and positron, which then release two additional photons (0.511 MeV each) via annihilation reaction. **Adds scatter** and widens margin around target

X-ray	Energy	Depth	Interaction	Uses
Diagnostic	20-150 kV	—	PE, Compton	Imaging
Superficial	50-200 kV	0-5 mm	Compton	Skin
Orthovoltage	200-500 kV	4-6 cm	Compton	Skin, ribs
Megavoltage	1-25 MV	1-30 cm	Compton, PP	Deep tissues

- Energy to produce an ion pair in gas: 33.97 eV
- Bremsstrahlung: Inelastic interaction between e^- and nucleus releases photon. Produces x-rays in x-ray tubes and linacs.

IMAGING AND RADIOLOGY

AARON JOSEPH GROSSBERG • CLIFTON DAVID FULLER

Imaging Radiation Basics

kVp: Peak x-ray energy (kV). Photons generated will have a range of energies with E_{max} = kVp.

mAs: E-current (milliamps) × time (seconds)

Quantity of x-rays produced in an exposure $\propto$ ***mAs*** × ***kV***^{2}

X-ray exposure that passes through patient to film $\propto$ ***mAs*** × ***kV***^{4}

- *Exposure of film/detector is very dependent on kV*

Imaging Examination	Approx. Effective Dose (mrem)	Lifetime Fatal Cancer Risk (per Million Persons)	Time for Equivalent Dose From Background Radiation
CXR	8	3	10 d
Lumbar spine film	127	51	155 d
Upper GI film	244	98	297 d
KUB	56	22	68 d
Pelvis	44	18	54 d
Barium enema	870	348	2.9 y
CT Head	180	72	219 d
CT Abdomen	760	304	2.53 y

Adapted from Dixon RL, Whitlow CT. In: Chen MYM, Pope TL, Ott DJ, eds. *Basic Radiology*. 2nd ed., 2011.

X-Ray Radiography

Production of two-dimensional images using (15-150 kV) low-energy x-rays

Use: Plain films (CXR, AXR, axial skeleton, extremities, etc.), mammography, kV IGRT

Physical interaction: Photoelectric (dominant) and Compton. Because interaction (P) $\propto$ atomic number $(Z)^3$/photon energy $(E)^3$, interactions are more likely with higher Z material (bone, metal) and lower kVp x-ray.

X-ray generation:
Bremsstrahlung (energy-dependent) and characteristic (anode material-dependent)

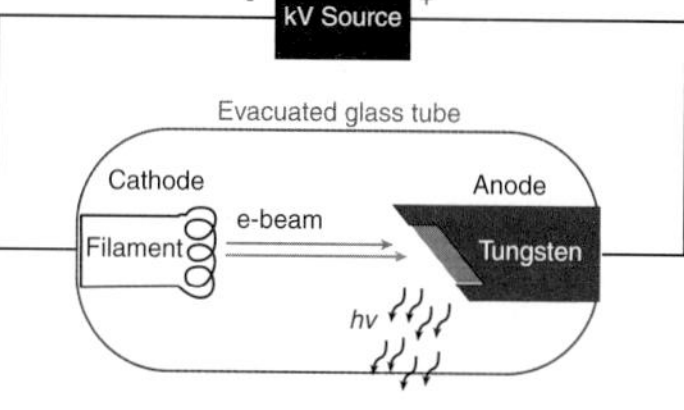

X-ray tube:

- ↑ kV: ↓ contrast, ↓ pt exposure (dose), ↓ exposure time (lower likelihood of interaction)
- ↑ mAs: ↓ exposure time
- ↑ size of focal spot (anode): ↑ penumbra, ↓ sharpness

Noise: Randomness of interactions within tissue. Compton interactions cause scatter electrons and increasing noise (energy independent in diagnostic range).

Mammography: To resolve glandular tissue or microcalcifications from fat, very low energy photons are needed. This is typically resolved by using an anode made from molybdenum (17.5 and 19.5 keV) or rhodium (20.2 and 22.7 keV), which emit characteristic x-rays of lower energy than tungsten (60-70 keV). Beryllium replaces glass as window of x-ray tube as it is lower Z and less attenuating.

Computed Tomography

Computer-processed combinations of multiple x-ray measures taken circumferentially around the patient to produce cross-sectional images (tomography). Because attenuation is closely related to tissue density and the probability of a Compton interaction is proportional to tissue density, CT number is used to calculate RT dose deposition.

Contrast: Dependent on differential attenuation, which reflects **physical density**. CT uses higher kVp and filtration (beam hardness), so interactions are mostly Compton scattering.

- **Hounsfield units (HU):** Linear CT contrast scale that normalizes the original linear attenuation coefficient measurement to the radio densities of water and air.

$$HU = 1000 \times \frac{\mu - \mu_{water}}{\mu_{water} - \mu_{air}}$$

- **Window (width) = range** of HU to be displayed
- **Level = midpoint** of the window

Substance	HU
Air	−1000
Water	0
Soft tissue	+100 to +300
Bone	+200 to +3000
Fat	−120 to −90
Blood	+13 to +50
Clotted blood	+50 to +75
Lung	−700 to −600
Liver	+55 to +65
Kidney	+20 to +45
Lymph nodes	+10 to +20
Muscle	+35 to +55
Gray matter	+37 to +45
White matter	+20 to +30
Gold, steel, brass	Up to 30 000

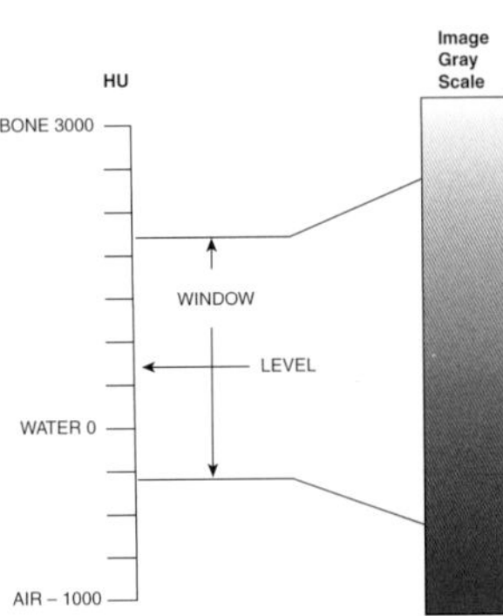

Image noise

Noise (graininess) is due to low number of x-rays contributing to each detector measurement.

- **↑ mAs → ↑ number of x-rays → ↓ noise**; can be impacted by changing mA or scan time(s)
- **↑ slice thickness → ↑ number of x-rays → ↓ noise** but decreased spatial resolution
- **↑ kVp → ↑ number of x-rays → ↓ noise** but decreased contrast (slightly)
- **↑ patient thickness → ↓ number of x-rays → ↑ noise**

Artifact: Any structure seen on an image that is not representative of actual anatomy

- **Shading artifact:** Lower than expected HU in regions downstream from high-density material—most commonly due to beam hardening that exceeds correction
- **Ring artifact:** Arise from errors, imbalances, or calibration drifts in part of the detector array. Errors are back projected along ray path to that detector, creating a ring.
- **Streak artifact:** Causes include bad detector measurement, motion, metal, insufficient x-ray intensity, partial volume effects, and tube arcing or system misalignment.

Additional limitations include bore size and field of view (FOV). Patient must be able to fit within the bore. FOV is always smaller than bore size. Contact with the CT bore or FOV limit, can cause incomplete scanning and artifact that impact dose deposition calculations.

Special CT protocols

Head and neck: Thin-slice (<3 mm) IV contrast-enhanced with single phase collected ~70 seconds after contrast injection +/− upper and lower angles (in which case ½ the contrast is used for the angle scans)

Pancreatic (3-phase): Thin-slice (<3 mm) multidetector CT with triple-phase IV contrast and low-density/water oral contrast. Arterial phase (<30 seconds) shows arterial anatomy/involvement; parenchymal phase (45-50 seconds) shows parenchymal masses as hypointense lesions (PDAC) vs isodense (neuroendocrine); portal venous phase (75 seconds)—delineates venous structures and liver metastases.

Liver (3 phase): Includes late arterial phase (20-35 seconds after contrast administration), portal venous phase (60-90 seconds), and delayed phase (>3 minutes). Hypervascular tumors identified during arterial phase, hypovascular tumors during portal venous phase, washout evaluated during delayed phase

4DCT: Continuous CT scan collected during breathing cycle. Tumor and normal tissue can be identified throughout breathing cycle, and the degree of movement can be represented on their simulation planning scan. Requires some level of respiratory management to ensure even, full breathing cycle during scan. The pitch of the scan is adjusted per the patient's respiratory rate.

Magnetic Resonance Imaging

Measures magnetic resonance: Frequency of energy released by protons as they "relax" from an energy pulse in a different direction from bore of the magnet (B_0). The local environment of each proton after excitation influences its return to alignment with B_0, yielding contrast. By changing the magnetic sequences and measured parameters, one can image different tissue characteristics.

T1: (spin-lattice relaxation) Time taken for spinning protons to realign with B_0 after 90 degrees pulse. "Longitudinal relaxation time." Dependent upon energy exchange with surrounding material

- Fat is bright; fluid (CSF) is dark.
- White matter is lighter than gray matter.
- Gadolinium increases brightness of blood/fluid by improving energy exchange (T1 + C = T1 with contrast).

T2: The component of T2* (transverse relaxation time) that is due to proton-proton interactions and thus tissue dependent. "Spin-spin relaxation"

- Fat is intermediate-bright, fluid (CSF) is bright.
- White matter is darker than gray matter.
- Gadolinium shortens T2 relaxation time → hypointense signal of blood/fluid.

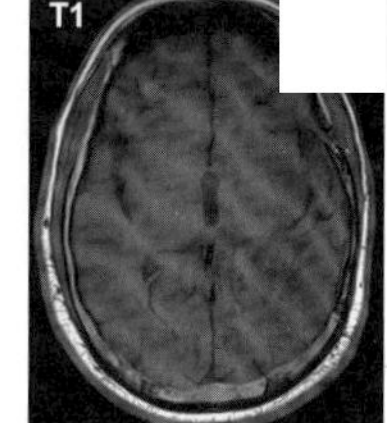

A

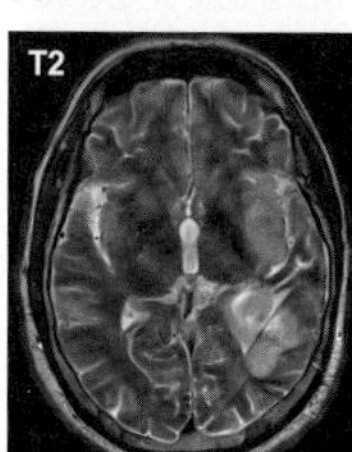

B

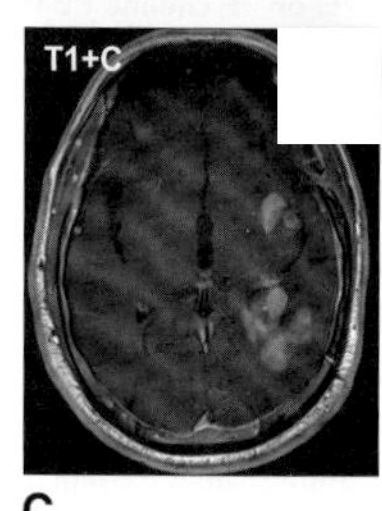

C

Special MRI sequences

- **STIR:** Short T1 inversion recovery. Used for fat suppression in T2-weighted images. Lower signal, poorer signal-to-noise, therefore often run at poorer spatial resolution to compensate
- **FLAIR:** Fluid-attenuation inversion recovery. Usually used in T2-weighted brain images to suppress CSF signal and improve sensitivity to pathology.
  - Fat is dark; fluid (CSF) is dark.
  - White matter is darker than gray matter.
- **Diffusion-weighted imaging: detects random movements of water** protons by adding sequential diffusion gradients in opposing directions to T2-weighted sequences. Diffusion weighting depends on:
  1. Gradient amplitude
  2. Gradient pulse application time
  3. Interval between gradients
- **Apparent diffusion coefficient (ADC):** Calculated by comparing multiple diffusion-weighted scans with different *b*-values (a measure of the strength and duration of applied gradients). Areas of low diffusion lose the least signal on high *b*-value images (small ADC). Areas of fast diffusion appear bright (lose more signal on high *b*-value images).

Positron Emission Tomography

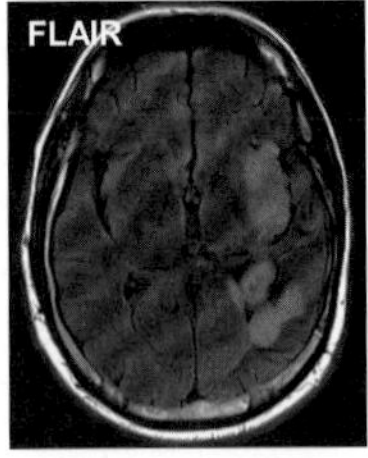

D

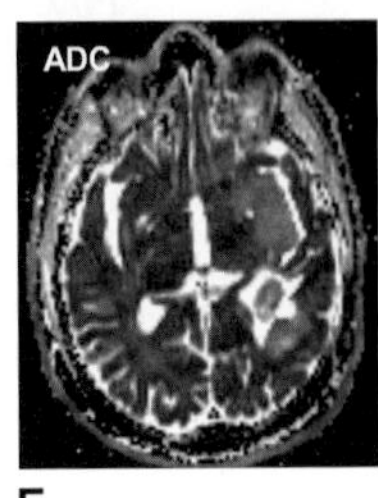

E

Allows imaging of biological uptake of radiolabeled tracer that emits positrons. Positron annihilation results in pairs of 511 keV photons at 180 degrees, which are detected by coincidence detection allowing for back calculation of location in 2D space in each slice.

- **Coincidence detection:** Photons released by positron annihilation detected at same time by detectors at 180 degrees from each other. Detection within 6-12 ns considered "in coincidence." Majority (~99%) of photons are thus excluded from results.
- ↑ **accumulated tracer → ↑ signal**

^{18}FDG-PET images glucose uptake (non-metabolized glucose analog builds up in metabolically active cells). Most common use for PET imaging

- **SUV:** Standardized uptake value. FDG uptake in a region/tumor/tissue normalized to the injected radiotracer and patient's weight
  - SUV more accurate if normalized to patient's lean body mass or body surface area, but this is not standard practice
  - Normal tissues: SUV 0.5-2.5, tumor—SUV > 2.5 (usually)

Patient preparation

- NPO 4-6 hours: FDG-PET to enhance FDG uptake by tumors. No caffeine/alcohol either. Blood glucose at time of injection <150 mg/dL
- No strenuous activity prior to imaging
- Typical dose of FDG **10 mCi**. Imaging initiated **60 minutes** after tracer injection
- Position: For HN, arms down; if below neck, arms above the head (decrease beam hardening during CT). Patient must be comfortable enough to lie for 45 minutes and instructed not to move.
  - PET can be done in treatment position (with immobilization) for better treatment planning image fusion. This is particularly important for INRT in lymphoma management.
- Duration: PET scanning typically takes 30-45 minutes.

Other PET tracers

- **Na^{18}F:** Images blastic and lytic bone lesions (alternative to traditional ^{99m}Tc bone scan)
- **^{11}C acetate PET:** Ketone body uptake. Related to enhanced lipid synthesis in prostate cancer tumor cells. Not cancer specific—also accumulates in BPH. 71% accuracy (*Jambor J Nucl Med* 2010)
- **^{11}C or ^{18}F choline PET:** Choline is used in cell membrane synthesis, which is increased in cancer cells. Highly sensitive for lymph node involvement or metastasis. High levels of uptake in liver, spleen, kidneys, pancreas, and salivary glands. Inflammation can confound interpretation of increased uptake.
- **^{18}F fluciclovine (Axumin) PET:** Analogue of L-leucine. Uptake increased in prostate cancer. No physiologic accumulation in urinary tract or brain allowing for sensitive detection of localized and metastatic disease. Used for metastatic or recurrent disease, proven by rising PSA
- **^{11}C metomidate:** 11β-hydroxlase inhibitor, key enzyme in biosynthesis of cortisol and aldosterone. Used for detection of adrenocortical tumors

Other Nuclear Medicine Imaging

- **Bone scan:** ^{99m}Tc with methylene diphosphonate (MDP). MDP adsorbs to bone hydroxyapatite, which is present at sites of bone growth/increased turnover. Patient is typically injected with 740 MBq of tracer and scanned with a gamma camera (planar images).
- **Myocardial perfusion:** ^{99m}Tc tracers include teboroxime and sestamibi. Evaluates areas of infarction, ischemia, or reduced blood flow

- **Renal scan:** aka renogram or MAG3 scan. May use ^{99m}Tc-conjugated mercaptoacetyltriglycine (MAG3) or diethylenetriaminepentaacetate (DTPA) injected intravenously. Progress through renal system tracked with gamma camera. Measures effective renal plasma flow. 40%-50% of MAG3 (20% of DTPA) is removed by the proximal tubules during each pass.
- **V/Q scan:** Evaluates circulation of air and blood within patients' lungs. Used for pre-op/pre-RT estimate of lung function pts with lung ca. or mesothelioma. For the ventilation scan, aerosolized radionuclides are inhaled by the patient through nonrebreathing mask. Perfusion scan is ^{99m}Tc microaggregated albumin.
- **MIBG:** Metaiodobenzylguanidine labeled with ^{123}I or ^{131}I. Localized to adrenergic tissue and can be used to identify pheochromocytomas and neuroblastomas. Use of ^{131}I allows for treatment as well as imaging. Must undertake thyroid precautions by pretreating with potassium iodide
- **Sentinel node identification:** Injection of ^{99m}Tc-labelled sulfur colloid or albumin colloid injected 2-24 hours prior to operation. Preoperative lymphoscintigram is obtained to map axillary drainage patter from tumor. Intraoperatively, a gamma counter is used to find the area of highest radioactivity.
- **^{123}I iodine scan:** Supplied as Na^{131}I and administered orally vs IV Iodine is taken up by the thyroid and images obtained by gamma camera.
- **^{131}I iodine scan:** Like ^{123}I, it is taken up by the thyroid. 90% of decay is by β-decay, allowing for short-range therapeutic effects, with the remaining 10% via gamma decay, allowing for detection using gamma camera. Dose ranges from 2220 to 7400 MBq. Patients cannot be discharged until activity falls below 1100 MBq. Patients advised to collect urine, wear clothes and socks, and to regularly clean toilets, sinks, etc. Patients who undergo treatment may trigger airport radiation detectors up to 95 days after tx.

Image-Guided Radiation Therapy (IGRT)

Goal of IGRT is to minimize geometric uncertainty during treatment.

Sources of geometric uncertainties

- **Intrafraction**
  - Seconds: Cardiac cycle, breathing
  - Minutes: Patient movement, setup variation
- **Interfraction**
  - Hours: Patient movement, setup variation
  - Days to months: Anatomic changes, tumor response, normal tissue response

Corrections

Remember that you are moving the patient, not the imager. Often corrections involve moving patient in *opposite* direction to apparent misalignment.

- Isocenter too superior (target too inferior on daily imaging): Move patient *in*
- Isocenter too inferior (target too superior on daily imaging): Move patient *out*
- Isocenter too far on patient's left (target too far on patient's *right* on daily imaging): Move patient *left*
- Isocenter too far on patient's right (target too far on patient's *left* on daily imaging): Move patient *right*

IGRT approaches

- **Surface markers:** Use surface anatomy to infer internal anatomy. Usually in conjunction with immobilization devices. Establish position of multiple surface markers at simulation and in treatment room (relative to isocenter or ODI). *Not a good approach for mobile internal targets*
- **Stereotaxy:** 3D localization of structures using mechanical frame and precise coordinate system. Allows for reduction in PTV. Most commonly used for intracranial targets (1-2 mm PTV). Concepts have been adapted using 4DCT simulation and full-body immobilization to apply stereotaxy to extracranial sites, including lung cancer (~5 mm PTV).
- **MV electronic portal imaging devices (EPIDs):** Creating of radiographic images using RT x-ray beam. Advantage is that imaging represents actual treatment field. Disadvantage is that MV imaging exhibits negligible photoelectric effect, limiting contrast to detect only bony anatomy. Very difficult to align to soft tissue
- **Single exposure:** Only images treatment field
- **Double exposure:** Treatment field and open field both imaged for better anatomy
- **Localization film:** A few cGy for imaging verification of setup
- **Verification film:** Full fraction (~2 Gy) of exposure

- **kV imaging:** Most new teletherapy machines have built in x-ray tube and EPID orthogonal to treatment ray. *Advantage* is that it offers increased contrast compared to MV. Also frequently incorporate fluoroscopy for real-time monitoring. Due to increased contrast detection due to greater influence of photoelectric effect, can also be used to localize implanted radiopaque markers. Excellent translational (*x*-, *y*-, and z-axis) resolution. *Disadvantage* is that images are not collected from treatment beam, so there is an opportunity for misalignment between kV imager and treatment beam. Insensitive to rotational error. Other vendors, including ExacTrac, offer floor-to-ceiling noncoplanar imaging that can be compared to on-board imaging in real time to detect intra- or interfraction motion.
- **Ultrasound:** Allows for soft tissue imaging with the transducer calibrated and coregistered with the isocenter, both in the CT scanner and in treatment rooms. Most commonly transabdominal ultrasound used for prostate cancer treatment setup. Bladder ultrasounds can also be used to assess bladder fullness during treatment for pelvic malignancies (uterus, prostate, cervix, and bladder cancers). *Advantages* are that it is relatively inexpensive and shows soft tissue contrast for targets that do not reliably align to bone. *Disadvantages* are that it requires technical skill, pressure may displace target or OARs, and that it cannot image through bone or air cavities.
- **Cone beam CT (CBCT):** Allows for volumetric imaging on conventional linac using onboard orthogonal x-ray tube and detector. CT reconstructions are acquired in the treatment position just prior to treatment. Images may be acquired in whole-fan or half-fan mode. FOV can approach 50 cm in the transverse plane ×25 cm in the craniocaudal plane, but may not include full thickness of patient. Total dose delivered is usually <3 cGy. *Advantages* include the ability to align soft tissue with good contrast in the treatment position, can see inter- and intrafractional changes in tumor and patient anatomy, and six-directional image verification. *Disadvantages* include limited FOV, which may not show patient to surface; slow image acquisition, making it susceptible to motion artifact and difficult to use with respiratory gating; and relatively high radiation dose delivered.
- **CT on rails:** Conventional CT scanner located in treatment room moves over patient and treatment table "on rails" to acquire images. Typically treatment table is rotated 180 degrees from treatment position for scanning. Treatment table is made of special low-attenuation material. *Advantages* include faster CT imaging, allowing for verification of intrafractional immobilization (eg, breath hold). *Disadvantages* include the need for extra equipment, relative scarcity of CT on rail-enabled treatment vaults, and requirement to rotate table out of treatment position for verification scans, introducing potential new source of error.
- **Tomotherapy imaging:** Tomotherapy devices include MV CT image system that uses a fan beam and helical acquisition. Images are acquired using a 3.5-MV x-rays with suppressed photon output. Typically imaging administers dose of 0.5-3 cGy. *Advantages* include images collected in treatment position and MV imaging not susceptible to artifact. *Disadvantages* include low contrast in MV images.
- **Electromagnetic 4-D tracking:** Electromagnetic transponders implanted in the target tissue for improving both intrafraction motion of the tissue and interfraction setup error. Includes beacons, electromagnetic console, receiver array, and three ceiling-mounted infrared optical cameras. Currently in use for prostate radiotherapy (Calypso). Less than 2 mm accuracy
- **Optical (surface) imaging:** Optical, often infrared camera system tracks patient surface during actual treatment. Used to monitor intrafraction motion. Current systems include AlignRT and C-Rad Sentinel. *Advantages* include speed, ability to monitor respiratory motion, and absence of ionizing radiation. *Disadvantages* include inability to use for tumors that poorly correlate to patient surface.
- **Magnetic resonance imaging:** Uses hybrid MRI/radiation units to provide continuous real time assessment of internal soft tissue anatomy and motion. *Advantages* include excellent soft tissue contrast, no ionizing radiation exposure, and excellent resolution. *Disadvantages* include inability to use for patients with metal implants or pacemakers and susceptibility to motion artifact.
- **Incorporating IGRT into margination:** ICRU 50 & 62 define target (PTV) and avoidance (PRV) volumes to account for setup and organ positional uncertainty. IGRT can be used to minimize magnitude of both random and systematic error, allowing reduced PTV margin.

Systematic Error

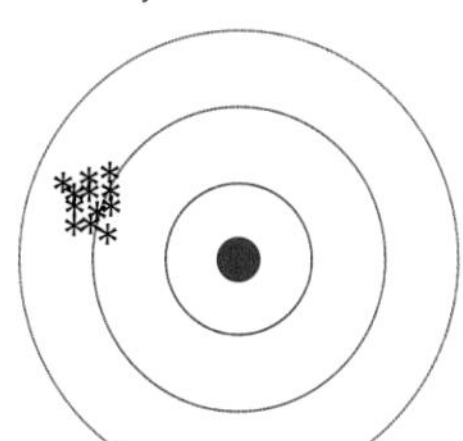

Random Error

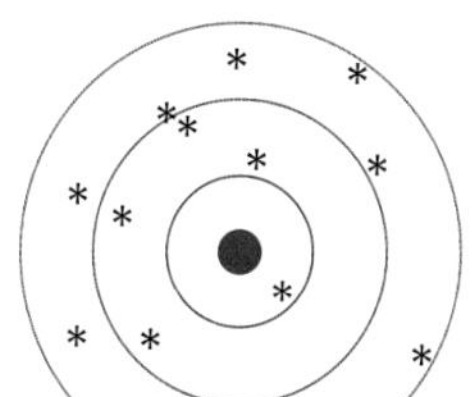

- **Random error, σ:** Fluctuations in patient position due to unknown and unpredictable factors (eg, changes in organ positions, bladder filling, minor fluctuations in immobilization devices). *Execution Errors*. Equal in all directions
  - Root mean square of SDs of measured fluctuations from all patients = σ
- **Systematic error, Σ:** Error in patient setup due to incorrect positioning information (eg, inaccurate isocenter determination, laser positioning, or setup documentation). *Preparation Errors*. Typically in a specific direction
  - SD of means per patient of observed fluctuations = Σ
  - Require 3-4x more margin than random errors
  - Can be minimized using multimodality imaging, clear delineation protocols, and electronic portal imaging with decision rules
- **Margin recipes**
  CTV *Margin* $= 2.5 \times \Sigma + 0.7 \times \sigma$ (*van Herk et al. IJROBP* 2000)
  * Minimum dose to CTV is 95% for 90% of patients.
  OAR *Margin* $= 1.3 \times \Sigma + 0.5 \times \sigma$ (*McKenzie et al. Radiother Oncol* 2002)
  *DVH of PRV will not underrepresent high dose to OAR for 90% of patients.

CHEMOTHERAPY AND IMMUNOTHERAPY

AARON JOSEPH GROSSBERG • CHAD TANG

Concurrent Chemoradiation

- Chemotherapy delivered concurrently with radiotherapy to increase efficacy
- Preclinical synergy with XRT: Gemcitabine, cisplatin, bleomycin, 5-FU, MMC, bevacizumab, cetuximab, PARP inhibitors, doxorubicin, dactinomycin, dacarbazine
- Associated with increased and earlier toxicity
- Rule of thumb: OAR dose constraints often **reduced by ~10%**

Head and Neck—*NPX, OPX, Supraglottic Larynx, Post-op*			
Drug	**Dose**	**XRT Rx**	**Notes**
Cisplatin	40 mg/m^2 qwk ×6 or 100 mg/m^2 q3wk ×2	70 Gy/33 fx	Total dose >200 mg/m^2
Cetuximab	400 mg/m^2 loading→ 250 mg/m^2 qwk ×6	70 Gy/33 fx	OPX, p16+, <N2b, <10 pk-yr G2+ acneiform rash = ↑ OS
Small Cell Lung Cancer (Limited Stage)			
Cisplatin	60 mg/m^2 d1 q3wk	45 Gy/30 fx *bid*	Start XRT during 1st two cycles of chemo (*De Ruysscher Ann Oncol* 2006)
Etoposide	120 mg/m^2 d1, 2, 3 q3wk		

Non–Small Cell Lung Cancer			
Cisplatin	50 mg/m^2 d1, 8, 29, 36	66 Gy/30 fx	Other platinum doublets used as well
Etoposide	50 mg/m^2 d1-5 and 29-33		
Esophageal			
Cisplatin 5-FU	20 mg/m^2 d1, 8, 15, 22, 29 300 mg/m^2/d CI	50.4 Gy in 28 fx	Oxaliplatin or capecitabine may be used as well
Carboplatin Paclitaxel	AUC2 mg/m^2 d1, 8, 15, 22, 29 50 mg/m^2	50.4 Gy in 30 fx	Other platinum doublets used as well
Gastric			
Capecitabine	825 mg/m^2 bid	45 Gy in 25 fx	Pre-op or post-op
5-FU	200 mg/m^2/d CI	45 Gy in 25 fx	
Pancreatic			
Capecitabine	825 mg/m^2 bid	50.4 Gy/28 fx	Pre-op or post-op
Gemcitabine	400 mg/m^2 qwk	50.4 Gy/28 fx	
Bladder Cancer			
Cisplatin and 5-FU	75 mg/m^2 d1 1000 mg/m^2 d1, 4	50-58 Gy at 2 Gy/fx	Many other concurrent bladder cancer regimes
MMC 5-FU	12 mg/m^2 d1 500 mg/m^2/d CI given on 1-5 fx, 16-20 fx	55 Gy at 2.75 Gy/fx or 64 Gy at 2 Gy/fx	
Anal			
Cisplatin 5-FU	20 mg/m^2 d1, 8, 15, 22 300 mg/m^2/d CI	50-58 Gy at 2 Gy/fx	XRT dose depends on T- and N-stage
MMC 5-FU	10 mg/m^2 d1, 29 300 mg/m^2/d CI	50-58 Gy at 2 Gy/fx	
Rectal			
Capecitabine	825 mg/m^2 bid	50.4 Gy in 28 fx	Boost to 54 Gy post-op
5-FU	225 mg/m^2/d CI	50.4 Gy in 28 fx	
Gynecologic Cancers (Cervix/Uterine/Vulvar/Vaginal)			
Cisplatin	40 mg/m^2 qwk	Variable	Final cis with 2nd ICBT
Glioblastoma			
Temozolomide	75 mg/m^2 daily	60 Gy/30 fx	Adjuvant dose 150-200 mg/m^2 d1-5 q4wk × 6c (or indefinitely)
Medulloblastoma (Pediatric)			
Vincristine	1.5 mg/m^2 qwk	54 Gy/30 fx	Followed by adjuvant PCV
Rhabdomyosarcoma (Pediatric)			
Vincristine	1.5 mg/m^2	36-50.4 Gy/30 fx	XRT dose and timing depends on risk stratification. Complex timing of concurrent chemo
Cyclophos-phamide	1.2 g/m^2		
Irinotecan	50 mg/m^2		

CHEMOTHERAPY AGENTS AND TOXICITIES

Underline = dose limiting toxicity

Alkylating Agents: Add alkyl group to 7-N guanine → DNA cross-link and strand breaks. Inhibit DNA repair and/or synthesis.

Cisplatin (Platinol) (20-100 mg/m^2 d1-5 q3-4wk; 40 mg/m^2 qwk—CCRT): N/V, nephrotox, ototox (irreversible), neuropathy (reversible), ↓PLT, anemia, taste changes

Carboplatin (Paraplatin) (AUC 3-7.5 q3-4wk; AUC2 qwk—CCRT): Myelosuppression (nadir 3-4 weeks), N/V, nephrotox, ototox, neuropathy, ↑LFTs

Oxaliplatin (Eloxatin) (85-140 mg/m² q2-3wk): Neurotox, neuropathy, fever, ↑LFTs, nephrotox

Bendamustine (Treanda, Bendeka) (70-120 mg/m² ×2d q3-5wk): Myelosuppression (nadir 3 weeks), N/V, fever, edema, rash, diarrhea

Cyclophosphamide (Cytoxan) (1-5 mg/kg/d po or 250-1800 mg/m² q3-4wk): Myelosuppression (recovery 1 week), hemorrhagic cystitis, nephrotox, N/V, cardiotox, infertility, alopecia

Chlorambucil (Leukeran) (0.1-0.2 mg/kg/d): Myelosuppression (nadir 3 weeks), hepatotox, rash, CNS tox, 2° malignancy

Melphalan (Alkeran) (2-10 mg/d PO): Myelosuppression (nadir 4 weeks), mucositis, diarrhea, pulm fibrosis, 2° malignancy

Ifosfamide (Ifex) (1200-3000 mg/m²/d ×3-5d q2-3wk): Myelosuppression (nadir 1-2 weeks), hemorrhagic cystitis, nephrotox, reversible neurotox N/V, alopecia

Mechlorethamine (Mustargen, Valchlor) (0.1-0.4 mg/kg/d): Myelosuppression, N/V, alopecia, mucositis, infertility, CNS tox

Carmustine (BCNU, Gliadel) (150-200 mg/m² q6-8wk): Myelosuppression (nadir 4 weeks), N/V, hepatotox, hypotension, pulm fibrosis

Lomustine (CCNU, Gleostine) (100-130 mg/m² q6wk): Myelosuppression (nadir 4 weeks), N/V, hepatotox, nephrotox, pulm fibrosis ***Crosses BBB*

Busulfan (Busulfex, Myleran) (1.8 mg/m²/d): Myelosuppression, N/V, diarrhea, anorexia, mucositis, infertility

Dacarbazine (375 mg/m² d1 and 15 q4wk): N/V, myelosuppression, flulike symptoms, inj site pain

Temozolomide (Temodar) (100-200 mg/m² d1-5 q4wk; 75 mg/m²/d—CCRT): Myelosuppression (nadir 3 weeks), N/V, HA, fatigue, constipation, edema

Antimetabolites: Replace building blocks in DNA synthesis. Groups include nucleotide analogues (5-FU, -MP, Ara-C, fludarabine), folate antagonists (MTX, pemetrexed), ribonucleotide reductase inhibition (hydroxyurea)

5-FU (Adrucil) ([IVP] 325-425 mg/m² × 5d q4wk or [CI] 750-1000 mg/m² × 5d q4wk): Diarrhea, mucositis, N/V, marrow suppression, alopecia, nail changes, hand-foot

6-MP (Purinethol) (1.5-2.5 mg/m²/d): Myelosuppression, jaundice, N/V, diarrhea, infxn

Capecitabine (Xeloda) (1000-1250 mg/m² bid ×2 wk q3wk; 825-1000 mg/m² BID-CCRT): diarrhea, hand-foot, mucositis, neurotox, coronary vasospasm, XRT recall

Cytarabine (Ara-C) ([CI] 100-200 mg/m²/d ×5-7d; high dose: 1500-3000 mg/m²/d ×3d): Myelosuppression (nadir 7-9 days/15-24 days), N/V, diarrhea, neurotox, ↑LFTs ***Crosses BBB*

Fludarabine (20-30 mg/m²/d ×3-5d q4wk): Myelosuppression (nadir 10-14 days, recovery 5-7 weeks), fever, infxn, weakness, cough, anorexia

Gemcitabine (Gemzar) (1000 mg/m² qwk or 800-1250 mg/m² d1, 8 q3wk): Myelosuppression, edema, flulike symptoms, fever, fatigue, N/V pneumonitis, ↑LFTs

Hydroxyurea (Droxia, Hydrea) (20-30 mg/kg/d): Myelosuppression (2-5 days), GI ulcer, rash, squamous cell ca., XRT recall

Methotrexate (MTX, Trexall) (range from 30-40 mg/m²/wk to 100-12 000 mg/m² × 1): Myelosuppression, mucositis, N/V, neurotox, nephrotox, ↑LFTs

Pemetrexed (Alimta) (500 mg/m² q3wk): Myelosuppression, mucositis, hand-foot, anorexia, fatigue, ↑LFTs

Plant alkaloids: Inhibit enzymes used in DNA replication, mitosis, or cell division. Includes antimicrotubular agents (docetaxel, paclitaxel, vincristine, vinblastine, vinorelbine) and topoisomerase inhibitors (irinotecan, etoposide, topotecan)

Docetaxel (Taxotere) (60-100 mg/m² q3wk): Myelosuppression (7 days), neuropathy, edema, alopecia, nail changes, N/V, XRT recall

Paclitaxel (Taxol) (60-250 mg/m² q1-3wk; 50 mg/m² qwk—CCRT): Myelosuppression (11 days), alopecia, neuropathy, arthralgias, N/V, diarrhea

Nab-paclitaxel (Abraxane): Myelosuppression, alopecia, ECG changes, neuropathy, arthralgias, N/V, weakness, fatigue

Vincristine (Oncovin) (0.5-1.5 mg/m² qwk; 1.5 mg/m² qwk—CCRT): Neuropathy, alopecia, constipation, N/V, weight loss ***Crosses BBB*

Vinblastine (Velban) (3.7-6 mg/m^2 qwk): Myelosuppression (~1 week), constipation, HTN, alopecia, bone pain, N/V

Vinorelbine (Navelbine) (25-30 mg/m^2 qwk): Myelosuppression (~1 week), N/V, alopecia, diarrhea, neuropathy

Etoposide (Toposar) (50-120 mg/m^2 ×3d q3-4wk): Myelosuppression (1-2 weeks), menopause, infertility, N/V, hypotension, rash, ↑LFTs, XRT recall

Irinotecan (Camptosar) (240-350 mg/m^2 q3wk): Diarrhea, abdmnl cramping, myelosupp, N/V, alopecia, wt. loss, weakness

Topotecan (Hycamtin) (1.5 mg/m^2 ×5d q3wk): Myelosuppression (1-2 weeks), N/V, alopecia, diarrhea, fever, rash, weakness

Antibiotics: *Streptomyces* antibiotics that interfere with cell cycle or DNA replication. Anthracyclines (-rubicin) and actinomycins inhibit topoisomerase II by intercalation. Bleomycin and mitomycin generate free radicals causing DNA breaks. Commonly cause radiation recall.

Actinomycin D (Cosmegen) (400-600 μg/m^2/d ×5d): Myelosuppression (nadir 14-21 days), alopecia, N/V, fatigue, mucositis, hepatotox, diarrhea, infertility, *XRT recall*

Daunorubicin (Cerubidine) (30-60 mg/m^2/d ×3d): Myelosuppression (nadir 10-14 days), alopecia, dark urine, N/V, mucositis, pain, cardiotox. *Max lifetime cumulative dose = 550 mg/m^2*

Doxorubicin (Adriamycin) (20 mg/m^2 qwk or 40-60 mg/m^2 q3wk): Myelosuppression (nadir 10-14 days), cardiotox, N/V, mucositis *XRT recall*, 2ndary leukemia, tumor lysis. *Max lifetime cumulative dose = 500 mg/m^2, less if >65, mediastinal XRT, heart disease or cyclophosphamide*

Epirubicin (Ellence) (100-120 mg/m^2/d q3-4wk, 50 mg/m^2 q3wk): Myelosuppression (nadir 10-14 days), alopecia, hot sweats, N/V, diarrhea, cardiotox. *Max lifetime cumulative dose = 1000 mg/m^2*

Bleomycin (Blenoxane) (5-15 units/m^2/wk ×3wk): Pulmonary tox/pneumonitis, skin rxn, mucositis, hypotension, hypersensitivity rxn, *XRT recall*

Mitomycin-C (Mutamycin) (10-15 mg/m^2 q6-8wk or 20-40 mg qwk or 10-15 mg/m^2 q4wk-CCRT): Myelosuppression (nadir 4-6 weeks), mucositis, rash, interstitial pneumonitis, HUS

Targeted Therapies

Naming Guide	
Monoclonal antibodies (-mab)	
Target	*Source*
• cir(r), circulatory system	• ximab, chimeric human-mouse
• li(m), immune system	• zumab, humanized mouse
• t(u), tumor	• mumab, fully human
Small molecules (-ib)	
• tinib, tyrosine kinase inhibitor (TKI)	
• zomib, proteasome inhibitor	
• ciclib, cyclin-dependent kinase inhibitor	
• parib, PARP inhibitor	

Adapted from: Abramson, 2017 Overview of Targeted Therapies for Cancer.

Common Nonchemotherapy Systemic Agents

Drug	Target	Indications	Side Effects
Erlotinib (Tarceva) **Afatinib (Gilotrif)** **Gefitinib (Iressa)** **Osimertinib (Tagrisso)**	EGFR	Lung adenoca, PDAC *EGFR ex19del; ex21mut*	**Rash, diarrhea**, fatigue, anorexia, neutropenia (osimertinib)
Cetuximab (Erbitux)	EGFR	HNC, mCRC	**Acneiform rash**, infusion rxn, anaphylaxis, N/V, ↓BP
Panitumumab (Vectibix)	EGFR	mCRC	Rash, N/V, diarrhea, hypoMg, keratitis

Drug	Target	Indications	Side Effects
Bevacizumab (Avastin)	VEGF-A	mColorectal, lung adenoca, mBreast, GBM, RCC	Weakness, pain, N/V, GI perf, hypertensive crisis, nephrotic syndrome, CHF
Ramucirumab (Cyramza)	VEGFR2	Gastric/GEJ, NSCLC, mColorectal	HTN, diarrhea, HA, bleeding, GI perf
Temsirolimus (Torisel) **Everolimus (Afinitor)**	mTOR	RCC, GI NETs	Lymphopenia, anemia, fatigue, rash, mucositis, hyperglyc, ↑TGs
Sunitinib (Sutent)	PDGFR VEGFR c-KIT RET	GIST, RCC, meningioma, neuroendocrine	Fatigue, diarrhea, N, hand-foot syndrome, stomatitis, rash
Sorafenib (Nexavar)	PDGFR VEGFR RAF	RCC, HCC, thyroid, desmoid	Lymphopenia, diarrhea, rash, hand-foot syndrome, N/V, fatigue
Pazopanib (Votrient)	PDGFR VEGFR c-KIT FGFR	RCC, sarcoma	N/V, diarrhea, changes in hair color, rash, myelosupp
Cabozantinib (Cabometyx, Cometriq)	VEGFR2 c-Met AXL RET	RCC, MTC	GI perf/fistula, bleeding, hand-foot syndrome, PRES, stomatitis
Regorafenib (Stivarga)	c-KIT PDGFR RAF RET VEGFR1-3	CRC, GIST, HCC	Anemia, ↑LFTs, fatigue, proteinuria, electrolyte abnl, ↓PLT, ↓WBC, wt loss
Axitinib (Inlyta)	VEGFR1-3 PDGFR c-KIT BCR-ABL	RCC, CML, ALL	Diarrhea, fatigue, hand-foot syndrome, N/V, fatigue, wt loss
Imatinib (Gleevec) **Dasatinib (Sprycel)** **Nilotinib (Tasigna)** **Bosutinib (Bosulif)**	BCR-ABL	CML, ALL, GIST, MDS	V, Diarrhea, muscle pain, edema, GI bleed, myelosuppr.
Trastuzumab (Herceptin) **Ado-trastuzumab emtansine (Kadcyla)**	Her2	Her2+ breast	Flulike, nausea, diarrhea, heart failure
Pertuzumab (Perjeta)	Her2	Her2+ breast	Diarrhea, joint pain, neutropenia, rash
Lapatinib (Tykerb)	Her2 EGFR	Her2+ breast	Hand-foot syndrome, N/V, diarrhea, ↑LFTs, heart failure, ↓RBC
Crizotinib (Xalkori) **Ceritinib (Zykadia)** **Alectinib (Alecensa)** **Brigatinib (Alunbrig)**	ALK ROS1- (crizotinib)	ALK-mutated NSCLC	Blurred vision, photophobia, N/V, diarrhea, pneumonitis, renal/hepatotox, marrow suppression, electrolyte abnl
Dabrafenib (Tafinlar)	BRAF	BRAFV600E mut melanoma and NSCLC	Hyperglycemia, hyperkeratosis, HA
Cobimetinib (Cotellic)	MEK	BRAFV600E mut melanoma	Nephrotoxic, myositis, ↑alk phos, N, diarrhea, lymphopenia, ↓Na

Drug	Target	Indications	Side Effects
Trametinib (Mekinist)	MEK	BRAFV600E mut melanoma and NSCLC	↑LFTs, rash, diarrhea, anemia, lymphedema
Olaparib (Lynparza) Niraparib (Zejula)	PARP	Ovary, peritoneal, BRCA-mut	Anemia, ↓PLT, ↓WBC, URI, N/V, fatigue, myalgia, ↑Cr
Tositumomab (Bexxar)	CD20	HNL	Marrow supp, fever, weakness
Vismodegib (Erivedge)	PTCH,SMO	Basal cell ca	Muscle spasms, wt loss, alopecia, abnl taste, N
Vorinostat (Zolinza)	HDAC	CTCL	Fatigue, diarrhea, nausea, dysgeusia, ↓PLT

Hormonal Therapy

Androgen

Enzalutamide (Xtandi) Androgen receptor signaling inhibitor
Indications: Metastatic castrate-resistant prostate cancer (mCRPC)
Dose: 160 mg po daily
Side effects: Edema, fatigue, HA, hot flashes, diarrhea, arthralgia, gynecomastia

Bicalutamide (Casodex) Nonsteroidal androgen receptor antagonist
Indications: Intermediate- to high-risk prostate cancer
Dose: 50 mg po daily × ≥14d w/ LHRH analogue or 150 mg daily (monotherapy)
Side Effects: Edema, constipation, hot flashes, diarrhea, bone pain, gynecomastia

Flutamide (Eulexin) Nonsteroidal androgen receptor antagonist
Indications: Intermediate- to high-risk prostate cancer; PCOS, congenital adrenal hyperplasia
Dose: 250 mg po tid
Side Effects: Hepatotoxicity (black box warning), hot flashes, bone pain, gynecomastia, N/V, diarrhea

Nilutamide (Nilandron, Anandron) Nonsteroidal androgen receptor antagonist
Indications: Intermediate- to high-risk prostate cancer; transgender hormone therapy
Dose: 300 mg PO daily ×30 d, then 150 mg po daily
Side Effects: Interstitial pneumonitis (black box warning), HA, hot flashes, insomnia, gynecomastia, impotence, breast tenderness, hepatitis

Apalutamide (Erleada) Nonsteroidal androgen receptor antagonist
Indications: Metastatic prostate cancer
Dose: 240 mg PO daily
Side Effects: Fatigue, nausea, vomiting, rash, bone fractures, seizures

Abiraterone (Zytiga) decreases production of androgen precursors by inhibiting CYP17A1
Indications: Used in combination with prednisone (5 mg daily) in mCRPC
Dose: 1000 mg po daily
Side Effects: Edema, HTN, hypokalemia, fatigue, ↑glucose, ↑TG, ↑LFTs, joint swelling, hot flashes, cough insomnia, UTI, diarrhea

Estrogen

Anastrozole (Arimidex) aromatase inhibitor; blocks conversion of androgens to estrogens in extragonadal tissues
Indications: Hormone receptor–positive breast cancer in postmenopausal women; breast cancer prophylaxis
Dose: 1 mg po daily
Side Effects: Decreased bone mineral density, flushing, HTN, fatigue, HA, hot flashes, mood disturbance, arthralgia, ↑CV risk, ↑cholesterol

Letrozole (Femara) aromatase inhibitor
Indications: Hormone receptor–positive breast cancer in postmenopausal women
Dose: 2.5 mg po daily
Side Effects: Decreased bone mineral density, flushing, weakness, edema, fatigue, HA, hot flashes, mood disturbance, arthralgia, ↑cholesterol

Exemestane (Aromasin) aromatase inhibitor
Indications: Hormone receptor–positive breast cancer in postmenopausal women
Dose: 25 mg po daily

Side Effects: HTN, fatigue, insomnia, HA, decreased bone mineral density, flushing, hot flashes, diaphoresis, mood disturbance, arthralgia

Fulvestrant (Faslodex) selective estrogen receptor degrader (SERD): Binds to ER and causes degradation

Indications: Hormone receptor–positive breast cancer in postmenopausal women

Dose: 25 mg po daily

Side Effects: Hot flashes, ↑LFTs, joint disorders, bone pain fatigue, HA, nausea, pharyngitis

Tamoxifen (Nolvadex, Tamifen, Genox) selective estrogen receptor modulator (SERM): Competitive inhibitor of ER

Indications: Hormone receptor–positive breast cancer in premenopausal women

Dose: 20 mg po daily

Side Effects: ↑uterine cancer, ↑VTE risk, flushing, hot flashes, nausea, wt loss, vaginal discharge, weakness arthralgia, amenorrhea

Raloxifene (Evista, Optruma) SERM: Competitive inhibitor of ER

Indications: Breast cancer prophylaxis

Dose: 60 mg po daily × 5y

Side Effects: ↑VTE risk, ↑CVA risk, edema, hot flashes, arthralgia, leg cramps

Gonadotropin-releasing hormone (GnRH)

Goserelin (Zoladex) GnRH agonist: Chronic activation leads to ↓LH/FSH and ↓steroidogenesis

Indications: Prostate cancer, breast cancer

Dose: 3.6 mg SC q4wk or 10.8 mg q12wk

Side Effects: Edema, fatigue, HA, hot flashes, mood disturbance, acne, ↓bone mineral density, ↓libido, vaginal dryness, ↑glucose

Leuprolide (Lupron) GnRH agonist

Indications: Prostate cancer, breast cancer

Dose: 7.5 mg q4wk/22.5 mg q12wk/30 mg q16wk/45 mg q24wk

Side Effects: Edema, fatigue, HA, hot flashes, mood disturbance, ↓bone mineral density, ↓libido, vaginal dryness, ↑glucose

Degarelix (Firmagon) GnRH antagonist

Indications: Prostate cancer; especially *h/o CV disease*

Dose: 240 mg loading dose SC × 1; then 80 mg SC q4wk

Side Effects: Hot flashes, ↑LFTs, wt gain, arthralgia

Bone-modifying Agents

Bisphosphonates inhibit bone resorption by osteoclasts

Drugs: **Alendronate (Fosamax), etidronate (Didronel), ibandronate (Boniva), risedronate (Actonel), pamidronate (Aredia), zoledronate (Zometa)**

Indications: Reduce risk of fracture and bone pain in metastatic solid tumors or multiple myeloma. May reduce mortality in MM, breast, prostate ca

Side Effects: Osteonecrosis of the jaw, GI irritation, esophageal erosion, muscle pain, ↓Ca

Denosumab RANKL inhibitor; inhibits osteoclasts

Drugs: **Xgeva, Prolia**

Indications: Prevention of bone loss and skeletal events in solid tumors

Dose: Xgeva—120 mg SC q4wk (prevention of skeletal events); Prolia—60 mg SC q6mo (bone loss)

Side Effects: Osteonecrosis of the jaw, rash, fatigue, peripheral edema, GI irritation, ↓Ca

Immunotherapy

Basic immunology

- **Innate immunity:** Immunogenic pattern recognition by macrophages, dendritic cells, and NK cells. Respond to pathogen-associated molecular patterns and damage-associated molecular patterns. Activation leads to cytokine production, recruitment of other immune cells, and phagocytosis. Antigen-presenting cells then present antigens, leading to activation of adaptive immune system
- **Adaptive immunity:** Lymphocyte-mediated (B and T cells) immune "memory" via activation of B-cell receptors and T-cell receptors. B-cell activation leads to humoral immunity (mediated by antibody production) in response to a Th2 response; T cells mediate cellular immunity in response to Th1 response (thought to be more important for cancer surveillance).
- **Cell types**
  - **Macrophages (MΦ):** Monocyte derived. Function as antigen-presenting cells (APCs), phagocytes (in response to Fc, complement, or mannose), and innate

immune surveillance/activation (activated by PAMPs, DAMPs). Often resident in tumor tissue (TAMs), where they can promote invasion and metastasis. Two subtypes with prognostic implications in cancer:
  - **M1:** "Antitumor"; produce tumoricidal TNF and NO; improved prognosis
  - **M2:** "Pro-tumor"; produce IL-10, arginase, TGF-β; prevent Th1 response
- **Dendritic cells:** APCs that respond to PAMPs, cytokines. Play role in activating tumor-specific cytotoxic T cells.
- **B Cells:** Lymphocytes that produce antibodies in response to B-cell receptor activation via Th2 response to antigens. Found in circulation, lymph nodes, spleen, MALT lymphoma
- **T Cells:** Thymus-conditioned lymphocytes that recognize antigen-MHC complex. Mediate cellular immunity
  - **CD4:** Helper T cells; activate immune depending on cytokine and antigen context. Required for activation of cytotoxic responses that underlie cancer immune surveillance. HIV immunosuppression via CD4 depletion → increased cancer incidence
  - **CD8:** Cytotoxic T cell; activated by MHC class I; produce IFNγ, IL-2. Can directly kill infected/tumor cells via Th1 cytokine response to tumor-expressed MHC class I. Tumor down-regulation of MHC-I is a common means of immune evasion. Activation requires coincident TCR-MHC and CD-28/B7 signals. Immune checkpoint receptors can inhibit or stimulate CD-8 activation. **Immunotherapeutics target checkpoint ligands/receptors**.
  - **Th17:** Produce IL-17 in response to IL-1, IL-6, and TGF-β. Regulate mucosal immunity and modulate inflammation. Pro- and antitumor effects
  - **Treg:** Maintain self-tolerance by inhibiting anti-self lymphocyte expansion. May play a role in suppressing antitumor immunity. Activated by IL-10 and TGF-β
  - **MDSCs:** Myeloid-derived suppressor cells. Immunosuppressive myeloid cells that can be found in tumor microenvironment and are associated with poor prognosis and outcome
- **NK Cells:** Cytotoxic innate immune lymphocytes activated by MΦ cytokines. Important for containing viral infections during adaptive immune activation. Key role in preventing relapse after BMT

Common Immunotherapy Agents

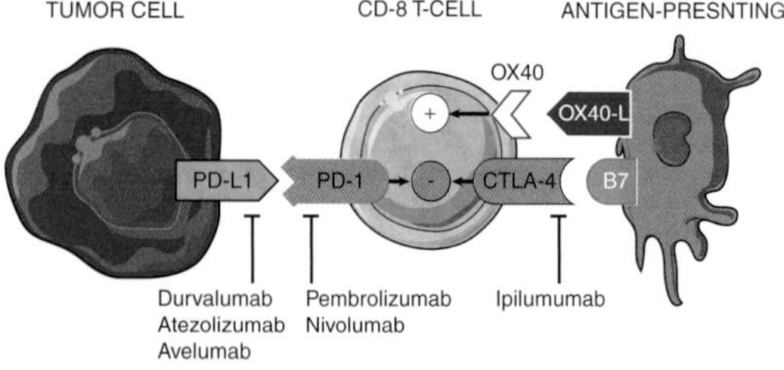

Drug	Target	Indications	Side Effects
Ipilimumab (Yervoy) **Tremelimumab**	CTLA-4	Melanoma	**Diarrhea, colitis, hypophysitis**
Pembrolizumab (Keytruda) **Nivolumab (Opdivo)**	PD-1	Melanoma, NSCLC, HNC, HL, RCC, **MMR or MSI tumors**	**Pneumonitis**, colitis, hypophysitis, thyroiditis, vitiligo
Durvalumab (Imfinzi) **Atezolizumab (Tecentriq)** **Avelumab (Bavencio)**	PD-L1	mUrothelial, NSCLC, Merkel	Rash, thyroiditis, hepatitis
MEDI6469	OX-40	Phase 1/2	Lymphopenia, fatigue, fever/chills, rash
Utomilumab (PF-05082566)	4-1BB	Phase 1	Fatigue, rash, hepatitis, diarrhea, neutropenia, ↑LFTs

Immunotherapy and Radiation

Several trials evaluated safety and effectiveness of radiation with immunotherapy.

- **XRT → ipilumumab**: Improved OS (not SS) in metastatic CRPC phase 3 trial (*Kwon Lancet Oncol* 2014)
- **Concurrent chemoRT → durvalumab**: **Increased PFS and OS** in stage III NSCLC in phase 3 PACIFIC trial (*Antonia NEJM* 2017 and *Antonia NEJM* 2018)
- **Concurrent WBRT or SRS + ipilumumab**: Phase I safe for melanoma patients with brain mets (*Williams IJROBP* 2017)
- **SBRT and ipilumumab**: Concurrent or sequential XRT/ipilumumab safe in metastatic solid cancers in phase I (*Tang Clin Cancer Res* 2017)

Several ongoing studies are evaluating possible synergy between radiation and immunotherapy in localized and metastatic solid cancer.

- Radiation may act as "tumor vaccine," exposing neoantigens after radiation-induced immunogenic cell death
- Thought to be most effective in the context of hypofractionated or stereotactic XRT

Immune Checkpoint Inhibitor–Associated Adverse Events

Side effects much different from cytotoxic therapy. Due to stimulation of autoimmunity.

General management principles:

- **Grade 1**: Local/symptomatic treatment (topical steroids, antidiarrheal)
- **Grade 2**: Rule out infection/disease progression; oral steroids (eg, dexamethasone 4 mg every 6 hours). Treat symptoms.
- **Grade 3-4**: Hold or discontinue Rx; IV steroids +/− additional immunosuppressants (eg, infliximab 5 mg/kg single dose)

Hypophysitis: Clinical hypopituitarism and radiographic pituitary enlargement. Symptoms—Headache, fatigue/weakness. Decreased thyroid, adrenal, gonadal hormones. DI and vision Δ rare. Rule out brain mets with MRI; full endocrine workup. Can resume immunotherapy with hormone replacement.

Pneumonitis: Rule out infection and hold treatment with G1. G2—add steroids; G3-4—d/c Rx; hospitalize with high-dose IV steroids

Diarrhea/Colitis: Diarrhea and radiographic changes such as diffuse bowel thickening or colitis. First rule out *Clostridium difficile* or other infection. In severe instances colonoscopy may help to diagnose. Treat diarrhea with antidiarrheal agents (eg, loperamide and atropine) and anti-immune medications (eg, steroids and infliximab).

Rash: Most common adverse event, occurring with 40%-50% of Pd-1 and CTLA-4 inhibitors. G1-2—supportive treatment with cold compresses, topical corticosteroids, and hydroxyzine, G3—hold treatment until return to G1. If G4 consider infliximab, mycophenolate mofetil, or cyclophosphamide. Rarely Stevens-Johnson syndrome/toxic epidermal necrolysis has been reported.

Adoptive T-cell Therapy

Transplantation of more effective antitumor T cells to induce direct tumor killing

- **Chimeric antigen receptor (CAR-T cells)** autologous or allogeneic T cells genetically engineered to express a chimeric T-cell receptor that includes tumor antigen–specific monoclonal Ab variable regions fused with the TCR and a costimulatory receptor (CD28). Activation is MHC independent, and response to antigen is supraphysiologic.
  - **Indications (FDA approved):** Pediatric ALL; refractory large B-cell lymphoma
  - **Adverse effects:** Cytokine release syndrome, off target effects (B-cell aplasia), cerebral edema, neurotoxicity; GVHD (if allogeneic T cells are used)
- **Engineered TCR** T cells are isolated from blood or tumor tissue and tumor antigen–responsive T cells are selected TCR from these cells are cloned and autologous lymphocytes are engineered to express selected tumor-specific TCR and infused into patient. Activation is MHC dependent.
- **Tumor-infiltrating lymphocytes (TIL)** lymphocytes are isolated from tumors, expanded in vitro in the presence of IL-2, and infused back into the patient after lymphodepletion with TBI or chemotherapy.
- **Donor lymphocyte infusion** Adoptive transfer of lymphocytes from a donor to a patient who has already received an HLA-matched transplant from the same donor. The goal is to augment antitumor immune response or ensure durable engraftment. Used to treat relapse after allogeneic SCT for CML, AML, and ALL
  - **Adverse effects:** Acute and chronic GVHD; bone marrow aplasia, immunosuppression

Oncolytic Viruses

Modified viruses that replicate preferentially in cancer cells. Many designed to stimulate immune system and induce antitumor immunity. Primary mechanism of action is virus replication in tumor cells causing oncolysis.

- **T-Vec (Imlygic)** modified HSV-1 expressing GM-CSF. Approved for inoperable melanoma. Delivered by intratumoral injection
- **Reolysin** unmodified human reovirus systemically administered oncolytic virus. Replicates in cells with activated Ras. Currently in phase III for HNSCC and CRC
- **JX-594 (Pexa-Vec)** attenuated vaccinia virus that expresses GM-CSF. Selectively replicates in cells with high levels of thymidine kinase (eg, p53 or Ras mutation). Currently in phase I-III clinical trials
- **DNX-2401 (Delta-24-RGD)** replication-competent adenovirus that selectively replicates in tumor cells with nonfunctional Rb pathway. Expresses RGD that enables uptake in tumor cells expressing integrins $\alpha_v\beta_3$ or $\alpha_v\beta_5$. Currently in phase I/II.
- **PVSRIPO**: Polio-rhinovirus chimera that recognizes the poliovirus receptor CD155, which is widely expressed in neoplastic cells of solid tumors. Recent phase I/II trial highlighted its use in recurrent glioblastoma, as it improved survival to 24-36 months, which is improved relative to historical controls (*Desjardins et al. NEJM* 2018).

Cytokines

- **GM-CSF (sargramostim)**
  - *Indications:* Chemo-induced neutropenia; myeloid reconstitution for HSCT
  - *Mechanism:* Stimulate expansion of myeloid cells (PMNs, DCs, MΦ)
  - *Side Effects:* Bone pain, myalgias, arthralgias, injection site rxn
- **G-CSF (filgrastim)**
  - *Indications:* Chemo-induced neutropenia; myeloid reconstitution for HSCT
  - *Mechanism:* Stimulate expansion of myeloid cells (PMNs)
  - *Side Effects:* Bone pain, myalgias, arthralgias, injection site rxn
- **IL-2 (aldesleukin)**
  - *Indications:* RCC, melanoma, adjuvant for autologous BMT
  - *Mechanism:* Expansion of lymphocytes (↑CD4, CD8, Treg, B cells, NK cells)
  - *Side Effects:* Capillary leak, shock, flulike symptoms

Vaccines

Induce immune response to shared or unique tumor antigens

Preventive vaccines: Vaccinate against cancer-causing viruses

- **HPV vaccines**: Inoculation of viruslike particles assembled from recombinant HPV coat proteins. Elicit virus-neutralizing antibody responses. 100% protection vs cervical CIN (*Harper Lancet* 2006)
  - **Gardasil and Cervarix** HPV types 6, 11, 16, and 18
  - **Gardasil-9** HPV types 6, 11, 16, 18, 31, 33, 45, 52, and 58
- **HBV vaccines**: Contain HBsAg, produced by yeast cells. Three vaccinations ~85%-90% protection
  - **Engerix-B and Recombivax HB**: HBV infection only (all ages)
  - **Twinrix** HAV and HBV (18 and older)
  - **Pediarix** infants whose mothers are negative for HBsAg (as early as 6 weeks old)

Therapeutic vaccines: Vaccinate against tumor-specific antigens to induce a T-cell response.

- Can be made from whole cells, modified whole cells (eg, express immunostimulatory molecules), peptides (HLA-restricted), DNA, DC conditioning, or Ag presentation in vectors (eg, virus) containing immunostimulatory molecules
- **Sipuleucel-T (Provenge)**: Dendritic cell vaccine FDA approved for metastatic prostate cancer. Stimulate immune response to prostatic acid phosphatase. Patient's DCs collected and cultured with PAP-GM-CSF, then reinfused. ↑OS in mCRPC by 4 months (*Kantoff NEJM* 2010)
- **Prostvac-VF**: Recombinant vaccinia virus encoding PSA and costimulatory molecule. ↑OS in mCRPC by 4 months in phase II (*Kantoff JCO* 2010)

CLINICAL STATISTICS

LAUREN ELIZABETH COLBERT • CLIFTON DAVID FULLER • BRUCE MINSKY

Basic Biostatistics

- **Statistical testing** requires defining a study hypothesis and thus a null hypothesis (H_o) to be tested. Applying the appropriate statistical test to this null hypothesis results in a **P-value** (α) → the probability of a result equal to or beyond that observed assuming H_o is true.
- The test, H_o, and thus the α can all be either **one sided** (only tests data on one side of the H_o) or **two sided** (tests data on both sides of the H_o).
- **Type I (or α) error** occurs when we conclude there is a difference when none exists; **Type II error (or β)** occurs when we conclude there is no difference when one exists; **Power (1-β)** is the probability of correctly rejecting H_o.
- **Sensitivity** and **specificity** are used to evaluate diagnostic tests. **Sensitivity** is ratio of True Positives/Actual Positives. Actual Positives includes True Positives + False Negatives. **Sensitivity** is the ratio of True Negatives/Actual Negatives. Actual Negatives includes True Negatives + False Positives.

$$\text{Refer to Figure 5.1: } \text{Sensitivity} = A/(A+C)$$
$$\text{Specificity} = D/(D+B)$$

- **Positive predictive value (PPV)** and **negative predictive value (NPV)** predict the likelihood of accuracy of a given test result. They both depend on the frequency of the disease in the underlying population. **PPV = True Positives/(True Positives + False Positives); NPV = True Negatives/(True Negatives + False Negatives).**

$$\text{Refer to Figure 5.1: } \text{PPV} = A/(A+B)$$
$$\text{NPV} = D/(D+C)$$

	Condition True	Condition False
+ Test	*A* (True Positive)	*B* (False positive, Type 1 error)
- Test	*C* (False Negative, Type 2 error)	*D* (True Negative)

Figure 5.1 2 × 2 contingency table showing expected test and condition results and their combinations.

Choosing a Statistical Test

Univariate analyses (one independent variable)

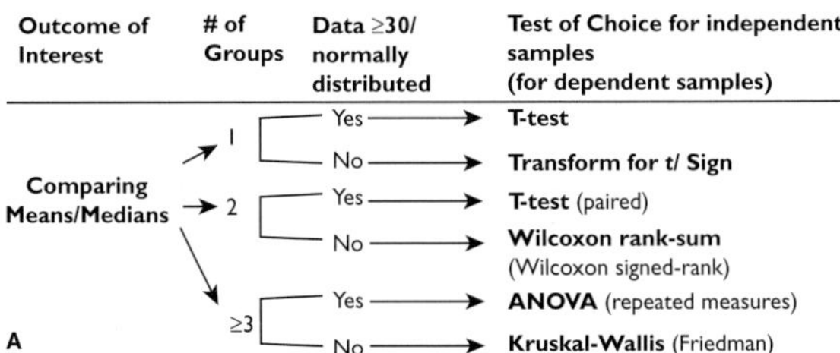

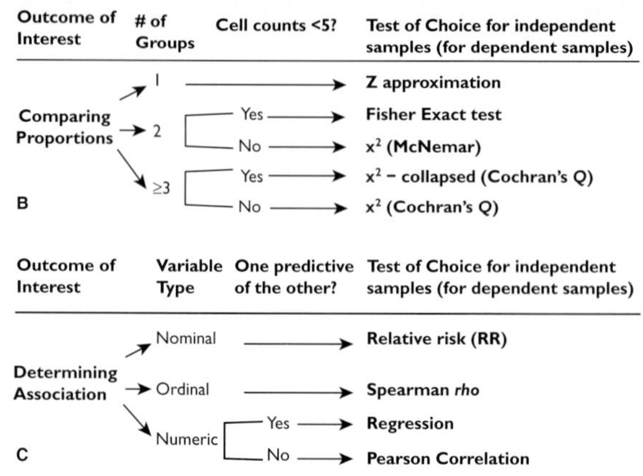

Multivariate analyses (two or more independent variables)

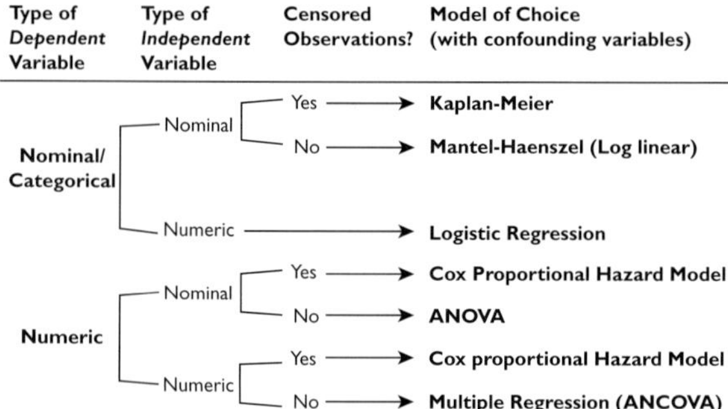

Note: A Cox multivariate analysis requires 10 events per variable analyzed. For example, if there are 100 local failures, then a total of 10 variables can be analyzed.

Clinical Trial Design

Phase 0	Proof of concept; first in human; testing pharmacokinetics, etc
Phase I	Primary objective is toxicity; can test pharmacokinetics, dose finding, toxicity, MTD studies
Phase II	Primary objective is efficacy; can also continue to test safety; can be single-arm or small multi-arm (either randomized or nonrandomized) trials; IIA often demonstrate clinical efficacy and IIB find optimum dose
Phase III	Primary objective is determining efficacy when compared against gold standard; often multi-institutional and/or randomized/controlled; typically single disease and well-defined patient population

IMPORTANT CONCEPTS—CLINICAL STUDIES

Phase I study designs

- **Traditional rule-based designs** (Classical 3 + 3, pharmacologically guided, accelerated titration)
    - **3 + 3 Design:** Based on traditional Fibonacci sequence. Cohorts of 3 patients are treated at a time and followed until specified time period before escalating. Once there is one patient with grade 3+ toxicity, a total of 6 are entered at that dose level. If a total of 2 or 3 of the 6 have grade 3+ toxicity, then that dose level is the maximal tolerated dose (MTD). The recommended dose level (RDL) for the phase II is one dose level below the MTD. **Advantages:** Simple and easy to follow/implement. **Disadvantages:** can be very slow and can treat unnecessary patients at below the MTD
    - **Accelerated titration (AT):** Allows escalating to next dose levels within cohort due to <3 patient cohorts (1 or 2). Only requires 3 patient cohort if a prespecified toxicity occurs. **Advantages:** Can increase pace of accrual and escalation. **Disadvantages:** Excessive/unsafe dose escalation may occur before toxicity is realized. May expose too many patients to toxic dose, particularly with radiation toxicities that may occur later
- **Model-based designs** (continual reassessment method [CRM, TITE-CRM], EffTox, Time to event, TriCR)
    - **Continual reassessment model (CRM):** Bayesian-based adaptive modeling accounts for *known prior probabilities* of toxicity including previously available data and previously accrued patients; adjusts dose as prior probabilities change. **Advantages:** May be more likely to treat patients at appropriate dose levels, does not throw out known data, may escalate more quickly. **Disadvantages:** Requires intensive statistical support and appropriate/trustworthy prior data.
    - **TITE-CRM** is a variety of CRM that incorporates time-to-event rather than only dichotomous toxicity data.
    - **EffTox** is a variety of CRM that incorporates both efficacy and toxicity into decision-making for dose assignment. Investigators set "rules" for requirements for efficacy and toxicity in order to escalate/de-escalate dose. **Advantages:** More efficient in diseases where some toxicity trade-off may be acceptable for increased efficacy (ie, pancreatic cancer, glioblastoma, diffuse intrinsic pontine glioma, etc.) or for extremely low toxicity studies (some RT studies). The Late Onset EffTox model (LOET) can be effective in radiation studies, where onset of toxicity may be later than in drug studies, for example.
- Phase I/II trials are designed to initiate a phase II trial at a prespecified criterion. Often the MTD identified in the phase I component of the trial is utilized in the phase II component.

Phase II study designs

- **Single-arm designs** generally compare only to known historical outcomes, with no built-in comparison arm. Outcomes may be response/no response, recurrence-free survival, or overall survival. **Advantages:** These require small sample size and allow for choice of comparison arm. **Disadvantages:** Historical comparisons are limited; comparisons may be biased.
- **Randomized phase II:** Two-arm studies that may be either comparative, with the intent to choose a winner for a phase III trial, or noncomparative. **Advantages:** Avoids limitations of historical comparison. **Disadvantages:** Require a much larger sample size. Allowed type I and type II error rates may be clinically futile given limitations in sample size.

Randomized phase II/III study designs

Patients are entered on the phase II portion and if an interim analysis meets a prespecified criterion (eg, does not show a difference between treatment arms), the trial continues as a phase III. The patients entered on the phase II become part of the phase III. **Advantages:** More efficient since there is only one trial. **Disadvantage:** The primary endpoint of the phase II must be different than the phase III. For example, the primary endpoint of the phase II could be local control whereas the primary endpoint of the phase III would be survival.

Phase III study designs

- **Randomized controlled trial (RCT)** represents "gold standard" of clinical testing. A double-blinded trial involves both the investigators and patients being blinded to treatment arm. Randomization can occur in many methods but involves randomly assigning patients to treatment arms. **Advantages:** Chance is only source of potential imbalance (eliminates selection and time biases), and randomization lends validity to statistical testing. **Disadvantages:** May require very large patient sample; not acceptable to some patients; administratively and financially complex. Placebo controls can be used for the control arm; this is difficult in radiation trials.
- **Superiority trials** are intended to show efficacy of a test treatment to be superior to that of a control (generally standard of care).
- **Noninferiority trial** is considered positive if efficacy is similar to a known effective treatment, and involves a one-sided statistical test (ie, an experimental arm is *not worse* by an allowable amount determined by investigators). **Equivalence trials** are similar, but require two-sided statistical tests. In general, an equivalence (and most noninferiority) trial requires about twice as many patients as a superiority trial.
- **Crossover design** trials allow patients to "cross over" from assigned arm to other arm. **Advantages:** Each patient can be his/her own control; more palatable to patients. **Disadvantages:** Difficult to interpret statistically; disease must be stable over time; one arm must not affect the other arm. Lastly, a crossover trial cannot use overall survival as the primary endpoint.
- **Two-by-two or "Factorial" design** involves more than one randomization or treatment arm assignment. **Advantages:** Allows testing of more potential treatments within one trial. **Disadvantages:** Difficult to analyze statistically; interactions between randomization factors may complicate interpretation; requires large patient sample sizes for reliability

---

Important Concepts

- **Odds ratio (OR)** represents the ratio of odds of an event (# currently with event/# currently without event) for the "exposed" cases divided by the "non-exposed" cases; often used in a case-control study.
- **Risk ratio or relative risk (RR)** is a measure of *incidence* (over time) and is expressed as ratio of cases who have or will develop an event in "exposed" group vs those in the "nonexposed" group.
- **Absolute risk reduction (ARR)** is the absolute difference between the RR in the experimental arm and the baseline RR of an event.
- **Number needed to treat (NNT)** is calculated as 1/Absolute risk reduction and represents the number of patients that would need to be treated to avoid one event.
- **Hazard ratio (HR)** is an Odds Ratio that compares risk over time instead of at a static time. It can be interpreted as the ratio of hazard of time in the "experimental" arm vs "baseline" arm.
- **Median overall survival (OS)** is calculated using actuarial methods and represents the time at which <50% of patients remain alive. It accounts for "time contributed" of patients lost to follow up.
- **Recurrence/relapse-free survival (RFS)** is calculated based on patients who survive without *either* recurring or dying.
- **Selection bias** occurs when the studied population does not represent the population of interest. **Classification bias** occurs when the variables are not clearly measured (have subjectivity) and misclassification affects outcome. **Confounding bias** occurs when the factor and outcome are erroneously linked, when they may be a confounding factor.
- **Randomization** attempts to eliminate selection bias by randomly assigning patients to groups. Clearly defining outcomes and variables up front can help eliminate classification bias. Some trials from the NSABP as well as the German Rectal Cancer Trial used "prerandomization." This approach increased enrollment; however, due to ethical concerns, it is no longer allowed.
- **Inclusion and exclusion criteria** are used to determine eligibility. Patients must meet all inclusion criteria and not meet exclusion criteria to be eligible.

- **An Institutional Review Board (IRB)** is generally institution specific and is responsible for ensuring that trials are safely and ethically conducted.
- **Intention-to-treat** analysis indicates that results were evaluated based on treatment arms originally assigned, even if patients change arms or do not complete therapy. An intention-to-treat analysis should be used whenever possible in a superiority study. **Per protocol analysis** analyzes only patients who were treated according to intended protocol arm (and completed therapy).
- **CONSORT guidelines** were designed to simplify and standardize reporting of parallel group controlled trials.

Levels of Evidence (per USPSTF)

Level I	Evidence from ≥1 properly designed RCT
Level II-1	Evidence from well-designed, nonrandomized trials
Level II-2	Evidence from well-designed cohort or case-control studies
Level II-3	Evidence from multiple time-based studies with or without intervention
Level III	Opinion-level evidence

Levels of Evidence (per NCCN)

Category 1	Based on high-level evidence, there is uniform NCCN consensus
Category 2A	Based upon lower-level evidence, there is uniform NCCN consensus
Category 2B	Based upon lower-level evidence, there is NCCN consensus
Category 3	Based on any evidence, there is major NCCN disagreement

BRACHYTHERAPY

ANNA LIKHACHEVA • CHAD TANG

Background

- **Definition:** Brachytherapy is a type of radiotherapy in which radioactive sources are placed inside or near target tissues.
- **Rationale:** Brachytherapy is arguably the most conformal form of radiotherapy. It can deliver ablative doses to the target while sparing adjacent uninvolved tissues.
- **Critical considerations:** Correct source placement is of outmost importance in brachytherapy. As opposed to EBRT where dose distribution is relatively homogenous, brachytherapy dose distribution is heterogenous with maximum doses inside the target being orders of magnitude higher than the prescription. 3D treatment planning is imperative.

Definitions of Dose Rate

LDR: 0.4-2 Gy/h
MDR: 2-12 Gy/h
HDR: >12 Gy/h
PDR (pulsed dose rate): HDR delivered in small fractions over a period of time typical for LDR implants. It is thought to mimic radiobiological quality of LDR, while providing the radiation safety of a remote afterloader and the 3D planning benefit of a stepping source. Generally requires inpatient admission

HDR BED calculation (*Nag and Gupta IJROBP* 2000): $N \times d\left(1+\frac{d}{\alpha/\beta}\right)$

LDR BED calculation (*Stock et al. IJROBP* 2006): $R/\lambda\left(1+\frac{R}{(\mu+\lambda)\times\alpha/\beta}\right)$

R (initial dose rate) = D90 × λ
λ (radioactive decay constant) = $0.693/t_{1/2}$
N = number of fractions, d = dose per fraction, and $t_{1/2}$ = half-life
μ = sublethal damage repair constant (typical values: prostate cancer = 0.693 h^{-1}, cervix cancer = 0.55 h^{-1})
α/β = characteristic parameter of the cell survival curve from the linear quadratic model (typical values: normal tissues = 2-4 Gy, tumors = 2-10 Gy)

Considerations for Invasive Procedures

- Screening colonoscopy within the last 3 years prior to prostate brachytherapy procedures
- Labs <7 days prior to procedure or after last cycle of chemo: Hct > 25, Plt > 50k for intracavitary and >100k for interstitial and for epidural/spinal anesthesia; coag panel
- NPO after midnight for conscious/deep sedation
- 1× antibiotic at procedure (eg, Ancef) with gram-negative coverage if preexisting orthopedic hardware (eg, gentamicin). Discharge 1-2 weeks of oral antibiotics (eg, fluoroquinolone).
- Stop Lovenox/heparin 12-24 hours prior, Xarelto/Eliquis/Fragmin/Arixtra 24-48 hours prior, Pradaxa 3-5 days prior, and 325 mg aspirin/Coumadin/Plavix/Effient/Pletal 5-7 days prior. If on Coumadin, bridge with heparin and hold heparin 24 hours prior. If ≤6 months from cardiac stent, discuss with cardiologist prior to stopping anticoagulation. Ok to continue 81 mg baby aspirin during procedure. Resume coagulation earliest next day and when signs of bleeding have ceased.
- Bowel prep for gyn and prostate: Clear liquid diet in the PM prior to procedure, two tabs of bisacodyl at 2 PM, bisacodyl suppository at night, saline Fleet Enema in AM

Common Brachytherapy Isotopes

	^{125}I	^{103}Pd	^{131}Cs	^{192}Ir	^{137}Cs	^{226}Ra	^{198}Au
Half-life	59.4 d	17 d	9.7 d	73.8 d	30 y	1600 y	2.7 d
Energy (kV)	27	21	29	380	662	830	412
HVL (mm-lead)	0.025	0.0085	0.022	2.5	6.2	14	3.3

Prostate Treatment Algorithms

• Low risk: cT1c-T2a, PSA < 10, Gleason Grade Group 1 • "Favorable" intermediate risk: only 1 intermediate risk factor, <50% cores positive (strongly recommend MRI to exclude patients with T3 disease)	Brachytherapy Monotherapy
"Unfavorable" intermediate risk	46 Gy/23 fx EBRT (to prostate + SVs) + brachytherapy boost
High risk	2 mo ADT → 46 Gy/23 fx EBRT (to prostate + SVs ± pelvic LNs) + brachytherapy boost → complete 12 mo ADT

- **Contraindications:** IPSS > 15-20 and postvoid residual >100 cc, large median lobe, gross ECE, seminal vesicle involvement, large-volume TURP, prostate volume >60 cc, IBD, or unable to undergo anesthesia

LDR Prostate Planning Metrics

Isotope	Loading Technique	Planning Metrics (PTV)	Monotherapy Prescription	Boost Prescription
I-125	Modified uniform	D90 > 140 Gy, V100 > 95%, V150 < 60%, V200 < 20%	144 Gy	100-110 Gy
Pd-103	Modified peripheral	D90 > 125 Gy, V100 > 95%, V150 < 75%, V200 < 45%	125 Gy	90-100 Gy
Cs-131	Modified peripheral with rectal modification	D90 > 115 Gy, V100 > 95%, V150 < 50%, V200 < 15%	115 Gy	75-85 Gy

- **Normal tissue constraints:** U150 = 0 cc and U125% < 1 cc. Rectal V100 < 1 cc
- **D0 evaluation metrics:** Consider the location of disease identified on pretreatment biopsy and MRI. Otherwise, D90 > 90% prescription dose and V100 > 90%. Immediate postimplant CT and/or MRI to evaluate dose distribution and confirm high-quality implant. Post-op day 30 evaluation if there is concern following day 0 dosimetry. Consider additional seed placement if inadequate coverage.
- **SIM:** 2-4 weeks prior to implant with MRI or endorectal US: (1) Identify the base and apex; (2) Obtain length; and (3) Evaluate pubic arch interference. If PAI, consider cytoreduction with 3 months Casodex + Lupron; make sure to obtain LFTs prior to initiation of Casodex
- **Target:** PTV depends on risk of ECE and imaging uncertainties. General expansion from CTV: 2-5 mm in all directions except 0-2 mm posterior (Fig. 6.1)

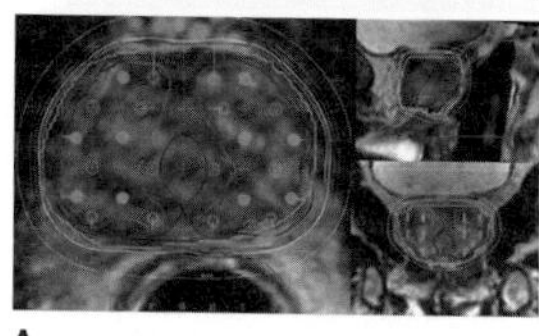
A

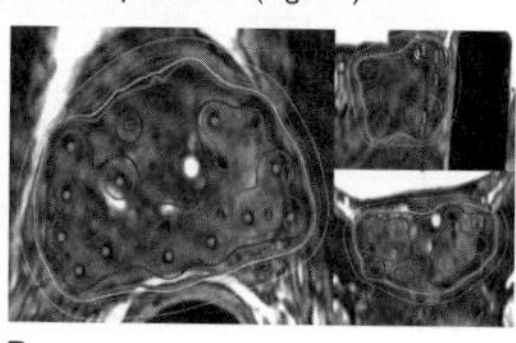
B

Figure 6.1 Example MRI LDR preplan **(A)** and D0 **(B)** plan for 144 Gy I-125 brachytherapy monotherapy implant to treat intermediate-risk prostate cancer. Showing the 100%, 150%, and 200% isodose lines. **See color insert.**

- **Side effects and management:**
  Infection: IV cefazolin and discharge home with PO ciprofloxacin
  Urinary (dysuria, hematuria, polyuria): Prophylactic use of alpha-blockers, discharge home with a Medrol Dosepak. If continued dysfunction, consider 2-week trial of ibuprofen 400 mg bid, increase alpha-blocker dose, or another Medrol Dosepak.

Urinary retention: If unable to urinate, acutely prompt placement of a Foley catheter is imperative. Consider other causes specifically postanesthesia (opioid-induced) retention.

Erectile dysfunction: Consider daily Cialis prior to and after treatment.

Proctitis and bleeding—steroid suppository → steroid enema → referral to gastroenterology → Argon plasma coagulation

- **Follow-up:** 1-month symptom phone call (and reevaluation if D0 implant concerns) → 6-month follow-up → regular intervals in the first 5 years with PSA and EPIC QOL. PSA bounce can happen 12-30 months after implant.

High-dose rate

- **Common indications:** Same as low dose rate
- **Contraindications:** IPSS > 20; prostate volume >60 cc can be overcome with a freehand technique. Proximal seminal vesicles can be implanted if involved. HDR is an option for patients with prior TURP if done >6 months prior and TURP defect can be well visualized. IBD is a relative contraindication. Colonoscopy within <3 years prior (*Hsu et al. Practical Radiation Oncology* 2014)
- **SIM:** Typically, no preplan is required. CT-based or US-based planning used. MR-based planning is under investigation.
- **Target:** Same as LDR, except can include ECE and proximal SV disease. No expansion from CTV to PTV if using real-time US planning (Fig. 6.2)
- **Evaluation metrics:** V100 > 97%, 105% < D90 < 115%; V150 < 35%; urethra V125% = 0; rectum V75% < 1 cc
- **Dose:**

  Boost: 15 Gy/1 fx or 19 Gy/2 fx.

  Monotherapy: 42 Gy/6 fx (two implants, 1 week apart), 38 Gy/4 fx (two implants, 1 week apart), 12-13.5 Gy/2 fx (one implant). All bid treatments should be delivered >6 hours apart.
- **Loading technique:** Start on a midgland slice. Peripheral catheter placement techniques (~2/3 peripheral, 1/3 central)
- **Side effects and management:** Same as LDR
- **Follow-up:** Regular intervals in the first 5 years with PSA and EPIC QOL. PSA bounce can happen 12-30 months after implant.

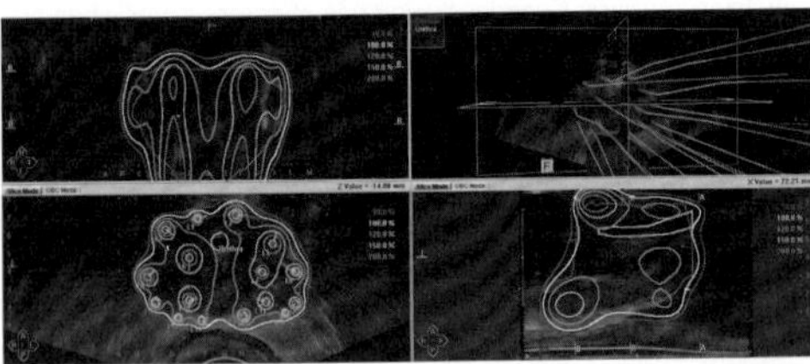

Figure 6.2 Example ultrasound HDR brachytherapy 15-Gy boost plan in a patient with high-risk prostate cancer after receiving 46 Gy/23 fx pelvic radiation.

GYNECOLOGIC

Endometrial (see Endometrial chapter)

- **Indications:** Early-stage high-intermediate risk cancer. Start 4-12 weeks post-op for brachy alone, within 2 weeks after EBRT. Examine the patient prior to placement to ensure adequate healing of vaginal cuff. Inoperable early-stage endometrial cancer
- **Technique:** Vaginal cuff dome HDR (Fig. 6.3)
- **SIM:** Place fiducial seed at vaginal cuff; size dome for largest diameter cylinder that patient can tolerate.
- **Target:** Top 2-3 cm of upper vagina
- **Dose:** 6 Gy × 5 fx (prescribed to mucosal surface) treated qod. for brachy alone; 5 Gy × 2 fx if post-EBRT
- **Dose constraints:** None
- **Follow-up:** q3mo for 2 years; q6mo until 5 years, then annually. Ca-125 if initially elevated

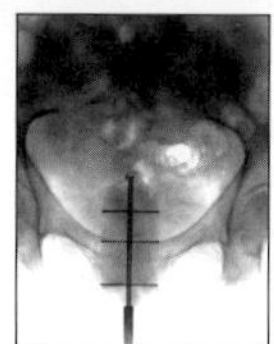

Figure 6.3 X-ray image of dome inserted in the vaginal cuff of an endometrial cancer patient ~6 weeks postoperatively. Note how the dome is up against the fiducial seed confirming adequate placement prior to HDR treatment.

Cervical (see Cervix chapter)

- **Indications:** Definitive treatment combined with EBRT and concurrent chemotherapy (total package time <8 weeks). Adjuvant/salvage
- **Technique:** Types of implants: intracavitary, interstitial, or hybrid. Ovoids/ring flush with cervix, tandem bisects ovoids, tandem 1/3 of the distance between the sacrum and pubic symphysis
- **SIM:** X-ray film immediately after device placement. CT simulation after device placement. MRI for at least first implant
- **Target:** (GEC-ESTRO definition)
  GTV = T2 lesion on MRI
  HR-CTV = GTV + cervix + any extension beyond cervix
- **Dose:**
  EQD2 dose to HR-CTV D90 = 80-90 Gy
  PDR: 40-45 Gy/0.5 Gy/h in two implants of 44-48 hours each
  HDR: 5.5-6 Gy × 5 fx; 7 Gy × 4 fx (in resource constrained environment)
- **Dose constraints:** ABS provides online Excel form for calculating combined EQD2 at https://www.americanbrachytherapy.org/guidelines/LQ_spreadsheet.xls
  Rectum, sigmoid, small bowel D2cc < 70 Gy
  Bladder D2cc < 80-90 Gy
- **Follow-up:** 1 month after treatment; q3mo for 2 years; q6mo until 5 years, then annually. PET/CT at 3 months; cervical cytology annually

Breast

- **Indications:** see **ESBC** chapter.
- **Target/technique:**
  - Multicatheter interstitial brachytherapy: PTV_EVAL = (surgical cavity + 15 mm), limited by 5 mm from skin surface and posterior breast tissue (excludes CW + pectoralis)
  - MammoSite brachytherapy: PTV_EVAL = (balloon + 10 mm) – balloon volume, limited 5 mm from skin surface and limited by posterior breast tissue
  - Conformal external beam APBI: PTV_EVAL = (surgical cavity + 25 mm), limited 5 mm from skin surface and limited by posterior breast tissue (see **ESBC** chapter)
  - Contura MLB: PTV_EVAL = (balloon + 10 mm) – balloon volume, limited 5 mm from skin surface and limited by posterior breast tissue
  - SAVI: PTV_EVAL = (SAVI device + 10 mm) – lumpectomy cavity volume, limited 2 mm from skin surface (or periphery of SAVI device if closer than 2 mm from skin surface) and limited by posterior breast tissue
- **SIM:** Thin-slice CT scan <3 days prior to first fraction
- **Dose:**
  HDR primary treatment: 34 Gy in 10 fractions; boost is 10 Gy in 2 fractions.
  LDR primary treatment: 45-50 Gy/0.5 Gy/h; boost is 15-20 Gy/0.5 Gy/h.
- **Evaluation metrics/dose constraints:**

	Interstitial	MammoSite	Contura MLB	SAVI
% of dose covering % of PTV_EVAL	≥90%/90%	≥90%/90%	≥95%/95%	≥95%/95%
V150	<70 cc	<50 cc	<30 cc	<50 cc
V200	<20 cc	<10 cc	<10 cc	<20 cc
Max skin dose	≤100%	<125%	<125%	<100%
Max rib dose	NA	<125%	<125%	<125%

Skin

- **Indications:** Early-stage nonmelanoma skin cancer (BCC and SCC). Contraindications, PNI (>0.1 mm), depth >3-4 mm, young age (<50), genetic disorders predisposing to skin cancer, previous RT or burn at treatment site
- **Technique:** Variable, including Ir-192 interstitial brachytherapy and superficial kV contact radiation.
- **SIM:** Clinical setup for fixed geometry applicators; thin-slice CT SIM for custom applicators
- **Target:** CTV = GTV + 4-10 mm (depending on size and histology)
- **Dose:**
  LDR: 60-70 Gy over 5 days
  HDR: 40 Gy (5 Gy/fx); 44Gy (4.4 Gy/fx) delivered twice or thrice per week, at least 48 hours apart (Fig. 6.4)
- **Dose constraints:** D_{min} > 95% and D_{max} < 135%
- **Follow-up:** H&P q3-12mo for 2 years, then q6-12; clinical photograph of treatment site at every visit

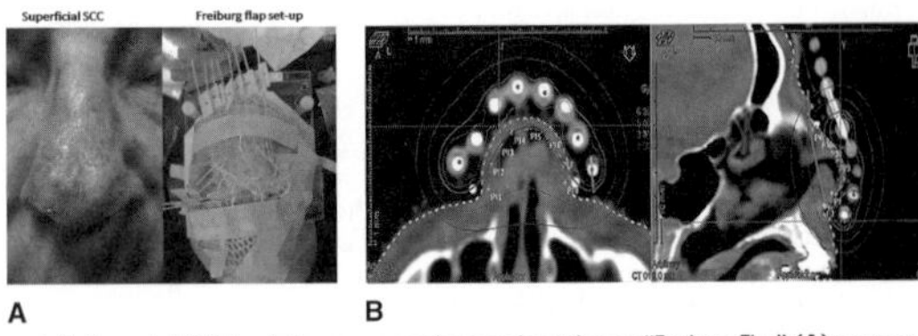

Figure 6.4 Example HDR brachytherapy monotherapy plan utilizing a "Freiburg Flap" **(A)** to treat superficial cutaneous squamous cell carcinoma involving the nose and bilateral ala. Patient was treated to 40 Gy **(B)** in 8 fractions given twice a week.

Notable Papers

Prostate brachytherapy boost improves outcomes for high-risk prostate cancer

- **ASCENDE-RT** (*Morris et al. IJROBP* 2017). Prospective randomized trial. 398 men with mostly high-risk disease randomized to 78 Gy in 39 fractions or 46 Gy in 23 fractions followed by LDR boost. Both arms received 12 months of ADT and pelvic radiation. The 5-, 7-, and 9-year b-PFS was 89%, 86%, and 83%, respectively, for the LDR-PB boost vs 84%, 75%, and 62% for the DE-EBRT boost (*P* < .001). No overall survival benefit
- *Kishan et al. JAMA* 2018. Retrospective multi-institution cohort study comparing RP, EBRT with ADT, EBRT + BT with ADT. 1809 patients with GS 9-10 treated in 12 tertiary centers between 2000 and 2013. 5-Year CSS better for EBRT + BT (97%) vs RP (88%) vs EBRT (87%). 5-Year DM rates were lower for EBRT + BT (8%) vs RP (24%) vs EBRT (24%). Adjusted 7.5-year all-cause mortality rates were lower for EBRT + BT (10%) vs RP (17%) vs EBRT (18%).

Brachytherapy for cervical cancer

- **RetroEMBRACE** (*Sturdaza et al. Radiother Oncol* 2016). Retrospective cohort study investigating 731 patients from 12 tertiary cancer centers treated with EBRT ± concurrent chemotherapy followed by IGBT followed by image-guided brachytherapy (IGBT) for locally advanced cervical cancer. Results demonstrated excellent LC (91%), PC (87%), OS (74%), CSS (79%) with limited morbidity. The 3/5-year actuarial LC, PC, CSS, OS were 91%/89%, 87%/84%, 79%/73%, 74%/65%, respectively. Actuarial LC at 3/5 years for IB, IIB, IIIB was 98%/98%, 93%/91%, 79%/75%, respectively. Actuarial PC at 3/5 years for IB, IIB, IIIB was 96%/96%, 89%/87%, 73%/67%, respectively. Actuarial 5-year G3-G5 morbidity was 5%, 7%, and 5% for the bladder, gastrointestinal tract, and vagina, respectively.

Breast brachytherapy

- *Strnad et al. Lancet* 2016. Randomized, noninferiority trial. 1184 patients with low-risk invasive and ductal carcinoma in situ treated with breast-conserving surgery randomized to either whole-breast irradiation (50-50.4 Gy in 25-28 fractions) or APBI using multicatheter brachytherapy (32 Gy/8 fx or 30.3 Gy/7 fx treated bid). At 5 years, local recurrence rates were similar between APBI (1.4%) and whole-breast radiation (0.9%). No difference in 5-year late skin toxicity, fibrosis, DFS, or OS

PROTON THERAPY

ALEXANDER F. BAGLEY • DAVID GROSSHANS

BACKGROUND

- **Brief history:**
  - 1946: First description of therapeutic protons
  - 1954: First patient treated with proton therapy at UC Berkeley synchrocyclotron
  - 1990: First hospital proton facility at Loma Linda University Medical Center, CA
  - 2006: MD Anderson Proton Therapy first to offer scanning beam capability
  - 2014: 15 active proton therapy facilities in the United States, 15 under construction, >110 000 patients treated with proton therapy with improved patient selection and advances in physics *(Mohan and Grosshans Adv Drug Deliv Rev 2017)*
- **Principles of proton therapy:**
  - *Interactions with matter*:
    - Three mechanisms: (1) Coulombic force with atomic electrons; (2) Coulombic force with atomic nuclei; (3) nuclear interactions (rare)
    - Linear energy transfer (LET): Stopping power or average rate of energy loss of particle per unit path length ($-dE/dx$); inversely proportional to square of particle velocity
    - Bragg peak: Protons lose energy at increasing rate as particle slows, with peak in dose deposition known as the Bragg peak just prior to stopping. Singular peak is referred to as "monoenergetic" or "pristine" Bragg peak (Fig. 7.1, below).
    - Spread-out Bragg peak (SOBP): Superposition of monoenergetic proton beams with differing intensities to sufficiently cover target volume (Fig. 7.2, next page)
  - *Biological effectiveness*:
    - Protons and photons assumed to be biologically similar
    - Relative biological effectiveness (RBE) proportional to linear energy transfer (LET). LET (and therefore RBE) continuously increases with depth.
    - Protons with estimated 10% higher average biological effectiveness relative to protons (RBE = 1.1)
    - Clinical approximation: Proton dose (Gy [RBE]) = 1.1 × photon dose (Gy)
    - Limitations of using fixed RBE 1.1:
      - Underestimates complexity of proton-tissue interactions
      - Based on limited in vitro and in vivo experiments under varied conditions in cell lines and tissues

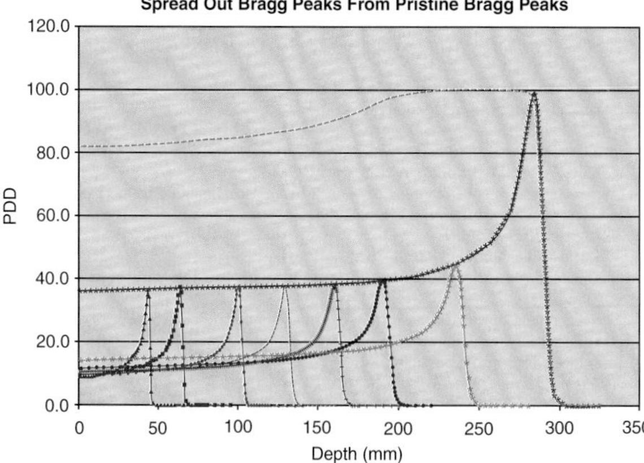

Figure 7.1 Summation of pristine Bragg peaks to generate a spread-out Bragg peak for proton therapy.

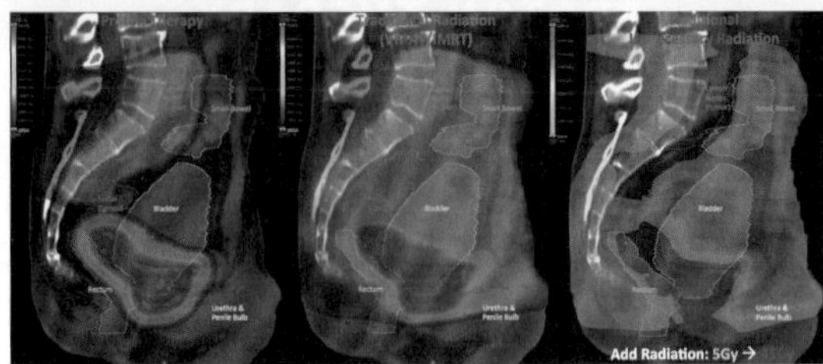

Figure 7.2 Comparative plan showing intensity-modulated proton therapy (*left*) vs a VMAT/IMRT plan (*middle*). Excess radiation dose (*right*) is calculated by subtracting the proton therapy plan from the VMAT/IMRT plan. **See color insert.**

        - For passively scattered beam, LET and RBE at end of range (distal portion of beam) may be higher than clinical approximation. This uncertainty necessitates consideration of proton beams direction so that Bragg peak ends proximal to critical structures.
        - For scanning beam, distal edge of beam does not conform to distal edge of target. RBE may differ significantly compared to passively scattered beam covering similar volume.
        - Variable RBE models in development; estimates range from <1.0 to >1.7.
- *Proton accelerators*:
    - Cyclotron:
        - Produces continuous stream of fixed-energy protons
        - More compact, higher beam intensity
        - Maximum energy 250 MeV; range ~38 cm in water
        - Uses energy degraders of varying widths in beam path to create lower energy beams for SOBP
    - Synchrotron:
        - Produces batches of protons at variable energies
        - Better energy flexibility and lower power consumption
        - Produces SOBP at any depth without energy degraders

Proton Therapy Technique

- **Passive scattering proton therapy (PSPT):**
    - More mature technology with greater clinical data available
    - Beam is spread laterally and longitudinally in the treatment head (nozzle).
        - Longitudinal: Using range modulators (ie, rotating modulator wheel) to create SOBP over the PTV; range compensator (eg, Lucite) to conform dose to distal edge of target
        - Lateral: Using dual scattering foils of high-Z materials; brass apertures to laterally conform dose to target
    - Limitation: SOBP is constant across field → no control of dose distribution proximal to target (*Mohan and Grosshans Adv Drug Deliv Rev* 2017)
- **Intensity-modulated proton therapy (IMPT):**
    - Increasing use of spot scanning or "pencil beam" scanning due to increased dose uniformity with preserved treatment range
    - Two categories of IMPT:
        - *Single-field optimization (SFO)*
            - Individual beams optimized by inverse planning to conform dose to target volume
            - Each field optimized separately to deliver uniform dose to target
            - Less sensitive to uncertainties
            - Integrated boost possible
        - *Multifield optimization (MFO)*
            - All beams simultaneously optimized to deliver homogeneous target dose
            - Multiple fields required to cover target
            - More sensitive to uncertainties
            - QA more demanding
            - Potential to place higher LET/RBE regions of proton beam within tumor volume for dose escalation with improved normal tissue sparing

- **Proton treatment planning and treatment**
  - Protons more sensitive to anatomy and beam direction due to (1) scattering properties; (2) sharp distal dose falloff; (3) range uncertainty
  - *Simulation*:
    - Position must be reproducible and provide adequate patient comfort.
    - Use proton-compatible immobilization devices.
    - Special considerations for high-Z materials. Generally, try to avoid placing these materials in the beam's path.
    - Use dual-energy CT for more accurate electron density mapping of tissues.
  - *Target delineation*: Use beam directions with short path to distal edge of target, minimal transit through heterogeneous tissue intensities, and avoidance of distal edge close to critical normal structures (increased RBE at end of proton beam).
    - Conventional "PTV" definitions for photons do not directly translate to protons due to range uncertainty (related to target depth and beam direction). Therefore, use of these terms in proton therapy literature should be interpreted with this understanding. At MDACC the STV ("scanning target volume") and ETV ("evaluation target volume") are analogous to the PTV for scanning beam and passive scatter, respectively.
    - Beam-specific PTV with different lateral margins and in each beam direction. See below for PTV margins in representative disease.
  - *Beam selection*: Use energy absorber (attached to the nozzle of the aperture) if target depth <3 cm, and avoid high–Hounsfield Unit materials.
  - *Dose and fractionation*: Use RBE adjustment as described above; RBE may vary from <1.0 to >1.7, but variable RBE models are not currently part of clinical treatment planning.
  - *Image guidance*: Use daily kV imaging or volumetric imaging during treatment to minimize setup variation, similar to conventional photon-based treatment.
    - Prompt gamma imaging (PGI): Formation of gamma-emitting nuclear isotopes after proton therapy used to approximate dose deposition; using "Compton cameras" or single gamma ray detectors
  - *Adaptive planning*: Consider verification simulation during 1st and 4th week of therapy and/or if any drastic changes in patient volume is noted during treatment.
    - Deformable registration with planning CT
    - Monitor weight loss and other anatomical changes that can alter dose distribution and DVH data.

PT 2-8

Clinical Indications

- **Standard indications (selected):**
  - *Craniopharyngioma* (Bishop et al. *IJROBP* 2014; Boehling et al. *IJROBP* 2012)
    - Target: GTV, operative cavity and residual disease; CTV, 2-5 mm customized margin; PTV, 3-mm uniform margin
    - Intent: Postoperative, definitive, salvage
    - Adverse effects: Endocrinopathy (hypopituitarism)
    - Considerations: PTV margin for lateral border especially close to optic apparatus and brainstem and CTV for proximal/distal borders
  - *Rhabdomyosarcoma* (Ladra et al. *JCO* 2014)
    - Intent: Postoperative
    - Adverse effects: Radiation dermatitis, mucositis
    - Considerations: Dose dependent on extent of residual tumor and primary site of disease (COG protocols)
  - *Atypical teratoid/rhabdoid tumor* (McGovern et al. *IJROBP* 2014)
    - Target: GTV, operative cavity and residual disease; CTV, anatomically constrained 1-cm margin; PTV, distal/proximal 3-mm margin
    - Intent: Postoperative
    - Adverse effects: Erythema, alopecia, cytopenia (with concurrent chemotherapy)
  - *Craniospinal* (Brown et al. *IJROBP* 2013; Barney et al. *Neuro Oncol* 2014)
    - Target: CTV, entire CSF (brain; upper, middle, and lower spine); PTV, posterior spine 7 mm (decreased 1-2 mm in c-spine)
    - Intent: Postoperative
    - Adverse effects: Myelosuppression, nausea, vomiting, dermatitis
    - Considerations: Junctions shifted 1 cm every 5 fractions; block anterior orbit, posterior neck, trachea, oral cavity

- *Prostate* (*Pugh et al. IJROBP* 2013; *Zhu et al. Radiat Oncol* 2014)
  - Target: CTV, prostate +/– seminal vesicles; ETV, uniform radial 6 mm margin except 5 mm posteriorly, 9-12 mm proximal/distally; STV, 12 mm lateral, 5 mm posterior, 6 mm all others to CTV
  - Intent: Definitive
  - Adverse effects: Bowel and urinary function, sexual function
  - Considerations: Use opposed R/L lateral beams.
- *Skull base—Chordoma/Chondrosarcoma* (*Grosshans et al. IJROBP* 2014)
  - Target: GTV, gross residual disease; CTV, 5-8 mm margin (to include areas of gross disease before resection) (CTV1—higher risk, CTV2—lower risk/surgical path); PTV, 2-3 mm
  - Intent: Postoperative, progression, recurrence
  - Adverse effects: Fatigue, nausea
  - Considerations: Use multiple CTVs: CTV1 = GTV + 5-8 mm margin (higher risk, higher dose), CTV2 = additional expansion to cover lower risk and surgical pathway; PTV with small margin to avoid optic chiasm, brainstem, temporal lobes
- *Seminoma* (*Haque et al. PRO* 2015)
  - Target: CTV (para-aortic and ipsilateral iliac vessels + 7 mm); GTV (involved LN + 10 mm); STV, uniform 5-mm margin for both CTV and GTV
  - Intent: Definitive
  - Adverse effects: Nausea
  - Considerations: Consider extended SSD technique and gantry rotation.

- **Sites under study (selected):**
  - *Nasopharynx, oropharynx, larynx* (*Frank et al. IJROBP* 2014; *Holliday et al. IJROBP* 2014)
    - Target: CTV1, gross disease; CTV2, high-risk nodal volume; CTV3, subclinical disease; PTV, 3-5 mm margin outside of critical structures
    - Intent: Definitive
    - Adverse effects: Xerostomia, mucositis
    - Considerations: Use three fields from three beam directions to treat bilateral neck (LAO and RAO with distal Bragg peaks lateral to spinal cord and single posterior beam with distal Bragg peak posterior to parotid).
  - *Esophageal* (*Lin et al. IJROBP* 2012)
    - Target: GTV, all disease present on PET and EGD; CTV, areas of potential spread; PTV, 1-1.5 cm margin
    - Intent: Preoperative, definitive
    - Adverse effects: Esophagitis, nausea, anorexia, radiation dermatitis
    - Considerations: AP/PA, PA/LLO, or 3-beam (RPO or PA, LL with LPO tilt, and LPO); brass blocks/Plexiglas compensators to deliver SOBP to encompass treatment volume
  - *Lung* (*Chang et al. Cancer* 2011; *Koay et al. IJROBP* 2012; *Liao et al. JCO* 2017)
    - Target: iGTV, envelope of motion of GTV on MIP image; iCTV, 8 mm isotropic margin
    - Intent: Definitive (with chemotherapy)
    - Adverse effects: Dermatitis, esophagitis, pneumonitis
    - Considerations: Use 4DCT for simulation/planning.
  - *Breast* (*Strom et al. IJROBP* 2014; *Strom et al. Pract Radiat Oncol* 2015)
    - Target: CTV, 15 mm expansion of tumor bed (including clips/seroma) with 5 mm contraction from skin and edited to exclude chest wall/muscle; PTV, radial 5 mm
    - Intent: APBI postoperative (see **ESBC** chapter)
    - Adverse effects: Radiation dermatitis
    - Considerations: Proximal/distal beam margins 3.5% of range + 1 mm from CTV
  - *Liver—unresectable hepatocellular carcinoma and intrahepatic cholangiocarcinoma* (*Hong et al. JCO* 2016)
    - Target: CTV, 10 mm expansion on GTV (depending on proximity of normal tissues), PTV 5-10 mm expansion
    - Intent: Definitive
    - Adverse effects: Thrombocytopenia, transaminitis, and liver failure
    - Considerations: Use 4DCT for simulation/planning.
  - *Postop prostate*
    - Target: CTV, prostate, and seminal vesicle fossa; ETV, uniform radial 7 mm margin except 5 mm posteriorly, 9-12 mm proximal/distally; STV, 12 mm lateral, 5 mm posterior, 6 mm all others to CTV
    - Intent: Postoperative/salvage
    - Adverse effects: Bowel and urinary function, sexual function
    - Considerations: Use opposed R/L lateral beams.

OLIGOMETASTATIC DISEASE

MICHAEL BERNSTEIN • DANIEL GOMEZ

Background

- **Definition:** First coined by Hellman and Weichselbaum representing a state of intermediate prognosis between localized disease and metastatic disease (*Hellman et al. J Clin Oncol* 1995). Number of metastases accepted as "oligo" are ≤5 in no more than 3 different organs.
- **Classification** (*Ricardi et al. J Radiat Res* 2016):
  - Oligometastatic (synchronous): ≤5 metastatic lesions in ≤3 organ systems at diagnosis
  - Oligoprogressive: Disease progression in ≤5 metastatic lesions in ≤3 organ systems
  - Oligorecurrent (metachronous): Disease recurrence with ≤5 metastatic lesions in ≤3 organ systems after definitive therapy for initially nonmetastatic disease
- **Biologic basis for oligometastatic disease** (*Reyes et al. Oncotarget* 2015):
  - Intermediate metastatic state, which manifests with limited sites of widespread metastatic disease. Numerous plausible rationales:
    - Environmental conditions in primary tumor forestalling clonal pressure
    - Sloughed-off cancer cells lacking properties (or genomic alterations) to survive circulation and invade target organ sites
    - Cancer cells landing in inhospitable target organs
- **Common oligometastatic subtypes:** Non–small cell lung cancer (NSCLC), breast, prostate, colorectal (CRC), and kidney
- **Common sites of treatment:** Brain, spine, lung, liver, lymph node, and bone

Local Therapy for Oligometastatic Sites

- **Rationale:** If primary site is controlled, or resected, and metastatic sites are ablated, prolonged disease-free interval, or cure, can be achieved (*Reyes et al. Oncotarget* 2015). Patients may never progress to widespread metastases.
- **Surgery (metastasectomy)**
  - Historically centered on hepatic resection in patients with primary CRC
  - 5-Year survival 53% after hepatic resection despite progression on chemotherapy (*Uppal et al. Eur J Surg Oncol* 2014)
- **Cryoablation**
  - 10% recurrence rate after treatment in largest series (*Littrup et al. J Vasc Interv Radiol* 2013). Sites included retroperitoneal, bone, head, and neck with average tumor size 3.4 cm.
- **Radiation therapy:** Stereotactic radiosurgery (SRS), stereotactic ablative body radiotherapy (SBRT)

Stereotactic Radiosurgery (SRS)/Stereotactic Ablative Body Radiotherapy (SBRT)

- Utilization of multiple beams originating from many directions/angles to converge on target
- Completed in 1-5 sessions, exceeding 5 Gy/fx with high level of conformity and sharp dose falloff
- Optimal regimen yet to be defined; however, general consensus that BED > 100 Gy is sufficient
- Local control rates between 70% and 90% for spinal (*Bhattacharya et al. J Clin Oncol* 2015), lung (*Huang et al. Radiat Oncol* 2014), and liver (*Aitken et al. J Clin Oncol* 2015) metastases have been achieved.

Patient Selection

Favorable prognostic factors include the following:

- Metachronous metastases (vs synchronous ones)
- Breast cancer histology may have significantly improved survival than nonbreast primaries (*Milano et al. Int J Radiat Oncol Phys* 2012).
- Time to recurrence >12 months
- Limited number of involved sites (1-3) (*Salama et al. Cancer* 2011)
- Higher performance status

Timing with Systemic Therapy

- Optimal therapy not known and likely variable with histology, but MDACC protocols generally prefer the following: neoadjuvant systemic therapy × 3-6 months > definitive local treatment > observation or maintenance systemic therapy.
  - Consider continuing systemic therapy during definitive local therapy if low chance of interaction. Otherwise, for newer systemic therapy or proven increased risk of toxicity, hold systemic therapy during local therapy.

Common MDA Dose/Fractionation Schemes for Oligomets

- Brain (stereotactic radiosurgery; all in 1 fraction, see **SRS** chapter): <2 cm, 20-24 Gy; 2-3 cm, 18 Gy; 3-4 cm, 15 Gy
- Spine (stereotactic spine radiosurgery; all in 1 fraction, see **SSRS** chapter): 24 Gy in 1 fraction (radioresistant), or 18 Gy in 1 fraction (radiosensitive)
- Lung: 50 Gy in 4 fractions (peripheral) or 70 Gy in 10 fractions (central)
- Liver: 50 Gy in 4 fractions
- Adrenal gland: 70 Gy in 10 fractions
- Lymph node: Varies by location; consider treating 46 Gy/23 fx or 50.4 Gy/28 fx to elective lymph node chain. Boost gross LNs to >55 Gy with conventional fractionation, variable fractionation for SBRT.
- Bone: Varies by location; consider 24 Gy in 1 fraction.

Notable Trials

Non–small cell lung cancer

- *De Ruysscher et al. J Thoracic Oncol* 2012: Single-arm prospective phase II trial examining radical treatment (surgery or radiation therapy) of 40 stage IV patients with <5 synchronous metastatic lesions. 95% had chemotherapy as part of primary therapy. Median overall survival (OS) was 13.5 months. Only two patients (5%) had local recurrence.
- *Gomez et al. Lancet Oncol* 2016: Multicenter randomized phase II study assessing role of aggressive local consolidative therapy (radiation or resection of all lesions) vs observation or maintenance therapy in patients with stage IV NSCLC with stable or responding disease involving ≤3 sites after neoadjuvant first line systemic therapy. 74 patients enrolled, and 49 patients were randomized. Median progression-free survival (PFS) in local consolidative group was significantly higher than that of observation arm (11.9 months vs 3.9 months, $P = .005$). Similar toxicity rates between arms
- *Iyengar et al. JAMA Oncol* 2017: Single-institution phase II randomized study investigating role of SBRT plus maintenance therapy vs maintenance chemotherapy alone in 29 patients with oligometastatic NSCLC (primary plus ≤5 metastatic sites) who exhibited stable or responding disease to prior first line systemic therapy. Significant improvement in PFS in SBRT-plus-maintenance chemotherapy arm compared to maintenance-alone arm (9.7 months vs 3.5 months, $P = .01$). No in-field failures and no difference in toxicities between arms

Colon cancer

- *Bae et al. J Surg Oncol* 2012: Retrospective analysis investigating efficacy of SBRT in 41 oligometastatic CRC patients with 1-4 metastatic lesions confined to 1 organ. Doses between 45 and 60 Gy in 3 fractions utilized to treat metastatic sites including lymph node, lung, and liver. 3-Year LC and OS were 64% and 60%, respectively.
- *Comito et al. BMC Cancer* 2014: Observational study examining safety and efficacy of SBRT in 82 patients with oligometastatic disease. 1-3 inoperable metastases confined to one organ (liver or lung) treated with doses ranging from 48 to 75 Gy in 3 or 4 consecutive fractions. 3-Year LC rates were 70% for lung and 85% for liver metastases, respectively. Median OS was 32 months. Difference in LC rates was significantly lower with doses <60 Gy vs >60 Gy.
- EORTC 40004 (*Ruers et al. JNCI* 2017): Randomized multi-institution phase II trial randomizing 119 oligometastatic CRC patients with liver-only metastatic disease with up to 10 metastatic lesions randomized to radiofrequency ablation +/– surgical resection followed by systemic therapy or systemic therapy alone. After a median follow-up of 9.7 years, median OS was significantly longer with upfront local therapy and systemic therapy vs systemic therapy alone (45.6 months vs 40.5 months, $P = .01$).

Other sites

- *Milano et al. Breast Cancer Res Treat* 2009: Prospective pilot study examining efficacy of SBRT in 40 patients with metastatic breast cancer with ≤5 metastatic foci treated with curative intent. 4-Year OS was 59%, LC 89%.
- STOMP (*Ost J Clin Oncol* 2017): Multicenter randomized phase II study assessing aggressive local therapy (radiation or resection of all lesions) vs surveillance in 62 prostate cancer patients with biochemical recurrence and ≤3 extracranial metastases. Aggressive local therapy associated with trend in ADT-free survival (median 13 months vs 21 months, $P = .11$). QOL of life was similar between groups. No grade 2-5 toxicities were observed.
- *Wong et al. Cancer* 2016: Prospective dose-escalation trial for 61 patients with solid tumors with ≤5 metastatic foci who received SBRT to all sites of disease. Median survival was 2.4 years. Longer time from initial cancer diagnosis to metastasis, longer time from diagnosis of metastasis to SBRT, and breast cancer histology were associated with improved overall survival.

STEREOTACTIC BODY RADIATION THERAPY

SAMANTHA M. BUSZEK • PENNY FANG • STEVEN J. FRANK

Background

- **Definition:** Stereotactic body radiation therapy (SBRT), also known as stereotactic ablative radiotherapy (SABR), refers to treatment of extracranial sites using >6 Gy/fx given over ≤5 fractions (ACR and ASTRO).
- Unique radiobiological characteristics cause dramatic tumor response ("ablative" RT).
- **Critical considerations:** High-resolution imaging, reproducible immobilization (acceptable daily error setup margin is <2 mm), breathing management, conformal radiation delivery techniques

Lung Cancer

- **Indication:** Stage I or II NSCLC—peripheral tumor (50 Gy/4 fx, plan for 60 Gy hot spot within GTV) or central tumor (70 Gy/10 fx, plan for 80 Gy hot spot within GTV) BED ≥ 100 Gy: Better local control and survival (*Onishi et al. Cancer* 2004)
- **SIM:** 4DCT. If tumor moves ≤1 cm, use free breathing—contour on MIP; otherwise, consider breathing management such as breath hold to reduce tumor motion if patient is able to hold breath.
- **Treatment setup:** Daily CBCT, daily MV, IMRT, or VMAT
- **Target:** iGTV: Gross tumor taking into account motion; no CTV; PTV = GTV + 0.5 cm
- **Dose constraints (for 50 Gy in 4 fractions):**
  Chest wall: V30 < 30 cc
  Spinal cord: D_{max} < 25 Gy, V20 < 1 cm^3
  Heart: D_{max} < 45 Gy
  Skin: V30 < 50 cc
  Major hilar or other great vessels: D_{max} < 49 Gy (NCCN)
  Brachial plexus: V30 < 0.2 cc, D_{max} 35 Gy
  Esophagus: V30 < 1 cm^3, D_{max} 35 Gy
  Spinal cord: V20 < 1 cm^3, D_{max} 25 Gy
  Total lungs: Mean < 6 Gy, V20 < 12%
  Ipsilateral lung: Mean < 10 Gy, V30 < 15%
- **Follow-up:** 1 month after treatment; q3mo for 2 years; q6mo until 5 years. CT of the chest for surveillance

Prostate Cancer per MDACC Protocol

- **Indication:** Low- and intermediate-risk prostate cancer (T1-T2b), pretreatment PSA < 10, Gleason score sum ≤ 7
- **SIM:** 3-4 gold fiducials placed in prostate via TRUS; noncon CT, supine, Alpha Cradle

- **Treatment setup:** Daily kV imaging with alignment on fiducials
- **Target:** GTV, prostate; no CTV; PTV = GTV + 3-4 mm posteriorly and GTV + 5-6 mm elsewhere
- **Dose:** 40 Gy/5 fx (qod); 95% of PTV getting 95%-110% of the prescription dose
- **Dose constraints:**
  Rectum: V20 ≤ 50%, V32 ≤ 20%, V36 ≤ 14%, V40 ≤ 5% (consider rectal spacing, eg, SpaceOAR, if constraints cannot be met)
  Bladder: V20 ≤ 40%, V32 ≤ 20%, V36 ≤ 15%, V40 ≤ 10%
  Femoral head: V16 ≤ 10%
  Small bowel: V20 ≤ 1%
- **Follow-up:** PSA q3mo for 2 years, PSA q6mo after 2 years

Hepatocellular Carcinoma and Cholangiocarcinoma

- **Indication:** Definitive treatment or bridge to liver transplant. If unable to meet dose constraints, consider hypofractionated regime (67.5 Gy/15 fx).
- **SIM:** Stereotactic cradle, MedTec Immobilizer, T-bar, 4DCT with breath hold, consider fiducial marker placement prior to SIM if difficult to visualize, IV contrast with delayed arterial phase
- **Treatment setup:** Daily CT-on-rails with alignment to fiducials if placed, daily MV port
- **Target:** GTV, hypodensity on CT; CTV = GTV + 0.5 cm; PTV = CTV + 0.5 cm
- **Dose:** 50 Gy/4 fx
- **Dose constraints:**
  Esophagus, large bowel: D_{max} 32 Gy
  Stomach, duodenum, small bowel: D_{max} 28 Gy
  Large bowel: D_{max} 30 Gy
  Spinal cord: D_{max} 18 Gy
  Kidney: Combined mean < 10 Gy
  Chest wall: V30 < 30 cc
  Gallbladder: D_{max} < 55 Gy
  Spleen: Mean < 6 Gy
  Common bile duct: D_{max} < 55 Gy
  Liver GTV: 700 cc spared < 15 Gy, Mean < 16 Gy
- **Follow-up:** Imaging and AFP q3-6mo for 2 years and then q6-12mo

Pancreatic Cancer per ALLIANCE A021501

- **Indication:** Locally advanced pancreatic cancer (T1-4N0-1 or NxM0); adenocarcinoma of the pancreatic head or uncinated process
- **SIM:** Fiducial markers in or within 1 cm of tumor placed prior to SIM; supine, arms above head; Alpha Cradle and wingboard; NPO 3 hours prior to CT SIM; IV and oral contrast highly recommended; 4DCT scan; expiratory phase gating (move OARs away)
- **Treatment setup:** Daily CBCT along with kV alignment to gold fiducials (placed by GI endoscopist within the target)
- **Target:** GTV = gross tumor on FB scan; iGTV = GTV; TVI = tumor vessel interface for each vessel, separately, at the level of the tumor; iTVI = TVI; PRV = planning risk volume = (duodenum + small bowel + stomach) + 3 mm
- **Dose:** 6.6-8 Gy × 5 fractions; PTV1 D_{min} > 22.5 Gy, PTV2 D_{min} > 29.7 Gy, PTV3 D_{min} > 32.4 Gy with max of 40 Gy within the GTV
  PTV1 = (iGTV + iTVI) + 3 mm = 25 Gy/5 fx
  PTV2 = PTV1 − PRV = 33 Gy/5 fx
  PTV3 = (iTVI + 3 mm) − PRV = 36 Gy/5 fx
- **Dose constraints:**
  Stomach, duodenum, bowel: V20 < 20 cc; V35 < 1 cc, D_{max} < 40 Gy
  Liver: V12 < 50%
  Combined kidneys: V12 < 25%
  Spinal cord: V20 < 1 cc
  Spleen: No constraint
- **Follow-up:** CA-19-9 and abdominal CT scans q16wk for 2 years

Oligometastases per NRG-LU002

- **Indication:** Stage IV NSCLC s/p 4 cycles of first-line systemic therapy with no evidence of progression and ≤3 discrete sites of extracranial metastatic disease (met locations—lung-peripheral, lung-central [GTV within 2 cm of proximal bronchial tree], mediastinal/cervical LN, liver [includes rib mets adjacent to liver], spinal/paraspinal [GTV arises within the vertebral bodies expanded by 1 cm], osseous, abdominal-pelvic)
- **Treatment setup:** Depending on organ targeted
- **SIM:** Proper immobilization; motion assessment (eg, fluoroscopy, 4DCT, beacon tracking, etc.), and motion control—strongly encouraged when GTV excursion is >1 cm in any direction. CT slice thickness ≤2 mm. IV contrast recommended. Ideally all mets will be treated in one treatment position.
- **Target:**
  Lung-central, lung-peripheral, liver, abdominal-pelvic, and mediastinal/cervical LN: CTV = iGTV; PTV axial = CTV + 0.5 cm; PTV craniocaudal = CTV + 0.7 cm
  Osseous: CTV = GTV; PTV = CTV + 0.3-0.5 cm
  Spinal: CTV = iGTV; PTV = CTV + 0.3-0.5 cm
- **Dose:** Depending on site. 1 or 3 fractions completed within 2 weeks of first SBRT dose; 5 or 15 fractions completed within 3 weeks of first SBRT dose
- **Dose constraints:** OAR should be contoured in their entirety if a portion of that organ is located within 10 cm of the metastasis.
- **Follow-up:** CT q3mo for 2 years, then q6mo for 3 years, and then annually

Head and Neck per MDACC Protocol (SOAR-HN—NCT03164460)

- **Indication:** Recurrent H&N cancer s/p RT or second 1° H&N cancer within previous RT field
- **SIM:** CT sim, supine, customized neck cushion, thermoplastic head, neck, and shoulder mask indexed to neck cushion, and customized bite block. Volumetric MRI, dual-energy CT with contrast, and PET/CT all in treatment position
- **Target:** GTV = tumor from all fused images (MRI, CT, PET); CTV = GTV + 0.8 mm; PTV = CTV + 0.2 cm for skull base or CTV + 0.3 cm if below C1
- **Treatment setup:** ExacTrac with daily bony alignment (verified and corrected in 6 degrees of freedom) and daily CBCT for treatment. ExacTrac before each arc
- **Dose:** 45 Gy to PTV in 5 fractions qod
- **Dose constraints:**
  Cochlea, optic nerve(s), temporal lobe: Max < 20 Gy
  Optic chiasm: Max < 18 Gy
  Brainstem: Max < 15 Gy
  Spinal cord: Max < 15 Gy
  Brachial plexus: Max < 25 Gy
  Parotid(s), carotid(s), and lingual artery: As low as possible. Goal is to maintain total max dose to <100 Gy.
- **Follow-up:** CT of the head and neck with contrast at 2 months and then q3mo

Notable Trials and Ongoing Protocols

Lung cancer

- **Pooled analysis of STARS (MDACC) and ROSEL (Dutch) trial** (*Chang et al. Lancet Oncol* 2015): 48 pts, T1-T2aN0M0 NSCLC, <4 cm diameter, randomized to SBRT vs surgery. STARS: SBRT 54/3 Gy peripheral, 50/4 Gy central over 5 days. ROSEL: SBRT 54/3 Gy peripheral (5-8 days), 60/5 Gy central lesions (10-14 days). Median follow-up 3.4 years. Outcomes: 3-year OS 95% (SBRT) vs 79% (surgery) *P* = .04. Toxicity: SBRT, grade 3 in 10%, no grade 4-5; surgery, grade 3-4 in 44%; 1 pt with grade 5. Conclusion: SBRT is better tolerated than surgery; SBRT might lead to better OS; SBRT could be an option for operable stage I NSCLC.

Prostate cancer

- UCLA/Stanford Phase II (*King et al. IJROBP* 2012): 67 low-risk prostate cancer patients treated with 36.25 Gy in 5 fractions; median follow-up 2.7 years. 4-Year relapse-free survival 94%. Toxicity: late GU grade 3 toxicity 3.5%, no grade 4 toxicity. No late GI grade 3 toxicity. Reduced grade 1-2 rectal (5% vs 44%, $P = .001$) and grade 1-2 urinary (17% vs 56%, $P = .007$) toxicities with qod vs daily treatments. Conclusion: Early and late toxicity and PSA response highly encouraging

Hepatocellular carcinoma and cholangiocarcinoma

- Princess Margaret Phase I (*Tse et al. J Clin Oncol* 2008): 41 pts, unresectable HCC ($n = 31$) or IHC ($n = 10$) with Child-Pugh A liver function and ≥800-cc uninvolved liver. SBRT with 6 fractions; dose dependent on NTCP calculations and was escalated throughout the trial. Median dose 36 Gy (24-54 Gy). 3-Month toxicity: no dose-limiting toxicity or RILD; 24% grade 3 liver enzymes, no grade 4/5; 23% progression to Child-Pugh B liver function. Late toxicity 6%. Outcome: median OS for HCC 11.7 months, intrahepatic cholangiocarcinoma 15 months. Conclusion: Individualized 6-fraction SBRT is safe.

Pancreatic cancer

- Stanford Retrospective (*Chang et al. Cancer* 2009). 77 pts with unresectable pancreatic cancer (58% locally advanced, 14% medically inoperable, 19% metastatic, 8% locally recurrent), ≤7.5 cm diameter. SBRT 25 Gy/1 fx. Prior EBRT 45-54 Gy in 21%. Median F/U 6 months. Outcome: 12-month LC 84%. 12-month PFS 9%. 12-month OS 21%. Grade ≥3 toxicities in 9% of patients
- ALLIANCE **A021501** Trial "Preoperative extended chemotherapy vs chemotherapy + hypofractionated RT for borderline resectable adenocarcinoma of the head of the pancreas" (*Katz et al.* 2017, Ongoing). Inclusion: borderline resectable adenocarcinoma of the pancreatic head. T1-4N0-1 or NxM0. Exclusion: prior chemo. Randomized to 8 cycles of systemic FOLFIRINOX vs 7 cycles of systemic FOLFIRINOX followed by short-course hypofractionated RT. RT with 6.6 Gy × 5 fractions. AIM: 18-month OS and R0 resection rate.

Head and neck cancer

- French Phase II (*Lartigau Radiother Oncol* 2013). 60 pts with inoperable recurrent or new primary head and neck tumor in previously irradiated area. SBRT with 36 Gy in 6 fractions to the 85% isodose line with concomitant cetuximab. Median follow-up 11.4 months. 3-month response rate of 58.4% and disease control rate 91.7%. 1-Year OS 47.5%. Grade 3 toxicities observed in 32% of patients and 1 grade 5 toxicity. Conclusion: Short SBRT with cetuximab is an effective salvage treatment with good response rate.

STEREOTACTIC CNS RADIOSURGERY

PENNY FANG • JING LI

Background

- Stereotactic radiosurgery (SRS) utilizes multiple beams to administer high doses to tumor while sparing normal brain tissue and can be given using Gamma Knife (192 individual Cobalt-60 sources) or through modern linear accelerators.
- Indications: Brain metastases, meningioma, pituitary macroadenoma, acoustic neuroma, trigeminal neuralgia
- For clinical considerations including patient selection for SRS vs other treatment modalities such as surgical resection, whole brain radiotherapy, and systemic therapies, consider multidisciplinary consultation and evaluation.
- **Local control rates:** 1-year local control 96.3% for lesions <2 cm and 87.3% for lesions ≥2 cm and <4 cm in diameter (*Likhacheva et al. IJROBP* 2013)

Workup

- **Imaging:** High-resolution, thin slice MRI imaging

SRS Day-of-Procedure (Gamma Knife)

Application of a Leksell invasive stereotactic headframe for rigid head fixation prior to simulation MRI (Fig. 10.1):

- **Simulation MRI:** Axial postcontrast 3D fast spoiled gradient echo images (1 mm slice thickness). Steps are as follows:
    1. Contrast administration: Intravenous MultiHance (gadobenate dimeglumine) injection at 0.1 mmol/kg (0.2 mL/kg)
    2. On import, check image quality.
    3. Discussion with neuroradiologist to identify all lesions
    4. Contour all lesions: Performed collaboratively by a radiation oncologist and neurosurgeon
    5. Place shots (see plan evaluation)
    6. Physics QA: On image import, check for fiducial definition errors, typically within 0.4 mm (mean) and 0.8 mm (max). Large deviations indicate stereotactic frame was incorrectly placed.
    7. Perform plan review including patient information, target coverage, prescription dose, collision checks, etc. For most cases, the minimum collision value should be >4 mm. Troubleshooting collision issues: Change angle, removal of a post from the stereotactic frame, and replacement of the stereotactic frame
    8. Consider giving a short course of dexamethasone to patients on treatment day who have large lesions and/or significant edema seen on MRI T2/flair sequence.

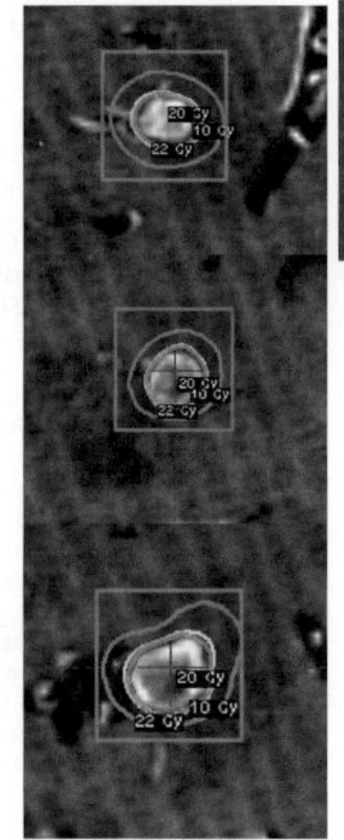

Figure 10.1 Representative axial, sagittal, and coronal images of a Gamma Knife plan to treat an intact brain metastasis.

SRS Dosing Strategy

MDACC approach to brain mets is adapted from RTOG 90-05 dose selection guidelines (Shaw et al. *IJROBP* 2000). *All treatments are given with a single fraction.*

- **Prescription isodose contour:** 50% isodose line
- Brain metastases (and postoperative cavity) SRS doses guidelines:
  Lesion diameter ≤2 cm: 20-24
  Lesion diameter 2-3 cm: 18 Gy
  Lesion diameter 3-4 cm: 15 Gy
- Meningioma: 12-16 Gy
- Pituitary adenoma: 22-24 Gy for secreting, ~15 Gy for nonsecreting
- Acoustic neuroma: 12-13 Gy
- Trigeminal neuralgia: See **Benign Disease** chapter.

Plan Evaluation

- Conformality index = prescription isodose volume/target volume (1 is perfect; ~1.2 is good)
- Gradient index = volume of 50% prescription isodose/volume of entire treatment isodose (~sharpness of dose fall off: want <3). Can turn on 25% isodose line when placing shots
- Heterogeneity index = maximum dose/prescription dose (~hot spots)
- **Dose constraints:**
  Brainstem: V12 Gy < 1 cc
  Optic apparatus: Max 8 Gy
  Brain: V12 Gy < 5-10 cc. For several lesions in proximity, minimize normal brain volume covered by 12-Gy isodose line.
  Cochlea: Max 4.2 Gy

Follow-up

- 4-Week follow-up post-SRS and then every 3 months with contrast-enhanced MRI at each visit

Notable Trials

Radiosurgery efficacy and toxicity

- **RTOG 90-05** (*Shaw et al. IJROBP* 2000): 156 pts with solitary nonbrainstem tumors ≤40 mm max diameter previously treated with partial or whole brain fractionated RT. Dose prescribed to the 50%-90% isodose line. Doses escalated as long as RTOG grade ≥3 CNS toxicity <20% within 3 months of SRS. Identified MTD to be 24 Gy for tumors ≤20 mm, 18 Gy for tumors 21-30 mm, and 15 Gy for tumors 31-40 mm
- **Alliance N0574** (*Brown et al. JAMA* 2016): 213 pts with 1-3 brain mets randomized to SRS +/– WBRT 30 Gy/25 fx. Primary endpoint cognitive decline >1 standard deviation from baseline on at least 1 cognitive test at 3 months. Identified less cognitive decline at 3 months after SRS alone (63.5% vs 91.7%, $P < .001$). Time to intracranial failure at 3 months worse with SRS (75% vs 94%, $P < .001$). No significant difference in OS
- ***Chang et al. Lancet Oncol* 2009:** Single-institution trial randomizing 58 pts with 1-3 brain mets to SRS +/– WBRT. Primary endpoint neurocognitive function as measured by deterioration in Hopkins Verbal Learning Test-Revised (HVLT-R) total recall at 4 months. SRS + WBRT significantly more likely (mean posterior probability of decline 52%) to be associated with a decline in learning and memory at 4 months vs SRS alone (mean posterior probability of decline 24%). At SRS + WBRT associated with improved 1-year intracranial control (27% vs 73%, $P < .001$).
- **JLGK0901** (*Yamamoto et al. Lancet Oncol* 2014): Multi-institutional prospective observation study enrolling 1194 patients with 1-10 new brain mets. Tumors <4 mL were treated with 22 Gy and 4-10 mL treated with 20 Gy. Overall survival was longer in patients with 1 brain met (median 13.9 months) compared with 2-4 and 5-10 (both median 10.8 months). New intracranial lesion recurrence was lower in patients with 1 brain met (23.9% at 6 months) compared with 2-4 (40% at 6 months) at 5-10 (46% at 6 months). Neurologic death, deterioration of neurologic function, was not different with respect to lesion number.

Benefit of postoperative SRS

- ***Mahajan et al. Lancet Oncol* 2017:** Single-institution phase III study randomizing 132 patients with completely resected 1-3 brain metastases to observation vs SRS demonstrated increased 12-month freedom from local recurrence (43% vs 72%, $P = .015$). No difference in OS
- **NCCTG N107C/CEC·3** (*Brown et al. Lancet Oncol* 2017): Multicenter phase III trial that randomized 194 patients with one resection cavity <5 cm to SRS vs WBRT 30 Gy/10 fx or 37.5 Gy/15 fx. Improved cognitive deterioration–free survival with SRS (median 3 months vs 3.7 months, $P < .001$). SRS associated with shorter time to intracranial tumor progression (median 6.4 months vs 27.5 months, $P < .001$) and lower frequency of 6-month surgical bed disease control (80.4% vs 87.1%, $P < .001$). No difference in OS

LOW-GRADE GLIOMAS

AHSAN FAROOQI • DEBRA NANA YEBOA • ERIK P. SULMAN

Background

- **Incidence/prevalence:** Estimated to be 2000 cases diagnosed per year. Low-grade gliomas are defined as WHO grade I and II gliomas (grade 3 and 4 are considered high grade).
- **Outcomes:** Median survival for low-grade *IDH* wild-type astrocytomas estimated at ~5 years. Median survival for low-grade oligodendrogliomas (1p19q codel) and *IDH* mutant astrocytomas is estimated at >10 years.
- **Demographics:** The median age of low-grade gliomas is estimated to be between 35 and 40 years. Males > Females
- **Risk factors:** Gliomas are largely sporadic without any clear risk factors aside from exposure to ionizing radiation.

Tumor Biology and Characteristics

- **Genetics:** Increased risk of developing low-grade astrocytomas in patients with NF1 and NF2. Tuberous sclerosis is associated with increased risk of developing subependymal giant cell astrocytomas. Increased risk also seen in Li-Fraumeni syndrome patients.
- **Pathology:** Historically, gliomas were classified based upon the histopathologic grade, although the diagnosis now includes molecular stratification (*WHO 2016 update; David et al. Acta Neuropathol* 2016). Grade I gliomas have low proliferation potential. Grade II gliomas are infiltrative, often recur, and have the potential to dedifferentiate into a higher grade (possibly by acquiring additional mutations). *TP53* mutations commonly seen in astrocytomas and 1p/19q codeletions seen in tumors with oligodendroglial histology. Recently, IDH mutations have been found in up to 80% of all low-grade gliomas and are associated with improved outcomes, independent of grade (*Ichimura et al. Neurooncology* 2009; *Olar et al. Acta Neuropathol* 2015).
- **Imaging:** Low-grade gliomas are typically lobar in location (most commonly in frontal or temporal lobes) and are contrast nonenhancing compared to high-grade gliomas. Because of the infiltrative nature of low-grade gliomas, they are associated with a hyperintense signal on T2 sequences, best seen on the T2/FLAIR sequence (FIG. 11.1).

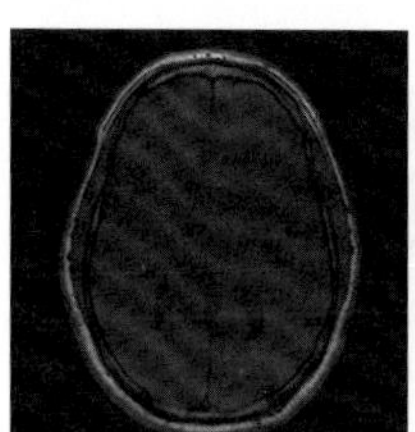

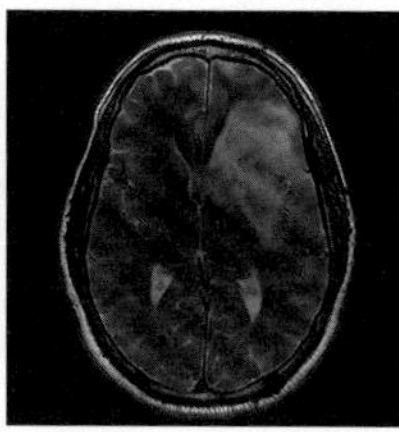

Figure 11.1 T1+contrast MRI image **(left)** shows an ill-defined non–contrast-enhancing hypointense lesion in the left frontal lobe without any necrotic features. The lesion is associated with a significant edematous component seen on T2-FLAIR sequence **(right)**, indicating associated edema and infiltrative pattern of spread.

Anatomy

LGGs typically arise from supratentorial cortex.

- **Frontal lobe:** Functions in regulating personality, behavior, emotions, and decision-making. Precentral gyrus (motor strip) lies anterior to central sulcus. Speech (Broca's)
- **Parietal lobe:** Interprets language, words, and sensory information Postcentral gyrus (sensory cortex) lies posterior to central sulcus.
- **Occipital lobe:** Vision

- **Temporal lobe:** Language comprehension (Wernicke's), memory, hearing, sequencing
- **Cerebellum:** Balance, movement, and spatial positioning

Workup

- **History and physical:** Including presenting symptoms, history of seizures (most common presenting symptom), and family history. Assessment of neurologic deficits and performance status important. Establish preoperative neurocognitive evaluation if applicable.
- **Labs:** CBC, CMP
- **Procedures/biopsy:** Neurosurgery evaluation for maximal safe resection or biopsy
- **Imaging:** MRI of the brain with and without contrast is the gold standard (FIG. 11.1) to evaluate location, grade, and extent of disease. Obtain postoperative MRI within 3 days of surgery to determine extent of resection and whether there is any residual disease. After 3 days, blood products make MRI interpretation difficult.

Staging/Grading

- **Grade I glioma:** Subependymal giant cell astrocytoma and pilocytic astrocytoma
- **Grade II glioma:** Pilomyxoid astrocytoma, diffuse astrocytoma, oligodendroglioma, and oligoastrocytoma. The 2016 WHO classification system (*WHO* 2016 update; *David et al. Acta Neuropathol* 2016) includes not just histopathologic grade but also molecular features. Specifically, mixed oligoastrocytomas are classified as either diffuse astrocytoma (1p19q noncodel) or oligodendroglioma (1p19q codel) to guide treatment decisions.

Treatment Algorithm

Grade I glioma	Maximal surgical resection → observation for all patients (RT only if clinical progression)
Grade II glioma <40 y of age[a]	Maximal surgical resection → immediate RT if STR, observation if GTR (RT at progression)
Grade II glioma >40 y of age	Maximal surgical resection → RT + adjuvant PCV or TMZ
Grade II glioma 1p19q noncodel *IDH* wt	Maximal surgical resection → RT ± concurrent TMZ → adjuvant TMZ

[a]Low-grade gliomas have multiple options and are managed with institutional variation. Important considerations for early radiation therapy may include large size (>5 cm), tumor crossing midline, astrocytic histology, neurologic symptoms/seizures (Pignatti criteria), or IDH wild-type molecular features in astrocytic histology.

Radiation Treatment Technique

- **SIM:** Supine, holding A-bar, aquaplast mask with isocenter placed at midbrain. MRI fusions—T1 + C sequence and T2 FLAIR sequences.
- **Dose:** 50.4-54 Gy in 28-30 fractions at 1.8 Gy/fx (can consider 2 Gy/fx)
- **Target:**
  GTV—surgical cavity
  CTV—GTV + 1 cm (+hyperintense signal on FLAIR sequence)
  PTV—CTV + 0.3 cm (daily kV) or 0.5 cm (weekly kV)
  Considerations: Limit CTV expansions to anatomic boundaries of disease spread (eg, bones, falx, brainstem, and ventricles).
- **Technique:** IMRT/VMAT. Consider use of protons on trial depending on anatomy and age.
- **IGRT:** Daily kV imaging
- **Planning directive:**
  Brainstem: V30Gy < 33%. Max < 54 Gy. If necessary may allow point max <60 Gy.
  Brain: V30Gy < 50%
  Optic chiasm: Max ≤ 54 Gy
  Cochlea: Max < 54 Gy. Mean < 30 Gy
  Lens: Max < 5 Gy
  Optic nerves: Max ≤ 54 Gy
  Pituitary: Mean < 36 Gy
  Eyes: Max < 40 Gy. Mean < 30 Gy
  Hippocampus (young patients, if concern): D100% < 9 Gy, Max ≤ 16 Gy
  Spinal cord: Max ≤ 45 Gy

Chemotherapy

- **Adjuvant:**
  Procarbazine, lomustine, vincristine (PCV) regimen (as per RTOG 9802)—procarbazine 60 mg/m^2 on days 8-21, lomustine 110 mg/m^2 on day 1, and vincristine 1.4 mg/m^2 on days 8 and 29. Cycle length is 8 weeks.
  Temozolomide (TMZ)—150-200 mg/m^2 daily for 5 days, every 28 days for 6 cycles.

Side Effect Management

- Nausea: First-line Zofran (4 mg q8h prn)
- Headaches/worsening neuro deficits: Likely due to increased edema. Consider treatment with dexamethasone at low dose (2 mg bid) with taper following resolution of symptoms.
- Scalp irritation/dryness: Aquaphor (OTC).
- Thrombocytopenia/lymphopenia/neutropenia: Likely due to PCV or TMZ. Refer to oncologist.

Follow-up

- Every 2-3 months with MRI of the brain w/ and w/o contrast for the first year following treatment, q4mo during years 2-4, and q6mo thereafter. Patients with age >40 years, large size (>5 cm), incomplete resection, astrocytic histology, and high proliferative index (MIB > 1%-3%) at high risk for recurrence (*Pignatti et al. JCO* 2002). Consider reirradiation on protocol or enrollment in investigational clinical trials at progression.

Notable Trials

Lack of improved efficacy with increasing RT doses

- EORTC 22844 ("Believer's Trial" *Karim et al. IJROBP* 1996)—Phase III randomized two-arm controlled trial. 379 patients underwent randomization following surgical resection to RT with either 45 Gy/25 fx or 59.4 Gy/33 fx. 5-year OS 58% for low-dose arm and 59% for high-dose arm (nonsignificant). 5-year PFS (47% vs 50%) also not significantly different between the two arms

RT timing

- EORTC 22845 ("Non-believer's Trial" *Van den Bent et al. Lancet* 2005). Phase III randomized two-arm controlled trial. 311 patients underwent biopsy, bulk, or GTR and were randomized to RT (54 Gy/30 fx) or observation (RT given when there is recurrence, ~65% of patients on this arm). RT arm had improved PFS vs observation arm (5.3 vs 3.4 years, $P < .0001$), but OS not significantly different. Importantly, early RT improved seizure control at 1 year (41% vs 25%).

Improvement in outcomes with chemotherapy

- RTOG 9802 (*Shaw et al. JCO* 2012; *Buckner et al. NEJM* 2016). Phase III randomized two-arm controlled trial. 251 patients aged >40 years or <40 with subtotal resection randomized to RT alone (54 Gy/30 fx) vs RT followed by adjuvant PCV (6 total cycles). Median OS 13.3 years in RT + PCV arm vs 7.8 years in RT alone (HR for death 0.59, $P = .003$). Median PFS was 10.4 years in RT + PCV arm vs 4.0 years in RT alone (HR for progression or death 0.50, $P < .001$). Histologic finding of oligodendroglioma favorable prognostic variable for both PFS and OS
- RTOG 0424 (*Fisher et al. IJROBP* 2015). Phase II trial of 129 high-risk (as defined by ≥3 high-risk factors) LGG treated with RT (54 Gy/30 fx) with concurrent and adjuvant TMZ. 3 year OS rate was 73.1% (95% CI 65.3%-80.8%), which was significantly improved compared to historical control of 54% ($P < .001$). 3 year PFS was 59.2%. Suggests adjuvant TMZ may offer similar OS and PFS benefit as PCV but randomized control trial between the two pending (CODEL trial)

HIGH-GRADE GLIOMAS

AHSAN FAROOQI • DEBRA NANA YEBOA • ERIK P. SULMAN

BACKGROUND

- **Incidence/prevalence:** There are ~20 000 new high-grade glioma (HGG) cases per year diagnosed in the United States. Of all malignant brain tumors, glioblastomas constitute ~60%.
- **Outcomes:** 5-Year OS rates for glioblastoma estimated between 5% and 10%. 5-Year OS rates for grade III gliomas estimated at 25%
- **Demographics:** The mean age at diagnosis of high-grade gliomas is 65 years. Males > females
- **Risk factors:** Gliomas are largely sporadic without any clear risk factors aside from prior exposure to ionizing radiation and genetic syndromes as noted below. There is no evidence that cell phone use leads to increased risk of developing gliomas.

TUMOR BIOLOGY AND CHARACTERISTICS

- **Genetics:** Associated with various familial genetic syndromes including Li-Fraumeni (germ-line mutations in *TP53*), neurofibromatosis type 1, and Turcot syndrome. Glioblastoma was the first cancer type to be systematically studied via The Cancer Genome Atlas (TCGA). P53, RB, and receptor tyrosine kinase (RAS) signaling pathways were found to be abrogated across nearly all glioblastomas (*Cancer Genome Atlas Network Nature* 2008). *TERT* promoter mutations, leading to increased expression and activity of telomerase, are also found in ~80% of glioblastoma (*Killela et al. Proc Natl Acad Sci* 2013). *IDH* and *ATRX* mutations are common among astrocytomas and are mutually exclusive with *TERT* promoter mutations. TCGA has now established four subtypes of glioblastoma: classical (EGFR mutated without *TP53* mutations), proneural (associated with *TP53 and IDH1* mutations), mesenchymal (associated with *NF1* mutations), and neural (resembling normal brain tissue) (*Verhaak et al. Cancer Cell* 2010). Methylation of the *MGMT* promoter leads to improved response to concurrent chemoradiation with temozolomide (*Monika et al. NEJM* 2005).
- **Pathology:** Historically, gliomas were all classified based upon the histopathologic grade, although the diagnosis now includes molecular data (*WHO* 2016 update; *David et al. Acta Neuropathol* 2016). Grade III astrocytomas and grade IV GBMs are highly cellular and infiltrative. Classically, glioblastomas are characterized by foci of microvascular proliferation and pseudopalisading necrosis. Consideration that *IDH* wt status may trump pathology when determining GBM diagnosis in the future
- **Imaging:** High-grade gliomas are contrast-enhancing on T1 scans with an associated edematous component best seen on T2-FLAIR sequences (Fig. 12.1). Additionally, glioblastomas commonly show a centrally necrotic pattern on imaging and can routinely cross midline ("butterfly" pattern).

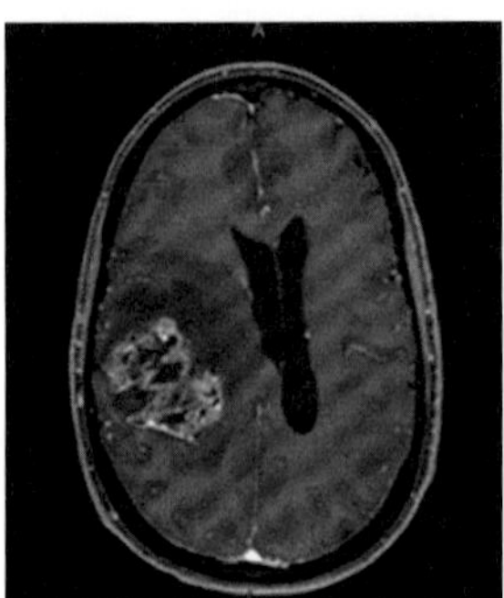

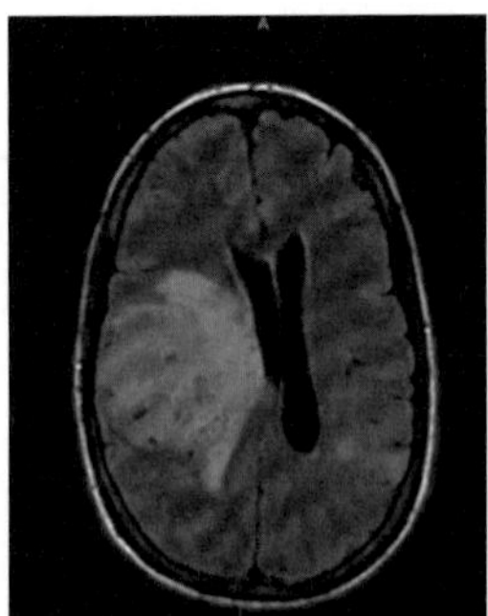

Figure 12.1 T1+contrast MRI image **(left)** shows large contrast-enhancing lesion in the right frontoparietal lobe with necrotic features consistent with glioblastoma. The lesion is associated with a significant edematous component seen on T2-FLAIR sequence **(right)**.

Anatomy

- Commonly present in the frontal lobe compared to parietal/temporal and occipital lobes. Infratentorial tumors are uncommon. See **LGG** chapter for review of neuroanatomy.

Workup

- **History and physical:** Including presenting symptoms, history of seizures, and family history. Assessment of neurologic deficits and performance status important. Important to ask about whether they are on steroids and whether their symptoms have improved
- **Labs:** CBC, CMP
- **Procedures/biopsy:** Neurosurgery evaluation for biopsy and/or resection
- **Imaging:** MRI of the brain with and without contrast is the gold standard (Fig. 12.1) to evaluate location, grade, and extent of disease.

Staging/Grading

- **Grade III gliomas:** Anaplastic astrocytoma, anaplastic oligodendroglioma, anaplastic oligoastrocytoma, and anaplastic ependymoma. 1p19q codeletion commonly associated with oligodendroglioma histologic subtype. *IDH* and *ATRX* mutations associated with anaplastic astrocytoma or mixed histologies. Cases with mutant *IDH* and/or 1p19q codeletion associated with improved prognosis compared to *IDH* wild-type tumors
- **Grade IV glioblastoma:** Important to assess IDH mutational status (if mutated, likely to be secondary as opposed to de novo). IDH mutant cases are associated with improved survival although inevitably these recur as well.

Treatment Algorithm

Grade III glioma	Maximal surgical resection → RT → adjuvant chemotherapy with TMZ or PCV. Consider concurrent chemotherapy if IDH wild-type
Grade IV glioblastoma[a]	Maximal surgical resection → concurrent chemoRT with TMZ → adjuvant TMZ + alternating electrical tumor-treating fields (TTF)
Grade IV glioblastoma Elderly with good PS[a]	Maximal surgical resection → concurrent hypofractionated chemoRT with TMZ → adjuvant TMZ + consider alternating electrical tumor-treating fields (TTF)
Grade IV glioblastoma Elderly with poor PS or MGMT methylation[a]	Maximal surgical resection → TMZ

[a]Elderly patients with glioblastoma have a multitude of options and can be treated with any of the above options. Important considerations include life expectancy, PS, methylation, and comorbidities.

Radiation Treatment Technique

- **SIM:** Supine, holding A-bar, aquaplast mask with isocenter placed at midbrain. MRI fusions (unless obtaining MRI SIM)—T1 + C sequence and T2/FLAIR sequences.
- **Dose and target:**

  High-Grade Glioma

  MDACC approach: **Simultaneous integrated boost (SIB) to CTV1 within CTV2.**

  CTV1: GTV (cavity + residual contrast enhancement)—57 Gy in 30 fractions at 1.9 Gy/fx

  CTV2: GTV + 1.5 cm (+uncovered hyperintense signal on FLAIR sequence)—50 Gy in 30 fractions at 1.66 Gy/fx

  Alternative RTOG approach, sequential radiation:

  CTV1: GTV (cavity + residual contrast enhancement) + 1 cm—59.4 Gy in 33 fractions at 1.8 Gy/fx

  CTV2: GTV (cavity + residual contrast enhancement) + 2 cm—50.4 Gy in 30 fractions at 1.8 Gy/fx

Alternative EORTC approach

PTV1: GTV (cavity + residual contrast enhancement) + T2/FLAIR + 1.5 cm—45 Gy in 30 fractions at 1.8 Gy/fx

PTV2: GTV + 1.5 cm—additional 14.4 Gy in 8 fractions of 1.8 Gy for a total of 59.4 Gy

Glioblastoma

MDACC approach: **SIB to CTV1 within CTV2 (Fig. 12.2).**

CTV1: GTV (cavity + residual contrast enhancement)—60 Gy in 30 fractions at 2 Gy/fx

CTV2: GTV + 2 cm (+uncovered hyperintense signal on FLAIR sequence)—50 Gy in 30 fractions at 1.66 Gy/fx

Alternative RTOG approach, sequential radiation:

CTV1: GTV (cavity + residual contrast enhancement) + edema on T2/FLAIR + 2 cm—46 Gy in 23 fractions at 2.0 Gy/fx

CTV2: GTV (cavity + residual contrast enhancement) + 2 cm—additional 14 Gy in 7 fractions at 2.0 Gy/fx for a total of 60 Gy in 30 fractions

Alternative EORTC approach

CTV: GTV (surgical cavity + residual enhancing tumor) + 2 cm—60 Gy in 30 fractions at 2.0 Gy/fx

Alternative hypofractionated regimes:

50 Gy/20 fx, 40 Gy/15 fx, 34 Gy/10 fx, or 25 Gy/5 fx if poor PS or elderly.

Considerations: Limit CTV expansions to anatomic boundaries of disease spread (bones, falx, brainstem), unless T2 hyperintense signal spreads beyond these barrier areas indicating probable disease.

For all high-grade gliomas, PTV expansions on CTV1 and CTV2 are generally 0.3 cm (daily kV) or 0.5 cm (weekly kV), at our institution.

- **Technique:** IMRT/VMAT. Consider use of protons on trial depending on anatomy and age.
- **IGRT:** Daily kV imaging.
- **Planning directive:**

Brainstem: V30Gy < 33%. Max < 54 Gy. If necessary may allow point max <60 Gy.
Brain: V30Gy < 50%
Optic chiasm: Max ≤ 54 Gy
Cochlea: Max < 54 Gy. Mean < 30 Gy

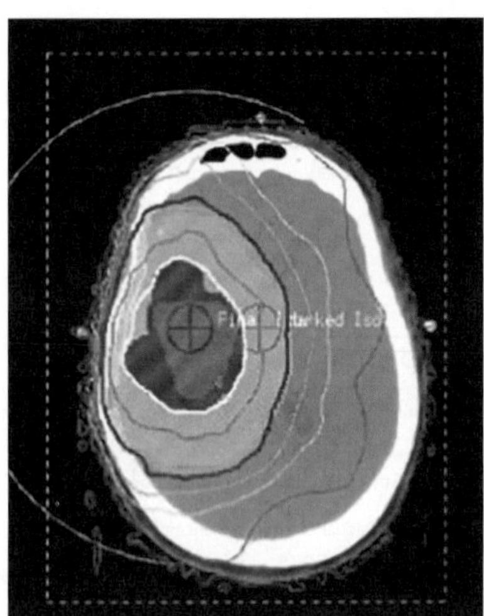

Figure 12.2 Representative plan for a patient with a grade IV glioblastoma. The 60-Gy isodose line (*white*) can be seen surrounding the red GTV/resection cavity (*red color wash*). The 50-Gy isodose line (*blue*) covers GTV + 2 cm (*tan color wash*), which is expanded to include hyperintense signal on T2-FLAIR sequence. **See color insert.**

Lens: Max < 5 Gy
Optic nerves: Max ≤ 54 Gy
Pituitary: Mean < 36 Gy
Eyes: Max < 40 Gy. Mean < 30 Gy
Hippocampus (young patients, if concern): D100% < 9 Gy, Max ≤ 16 Gy
Spinal cord: Max ≤ 45 Gy

Chemotherapy

- **Concurrent:** Temozolomide (TMZ) 75 mg/m^2 daily during RT, 7 days a week.
- **Adjuvant:** TMZ 150-200 mg/m^2 daily for 5 days, every 28 days for 6 cycles (or indefinitely). Procarbazine, lomustine, vincristine (PCV) regimen historically used in an adjuvant setting for grade III gliomas although most oncologists are now giving TMZ due to decreased toxicities and retrospective studies suggest equivalent efficacy.

Side Effect Management

See **LGG** chapter.

Follow-up

Every 2-3 months with MRI of the brain w/ and w/o contrast for the first year following treatment, q4mo during years 2-4 and q6mo thereafter. Offer NovoTTF to patients after they have completed RT if they are willing. Many patients will recur in the first year following treatment. Consider reirradiation on protocol or enrollment in investigational clinical trials.

Notable Trials

Glioblastomas

- EORTC 26981/22981-NCIC (*Stupp et al. NEJM* 2005; *Stupp et al. Lancet Oncol* 2009): Two-arm prospective randomized phase III trial. 573 patients underwent surgical resection (40% GTR) and then randomized to RT alone vs RT with concurrent TMZ, both followed by 6 cycles of adjuvant TMZ. Radiation dose was 60 Gy/30 fx. Median OS RT alone 12.1 months vs RT + TMZ 14.6 months, 2-year OS 10% RT alone vs 26% RT + TMZ (HR 0.63; $P < .001$). Grade 3 or 4 hematologic toxicity with TMZ 7%. *MGMT* methylation status greatest predictor for outcome and benefit from TMZ chemotherapy (*Stupp et al. Lancet Oncol* 2009)
- EF-14 NovoTTF (*Stupp et al. JAMA* 2015): Two-arm prospective randomized phase III trial. Glioblastoma patients randomized following completion of chemoradiation (2:1) to receive maintenance treatment with TTFields plus temozolomide vs temozolomide alone. TTFields treatment was delivered continuously (>18 h/d) via four transducer arrays placed on a shaved scalp. Interim analysis at median f/u of 38 months. Median OS in TTF + TMZ arm 20.5 vs 15.6 months (HR 0.64, $P = .004$).

Grade III gliomas

- EORTC 26951 (*Van den Bent et al. JCO* 2006, 2013). Two-arm prospective randomized phase III trial. 368 anaplastic astrocytoma and oligodendroglioma patients underwent surgical resection followed by RT (59.4 Gy/33 fx) and randomized to observation vs 6 cycles of PCV. 82% of patients in the observation arm received chemotherapy at progression. 38% of patients in RT→ PCV arm had discontinuation of chemotherapy due to toxicity. RT→ PCV arm had improved OS (42.3 vs 30.6 months, HR 0.75) and PFS.
- CATNON (*Van den Bent et al. Lancet* 2017). 2 × 2 factorial phase III randomized trial. 1p19q noncodeleted anaplastic glioma patients randomized to RT (59.4 in 33 fractions) alone, RT + adj TMZ, chemoRT, or chemoRT + adj TMZ. Interim analysis shows OS at 5 years improved with adj TMZ (55.9% vs 44.1%, $P = .0014$).

MENINGIOMA

HUBERT YOUNG PAN • DEBRA NANA YEBOA • ERIK P. SULMAN

BACKGROUND

- **Incidence/prevalence:** Meningioma is the most common benign brain tumor (1/3 of primary intracranial neoplasms), ~25-30 000 cases per year in the United States.
- **Outcomes:** Typically long natural history. Recurrence rate is strongly correlated with WHO grade (~10% for G1, 40% for G2, 70% for G3).
- **Demographics:** Female > male (2:1), incidence peaks in sixth to seventh decades
- **Risk factors:** Prior radiation at long interval (~20 years) from even low dose (1-2 Gy), NF2, MEN1, and long-term hormonal replacement usage are all identifiable risk factors.

TUMOR BIOLOGY AND CHARACTERISTICS

- **Genetics:** Loss of chromosome 22 is the most common alteration, associated with NF2 mutation (50%). Less common alterations include AKT1 (~10%), SMO, TRAF7 (~25%), and PI3KA.
- **Pathology:** WHO grading based on mitotic activity—Grade I (85%-90% of cases, benign histology), grade II (5%-10%, atypical, clear cell, choroid), and grade III (<5%, anaplastic, papillary, rhabdoid). Characteristically, psammoma bodies and calcifications are seen in grade I meningioma. Grade II is defined by ≥4 mitoses/10 HPF. And grade III is defined as ≥20 mitoses/10 HPF or the presence of carcinomatous, sarcomatous, and melanomatous features and/or with brain invasion. Subset expresses hormone receptors (progesterone and/or estrogen).
- **Imaging:** MRI is preferred as dural tail can be seen on 2/3 of cases (Fig. 13.1), typically T1 isointense, T2 hyperintense, and strongly enhancing. CT shows extra-axial mass displacing normal brain, isodense, with ~25% having calcification.

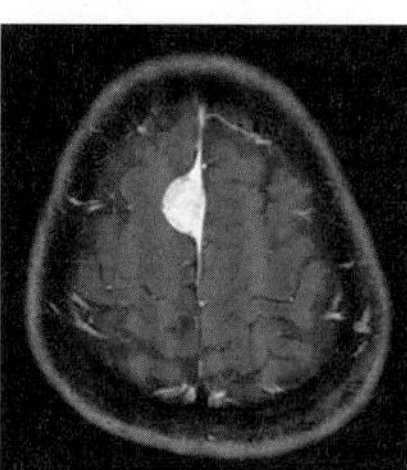

Figure 13.1 T1+C MRI sequence showing enhancing lesion with dural origin, consistent with meningioma. Note enhancing dural tail seen in ~2/3 of cases.

ANATOMY

- Meningiomas have dural origin, most commonly within the skull (90%) at sites of dural reflection (falx cerebri, tentorium cerebelli, venous sinuses) but can also present in the optic nerve sheath and choroid plexus. Common sites of presentation include cerebral convexity and parafalcine/parasagittal regions.

WORKUP

- **History and physical:** History with careful attention to neurologic deficits and exam
- **Labs:** CBC, CMP
- **Procedures/biopsy:** Neurosurgery evaluation for maximal safe resection and/or biopsy
- **Imaging:** Head CT and MRI of the brain to evaluate extent of disease. Evaluate for perilesional edema and/or bony invasion.

STAGING AND GRADING (SEE TABLE 13.1)

Table 13.1 Simpson Grading System for Meningioma

Grade	Description	10-Year Recurrence
1	GTR, including dural attachment and any abnormal bone	9%
2	GTR, with coagulation instead of resection of dural attachment	19%
3	GTR of meningioma without resection or coagulation of dural attachment	29%
4	Subtotal resection	44%
5	Tumor debulking or decompression only	N/A

TREATMENT ALGORITHM

Incidental/asymptomatic	Observation with MRI at 3, 6, and 12 mo (2/3 will stay stable)
Progressive/symptomatic	Surgery ± RT (unresectable, recurrent, grade II STR, any grade III)

RADIATION TREATMENT TECHNIQUE

- **SIM**: Supine, thermoplastic mask, scan vertex to shoulders. Isocenter placed at midbrain. MRI fusions (unless obtaining MRI SIM)—T1+C sequence and T2-FLAIR sequences.
- **Dose and target:**

WHO Grade	Dose	Target
Grade 1	50.4-54 Gy in 28-30 fx at 1.8 Gy/fx **or** SRS 14-16 Gy	Residual enhancing tumor
Grade 2 (or recurrent G1)	54-59.4 Gy in 30-33 fx at 1.8 Gy/fx **or** SRS 14-16 Gy	Tumor and/or resection bed + 1 cm CTV (restrain to dura)
Grade 3 (or recurrent G2)	CTV1: 60 Gy in 30 fx CTV2: 50-54 Gy in 30 fx (SIB with CTV1)	CTV1: Tumor and/or resection bed + 1 cm CTV2: Tumor and/or resection bed + 2 cm

- **Technique:** IMRT/VMAT. PTV 3 mm if daily kV, 5 mm if weekly kV. Consider SRS if G1, <3-4 cm size, with sufficient distance from critical structures, that is, optic apparatus (>2 mm). For SRS, prescribe 14-16 Gy to 50% isodose line, to be as conformal as possible.
- **IGRT:** Daily kV
- **Planning directive:**
  Fractionated EBRT
  Brainstem: V30Gy < 33%. Max < 54 Gy. If necessary may allow point max <60 Gy.
  Brain: V30Gy < 50%
  Optic chiasm: Max ≤ 54 Gy
  Cochlea: Max < 54 Gy. Mean < 30 Gy
  Lens: Max < 5 Gy
  Optic nerves: Max ≤ 54 Gy
  Pituitary: Mean < 36 Gy
  Eyes: Max < 40 Gy. Mean < 30 Gy
  Hippocampus (young patients, if concern): D100% < 9 Gy, Max ≤ 16 Gy
  Spinal cord: Max ≤ 45 Gy

For single-fraction SRS, limit dose to optic apparatus to 8 Gy (can push up to 10-Gy point dose). Can consider dose escalation to 16 Gy in single fraction if higher grade. We typically do not recommend SRS for grade 3 tumors.

Chemotherapy

Experience with systemic therapy is limited to observational studies in the recurrent setting with limited efficacy. Studied options include Sutent, hydroxyurea, somatostatin analogs (octreotide), and various inhibitors (progesterone, estrogen, PDGF, EGFR, VEGF).

Follow-up

Grade 1: MRI at 6 months and then annually
Grade 2: MRI q3-6mo × 1 year and then annually
Grade 3: MRI q3-6mo × 5 years and then q6-12mo

Depending on location of RT, important to assess for potential hormonal deficiencies (ie, pituitary hormones).

Notable Studies

- RTOG 0539 (*Rogers et al. J Neurosurg* 2018; *ASTRO abstract IJROBP* 2016): Phase II trial of risk-stratified postoperative management of meningioma. Only prospective trial for RT in meningioma that we have data for currently. Low risk (newly diagnosed G1) observed with 3-year PFS 92%, but 40% 5-year crude LF if STR (abstract). Intermediate risk (recurrent G1 or new G2 s/p GTR) received 54 Gy in 30 fractions with 3-year PFS 93.8% (P = .0003 when compared to 3-year PFS in historical control). High risk (any G3, recurrent G2, or new G2 s/p STR) received 60 Gy in 30 fractions with 3-year PFS 59% (abstract).

BENIGN CNS

CHRISTOPHER WILKE • CAROLINE CHUNG

Vestibular Schwannoma

Background

- **Incidence/prevalence:** Vestibular schwannoma (acoustic neuroma) accounts for 8% of adult intracranial tumors and 85% of cerebellopontine angle tumors. Incidence is ~1 per 100 000 person-years although true rate may be higher based upon incidental findings on autopsy and MRI studies. Almost always presents with unilateral involvement except for patients with NF2
- **Outcomes:** Typically slow-growing with long natural history. 40% will show no growth.
- **Demographics:** Median age of diagnosis 50 years. 1:2 M/F ratio
- **Risk factors:** NF1 and NF2 (bilateral lesions), acoustic trauma (loud noise), childhood exposure to low-dose radiation

Tumor biology and characteristics

- **Genetics:** Inactivation of NF2 gene (produces tumor suppressor schwannomin) is found in most sporadic schwannomas.
- **Pathology:** Benign (WHO Grade I) tumor arises from perineural elements of Schwann cell of the 8th CN with S-100+ on IHC. Malignant transformation is rare.
- **Imaging:** MRI with contrast is the gold standard and preferred, including mm sections through internal auditory canal (IAC), seen as well-circumscribed, heterogeneously T2 hyperintense, contrast-enhancing lesions (Fig. 14.1).

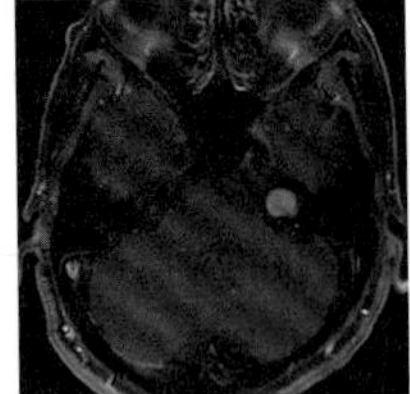

Figure 14.1 T1 + C MRI sequencing showing a 1.3 × 1.0 cm schwannoma on the left intracanalicular space. The tumor extends slightly into the left cerebellopontine angle.

Anatomy

- Schwannomas are the most common peripheral nerve sheath tumor and can involve other extracranial or intracranial (trigeminal, facial, jugular foramen) nerves. The internal acoustic canal is a short segment (~1 cm) in the temporal bone that contains CN VII and VIII; vestibular schwannomas typically affect the intracanalicular segment of the vestibular portion of CN VIII.

Workup

- **History and physical:** History with careful attention to neurologic deficits and exam (Weber and Rinne tests). If facial/trigeminal involvement, patients may present with altered taste and paresis
- **Procedures/biopsy:** Audiometry should be done to establish baseline. Neurosurgical evaluation for resection/biopsy
- **Imaging:** MRI of the brain w/ contrast. High-resolution CT if MRI not available

Koos grading scale for vestibular schwannoma

Grade	Description
I	Intracanalicular
II	Tumor extending into posterior fossa without touching brainstem
III	Tumor extending into posterior fossa, touching brainstem, no midline shift
IV	Tumor extending into posterior fossa, touching brainstem, with midline shift

Treatment algorithm

Small (<2 cm), no symptoms, no growth, elderly patients with comorbidities	Audiometry and MRI scans every 6 mo to 1 y
Large (>4 cm), symptomatic, recurrent or progressive after XRT	Surgical resection
Large, symptomatic, not surgical candidate	Definitive radiation

Radiation treatment technique

- **SIM:** Supine, thermoplastic mask. MRI fusions (unless obtaining MRI sim)—T1 + C sequence.
- **Dose, target, technique, IGRT:**

Technique	Dose	Target	IGRT
Standard fractionation preferred for lesions >2-3 cm	50.4 Gy in 28 fx	GTV + 3-5 mm PTV	Daily kV
Stereotactic radiosurgery (Fig. 14.2) preferred for smaller lesions, <3 cm in diameter	12-13 Gy to 50% IDL	GTV only	MRI
Hypofractionation (*Kapoor IJROBP* 2011) is preferred for smaller lesions that are not ideal SRS candidates owing to anatomic constraints	25 Gy in 5 fx	GTV + 3 mm PTV	Daily CBCT

- **Planning directive:**
  SRS
  Brainstem: 0.01 cc $\leq$ 12 Gy
  Optic nerves and chiasm: Max < 8 Gy
  Cochlea: Limit central cochlear dose to <4.2 Gy (*Kano et al. Neurosurgery* 2009).

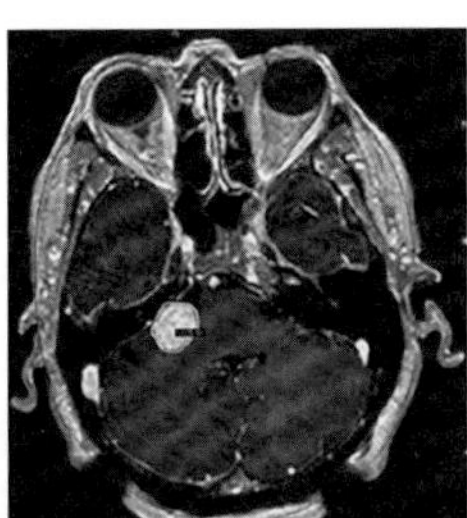

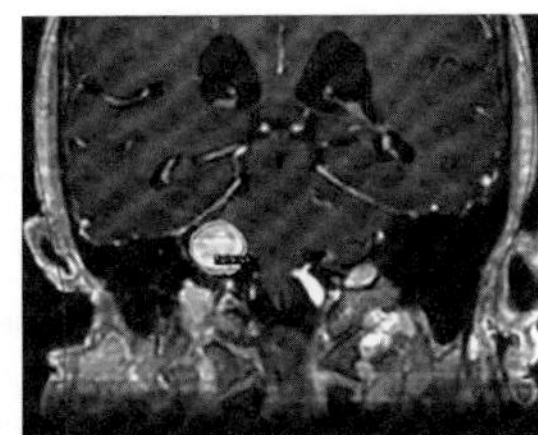

Figure 14.2 Axial and coronal sections demonstrating treatment of an acoustic neuroma with Gamma Knife SRS. A dose of 12.5 Gy was prescribed with 50% isodose.

- **Fractionated radiotherapy (1.8 Gy/fx):**
  Spinal cord: Max < 45 Gy
  Brainstem: Max < 54 Gy
  Optic nerves and chiasm: Max < 54 Gy
  Cochlea: Max < 35 Gy
  Pituitary: Max < 40 Gy

Follow-up

- First follow-up at 3-6 months and then annual MRI is typically recommended for 10 years with less frequent studies if no evidence of tumor progression
- All patients should undergo baseline audiology evaluation prior to treatment and regularly with follow-up posttreatment.

Surgery

- **Technique:**
  - Middle cranial fossa approach: Best suited for small tumors with focus on hearing preservation
  - Translabyrinthine approach: Usually reserved for larger tumors in patients who have already lost functional hearing, as this approach sacrifices hearing in the operated ear
  - Retrosigmoid (keyhole) approach: Most often used for moderate or large tumors in patients with functional hearing with the goal of hearing preservation
- **Outcomes:** Excellent if GTR, but about 15% LR if STR.

Notable studies

- German retrospective (*Combs et al. Int J Radiat Oncol Biol Phys* 2010): Prospective cohort study of 200 pts treated to median dose of 57.6 Gy at 1.8 Gy/fx or Linac-based SRS. No difference in 10-year LC of 96%. Hearing preservation of 78% at 5 years for standard fractionation and patients with SRS < 13 Gy
- Japan retrospective (*Hasegawa et al. Int J Radiat Oncol Bio Phys* 2013): Single-institution review of 440 pts using Gamma Knife SRS with median marginal dose of 12.8 Gy showed 10-year PFS of 92% and <5% rate of CN palsy.

Paraganglioma (Jugulotympanic)

Background

- **Incidence/prevalence:** Rare, typically benign, neuroendocrine tumor, which most commonly presents during the fifth to sixth decade of life
- **Clinical presentation:** Less than 5% of all paragangliomas present in the head and neck. Most symptoms result from mass effect of the tumor and may include pulsatile tinnitus, hearing loss, and cranial nerve palsies. Paragangliomas of the head and neck are more often non–catecholamine secreting compared with other organ sites.
- **Pathology:** Mutations in the succinate dehydrogenase enzyme complex have been shown to predispose to the development of head and neck paragangliomas (*Neumann et al. Cancer Res* 2009).
- **Imaging:** Reliably imaged with both CT and MR angiography. CT is beneficial for visualizing destruction of the temporal bone. Octreotide imaging has demonstrated a sensitivity of 94% in patients with head and neck paragangliomas (*Telischi et al. Otolaryngol Head Neck Surg* 2000).

Treatment

Observation

- Initial observation and close follow-up may be considered for small asymptomatic tumors.
- Median growth rate for head and neck paragangliomas is ~1 mm/y (*Jansen et al. Cancer* 2000).

Surgery

- Typically preferred for small tumors in which there is felt to be a low risk of serious complications or functional deficits
- Resection is also preferred for immediate relief of symptomatic tumors or catecholamine-secreting tumors.
- Local control rates with surgery alone exceed 80%-90% following gross total resection.

Radiotherapy

- Stereotactic radiosurgery:
  - Provides excellent local control (>95% at 3 years; *Guss et al. IJROBP* 2011) and is a good option for smaller tumors that are at high risk of potential surgical complications
  - Typically prescribed as 16 Gy to the 50%-80% isodose

- Fractionated radiotherapy:
  - Useful for larger tumors, which cannot be safely treated with SRS due to tumor volume and/or potential dose to critical structures
  - Doses of 45-50.4 Gy in 1.8 Gy/fx are associated with local control similar to surgical series.

Dose constraints

- **See dose constraints for vestibular schwannomas.**

Follow-up

- Imaging every 6-12 months for 3 years and then annually for 10 years
- Serum markers should be tested in secretory tumors.

Trigeminal Neuralgia

Background

- **Incidence/prevalence:** Annual incidence is ~5 per 100 000 person-years. Approximately 50% more prevalent among females vs males. Most commonly seen in patients aged 50 years and older.
- **Clinical presentation:** Brief, recurrent episodes of severe unilateral shooting/stabbing pain localized to one or more divisions of the trigeminal nerve in the absence of other neurologic deficits
- **Pathology:** Majority of cases are thought to be caused by compression of the trigeminal nerve root, which leads to demyelination and disrupted neuronal signaling.
- **Imaging:** Volumetric acquisitions with thin slice MRI/MRA are useful in the detection of neurovascular compression.

Treatment

Medical management

- Preferred as upfront treatment prior to consideration of surgery or radiotherapy
- Carbamazepine is the most commonly used agent for front-line therapy. Others shown to be efficacious include oxcarbazepine, baclofen, and lamotrigine.

Surgery

- Usually reserved for patients with medically intractable symptoms. Very effective for initial pain relief although efficacy tends to fall over time
- Surgical options include
  - Microvascular decompression to relieve the pressure of vascular structures off the trigeminal nerve
  - Rhizotomy with destruction of the gasserian ganglion by RF ablation, mechanical compression, or chemical lysis

Radiosurgery

- Mechanism of pain relief remains poorly understood although animal models have demonstrated axonal degradation, fragmentation, and edema following ablative SRS doses to the trigeminal nerve root (*Kondziolka et al. Neurosurgery* 2000).
- When performed using Gamma Knife SRS, a maximum point dose of 70-90 Gy is delivered using a single 4-mm isocenter targeting the proximal ipsilateral trigeminal nerve (Fig. 14.3). Several institutional series have also demonstrated efficacy of CyberKnife/Linac modalities with acceptable rates of toxicity.

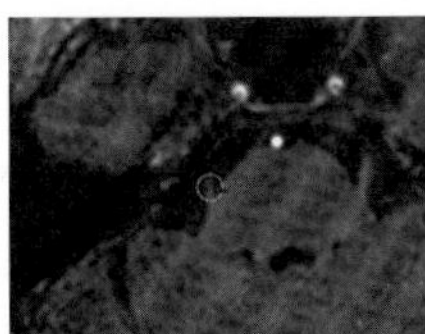
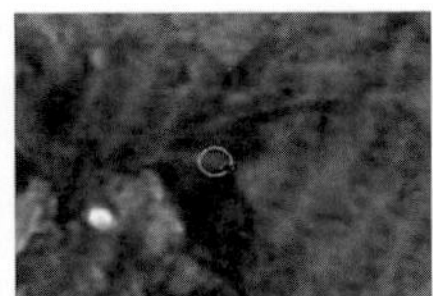

Figure 14.3 Axial and sagittal sections demonstrating treatment of a right-sided trigeminal neuralgia using Gamma Knife SRS. A maximum point dose of 80 Gy was delivered using a single shot with a 4-mm collimator.

- Prospective data demonstrate pain relief in a proportion of patients with low rates of toxicity (*Regis et al. J Neurosurg* 2006). However, the efficacy over time also declines similar to reported surgical series.

ARTERIOVENOUS MALFORMATION

Background

- **Incidence/prevalence:** Annual incidence of ~1 per 100 000 person-years. Median age at diagnosis of 30.
- **Clinical presentation:** Wide range of initial presentation from detection as an incidental finding to intracranial hemorrhage, seizures, headaches, and focal neurologic deficits. Most are supratentorial (90%) and present with a single lesion (90%). The presence of multiple AVMs is strongly associated with Osler-Weber-Rendu syndrome (hereditary hemorrhagic telangiectasia).
- **Pathology:** Abnormal communication between arteries and veins without usual intervening capillary network. The high flow rates can create vessel enlargement and both arterial and venous aneurysms.
- **Imaging:** Cerebral angiography is the gold standard for evaluating the location of feeding vessels and drainage patterns. Contrast-enhanced CT and MR angiography can also be useful for initial diagnosis.

Treatment

Medical therapy

- Historically, interventional therapy for AVMs has been favored due to the 2% annual rate of hemorrhage in patients with untreated lesions.
- The role of routine interventional therapy in asymptomatic patients has come into question with the results of the ARUBA trial demonstrating a significantly elevated risk of stroke and death following intervention as compared with those receiving medical management alone (*Mohr et al. Lancet* 2014).

Microsurgery

- Treatment of choice for patients felt to be at high risk of hemorrhage, as it provides immediate treatment of symptomatic AVMs and immediately reduces risk of hemorrhage postprocedure.
- The Spetzler-Martin grading system is used to assess the risk of postoperative neurologic complications and aids in treatment modality decision-making (*Spetzler and Martin J Neurosurg* 1986).

Embolization

- Endovascular embolization is commonly used to reduce the size of large AVMs prior to treatment with radiotherapy or surgery, but it can result in complete obliteration of the nidus in some instances.

Radiosurgery

- Usually reserved for lesions that are inaccessible or felt to be at very high risk with surgical intervention due to operative complications or medical comorbidities.
- Mechanism of action is thought to be induction of progressive thrombosis and fibrosis.
- Approximately 80%-90% of patients will have eventual obliteration of the nidus although the mean time to obliteration following SRS is ~2-3 years. The elevated risk of hemorrhage is not eliminated until complete obliteration of the AVM.
- A prescription dose of 20 Gy covering the nidus is associated with in-field obliteration rates in excess of 90% (*Flickinger et al. IJROBP* 1996).
- MRI/MRA can be used for posttreatment surveillance with cerebral angiography used to confirm resolution.

PITUITARY ADENOMA AND CRANIOPHARYNGIOMA

HUBERT YOUNG PAN • DEBRA NANA YEBOA • ERIK P. SULMAN

BACKGROUND

- **Incidence/prevalence:** The most common sellar mass is pituitary adenoma (90%-95%), which accounts for 10% of intracranial tumors. 12 000 cases per year in the United States (*Ostrom et al. Neuro Oncol* 2017). Female > males
- **Outcomes:** Long natural history as incidental imaging finding, endocrine abnormality, or local compressive symptoms; RT provides 90+% LC
- **Demographics:** Pituitary adenoma presents 30-50 years, craniopharyngioma bimodal (1/3 at 0-14 years, 2/3 at 45-60 years)
- **Risk factors:** MEN-1 (parathyroid, pancreas, pituitary), history of colorectal cancer

TUMOR BIOLOGY AND CHARACTERISTICS

- **Pituitary adenoma:** Classified by size (<1 cm microadenoma vs >1 cm macroadenoma, >4 cm giant adenoma), functional vs nonfunctional, and cell origin. 75% of pituitary adenomas are secretory (50% PRL, 25% GH, 20% ACTH, <1% TSH).
- **Craniopharyngioma:** Epithelial tumor derived from Rathke pouch, the embryonic precursor to anterior pituitary; adamantinomatous (Wnt activation) vs papillary (BRAF mutation)
- **Pathology:** Mallory trichrome staining helps differentiate functional vs nonfunctional adenomas.
- **Imaging:** Craniopharyngioma often presents with calcification (60%-80%) and mixed solid-cystic (75%) components. Adenomas appear hypointense in the early phase of dynamic contrast-enhanced MRI (due to poor vasculature relative to normal tissue).

ANATOMY

- **Pituitary fossa:** Located within the sphenoid bone, bounded by hypothalamus and optic chiasm (superior), sphenoid sinus (inferior), and cavernous sinus (lateral)
- **Pituitary gland:** Divided into anterior (GH, PRL, TSH, ACTH, FSH, LH) and posterior (oxytocin, ADH)

WORKUP

- **History and physical:** History with careful attention to potential endocrinopathies
- **Procedures/biopsy:** Neurosurgical evaluation for resection/biopsy. Endocrine evaluation if medical management desirable
- **Labs:** CBC, CMP, endocrine function tests (TSH, ACTH, cortisol, prolactin, IGF-1)
- **Imaging:** MRI of the brain w/ contrast

TREATMENT ALGORITHMS

- **Pituitary adenoma:**
  - **First line:** Medical management if functional (see Medical management section)
  - **Second line:** Surgical resection for all other functional and nonfunctional adenomas to relieve compression
  - **Third line:** Consideration for RT (if inoperable, persistent post-op hormone elevation, macroadenoma with STR, recurrent disease)
- **Craniopharyngioma:**
  - Maximal safe resection (shunt if hydrocephalus) → consideration for RT (if STR)
  - Consider observation for asymptomatic pituitary adenomas without lab abnormalities.

RADIATION TREATMENT TECHNIQUE

- **SIM:** Supine, thermoplastic mask, bite block, scan vertex to shoulders
- **Dose, target, and technique:**

	Target	External Beam	SRS
Nonfunctional pituitary adenoma	GTV or postoperative bed + 0.3-0.5 cm PTV (typically no CTV)	45-50.4 Gy in 25-28 fx	14-18 Gy
Functional pituitary adenoma		50.4-54 Gy in 28-30 fx	20-24 Gy
Craniopharyngioma		50.4-54 Gy in 28-30 fx	12-14 Gy

- **IGRT:** Daily kV, weekly-biweekly reimaging for craniopharyngioma to monitor changes in cyst shape/size, which may necessitate replanning
- **Considerations:** We favor fractioned EBRT for larger (>3 cm) tumors or for tumors close (<2 mm) to critical structures (ie, optic chiasm). Repeat imaging during treatment of craniopharyngioma to assess cyst volume changes. See **LGG** chapter for normal tissue constraints.

Surgery

- **Transsphenoidal resection:** Endoscope inserted through one nostril and opening made in the nasal septum and sphenoid sinus to access the sella. Fat graft placed in resection bed and cartilage craft to seal sella hole. Complications include diabetes insipidus, CSF leaks, and hemorrhage.
- **Pterional craniotomy:** Temporal craniotomy may be required to access extrasellar disease, particularly for craniopharyngioma.

Medical Management

Hormone	Labs	Symptoms	Medical Tx
PRL	Serum PRL	Galactorrhea, amenorrhea	Dopamine agonist (eg, cabergoline, bromocriptine)
GH	Serum GH, IGF-I	Acromegaly	Somatostatin analog (eg, octreotide) or GH antagonist (pegvisomant)
ACTH	24-h urine free cortisol	Cushing syndrome	Steroid synthesis inhibitor (eg, ketoconazole, etomidate)

Follow-up

- Endocrine evaluation and MRI q6mo, normalization of hormones can take years.

Notable Studies

- Pituitary adenoma UVA retrospective (*Sheehan et al. J Neurosurg* 2011). Review of 418 patients treated with Gamma Knife. LC 90%, median time to endocrine remission 48 minutes, new pituitary hormone deficiency in 24% of patients. Smaller adenoma volume correlated with improved endocrine remission rates
- Craniopharyngioma UCSF retrospective (*Shoenfeld et al. J Neurooncol* 2012). Review of 122 pts showed no difference in PFS (P = .54) and OS (P = .74) when treated with GTR vs STR + XRT but significantly shorter PFS if STR alone (P < .001). Additionally, GTR was associated with greater risk of DI (56% vs 13%, P < .001) and panhypopituitarism (55% vs 27%, P = .01) vs STR + XRT.
- Craniopharyngioma (*Bishop et al. Int J Radiat Oncol* 2014). Retrospective study of 52 children treated with protons (21) or IMRT (31) at two institutions. Of 24 pts with imaging during RT, 10 (42%) had cyst growth and 5 (21%) required change in treatment plan. Outcomes similar with IMRT and protons

MEDULLOBLASTOMA

SHANE R. STECKLEIN • ARNOLD C. PAULINO

BACKGROUND

- **Incidence/prevalence:** Second most common pediatric brain tumor. Most common malignant tumor in the posterior fossa. There are ~500 cases per year in the United States.
- **Outcomes:** 5-Year survival 80%-85% for average-risk disease and 60%-65% for high-risk disease.
- **Demographics:** Bimodal age distribution; peak incidence 6 years in children and 25 years in adults.
- **Risk factors:** Gorlin syndrome (nevoid basal cell carcinoma syndrome, due to mutations in *PTCH*, which regulates Sonic Hedgehog [SHH] signaling), Turcot syndrome (familial adenomatous polyposis [FAP] with brain tumors, due to mutations in *APC*, which regulates Wnt signaling)

TUMOR BIOLOGY AND CHARACTERISTICS

- **Pathology:** Small, round, blue cell tumor. Primitive neuroectodermal tumor (PNET) of the superior medullary velum (germinal matrix) of the cerebellum or cerebellar vermis. Classic histologic finding is the Homer-Wright pseudorosette (tumor cells concentrically arranged around a lumen containing neuropil).
- **Imaging:** Typically hypointense to isointense on T1-weighted images and generally shows avid enhancement on postcontrast sequences

ANATOMY

Tumors most commonly arise from the cerebellar vermis and often protrude into the 4th ventricle and may grow through the lateral foramina of Luschka and the posteromedial foramen of Magendie into the subarachnoid space. Midline tumors are most commonly associated with Wnt subtype, extensive anterior growth (including into the brainstem) is seen in Group 3/4 tumors, and lateral tumors are most likely to be SHH. Obstruction of the cerebral aqueduct can cause obstructive hydrocephalus.

SUBTYPES OF MEDULLOBLASTOMA (TAYLOR ET AL. ACTA NEUROPATHOL 2012)

Molecular Subtype	Histologic Subtype	Age[a]	Prognosis
Wnt	Classic, rarely large cell/anaplastic	C, A	Very good
SHH	Desmoplastic/nodular, MBEN	I, C, A	Good (I)/intermediate (C, A)
Group 3	Classic, large cell/anaplastic	I, C	Poor
Group 4	Classic, large cell/anaplastic	I, C, A	Intermediate

[a]I, infants; C, children; A, adults.

WORKUP

- **History and physical:** Patients should have baseline evaluations by endocrinology, ophthalmology, audiology, and neuropsychology. Neurologic examination may reveal cerebellum deficits including gait or truncal ataxia, cranial nerve deficits, or signs of increased intracranial pressure including papilledema and loss of vision. Postoperatively surgical resection associated with posterior fossa syndrome, which appears 1-2 days after surgery and includes mutism and emotional lability.
- **Labs:** General labs and CSF evaluation 10-14 days after surgery
- **Procedures/biopsy:** Lumbar puncture often contraindicated prior to surgery secondary to risk of herniation. Perform lumbar puncture 10-14 days after surgery.
- **Imaging:** Contrast MRI is the preferred examination. Preoperative and postoperative (within 48 hours of surgery) contrast-enhanced brain MRI. Spine MRI (if not done preoperatively) 10-14 days after surgery.

Staging and Risk Stratification

Modified Chang Staging	
M0	No subarachnoid or hematogenous metastases
M1	Microscopic tumor cells in the CSF
M2	Gross intracranial nodular seeding
M3	Gross spinal subarachnoid seeding
M4	Metastases outside the neuroaxis (rare; bone and bone marrow most common sites of extraneural spread)
Risk Stratification	
Average risk	≤1.5 cm² residual tumor after surgery, M0 by craniospinal MRI and lumbar puncture
High risk	Subtotal resection (>1.5 cm² residual tumor), M+

Treatment Algorithm

Average risk	Maximal safe resection; low-dose craniospinal irradiation (CSI) with tumor bed boost; adjuvant chemotherapy.
High risk	Maximal safe resection; high-dose CSI with tumor bed boost and boost to other sites of gross disease; adjuvant chemotherapy.
Infants <3 y	Maximal safe resection; consideration of chemotherapy intensification and deferment of CSI until 3 y of age or later.

All patients should be considered for a clinical trial.

Radiation Treatment Technique

- **SIM:** Supine on foam board, thermoplastic mask. Anesthesia often required for young children.
- **Dose:**
  - Average risk: CSI to 23.4 Gy in 17 fractions (1.8 Gy/fx), sequential boost to tumor bed plus margin to 54.0 Gy
  - High risk: CSI to 36.0 Gy in 20 fractions (1.8 Gy/fx), sequential boost to tumor bed plus margin to 54.0 Gy
- **Target:**
  - CSI:
    - Entire craniospinal axis
    - Ensure coverage of cribriform plate and thecal sac
  - Tumor bed boost:
    - Collapsed tumor bed and gross residual disease if present
    - 1.0-1.5 cm anatomically constrained expansion for CTV
- **Technique:** Passive scatter proton radiotherapy to spare anterior structures. RAO and LAO cranial fields (10-15 degrees from horizontal plane to reduce dose to contralateral lens; do not compromise cribriform plate coverage to spare lenses) and posterior spinal fields. Multiple ways to handle junctions, including junction shifts every 4-5 fractions to feather overlap at brain-spine and spine-spine junctions. For growing children, ensure coverage of entire vertebral body to prevent asymmetric growth and reduce risk of lordosis.
- **IGRT:** Daily kV.
- **Dose constraints:**

Spinal cord	Max < 50 Gy
Brainstem	Max < 57 Gy, V54 < 10%
Optic nerves	Max < 54 Gy
Optic chiasm	Max < 54 Gy
Retinas	Max < 45 Gy
Cochleae	Max < 45 Gy, mean < 26 Gy (can tolerate mean dose of 38 Gy for high risk)
Parotids	Mean < 10 Gy
Lacrimal glands	Mean < 26 Gy
Kidneys	V20 < 30%, V12 < 55%
Pituitary	Mean < 36 Gy

Chemotherapy

- Standard adjuvant regimens include cisplatin, vincristine, and lomustine (CCNU) or cyclophosphamide.
- Use of targeted agents (eg, vismodegib [Erivedge] for SHH medulloblastoma) emerging
- Some protocols (COG) include weekly vincristine given during radiotherapy.

Treatment of Medulloblastoma in Children <3 Years of Age

- Goal is to delay radiotherapy as long as possible to mitigate long-term toxicity.
- Standard approach is maximal safe resection followed by intensive chemotherapy (high-dose methotrexate followed by carboplatin, thiotepa, and etoposide) with autologous stem cell rescue.
- Focal radiotherapy to tumor bed may be considered in select cases, but patients are at significantly higher risk for failure at non–tumor bed-irradiated sites.

Follow-up

- MRI of the brain and spine 4-6 weeks after radiotherapy, then every 3 months for the 1st year, every 4 months for the 2nd year, every 6 months until year 5, and then annually thereafter
- Patients should have periodic evaluations by endocrinology, ophthalmology, audiology, nd neuropsychology to detect and manage long-term sequelae of treatment.

Notable Trials/Papers

Radiation dose and field in medulloblastoma

- CCG 9892 (*Packer JCO* 1999). Pilot study evaluating low-dose CSI (23.4 Gy) followed by posterior fossa boost to 55.8 Gy with concurrent vincristine and then adjuvant lomustine/vincristine/cisplatin in average-risk patients. PFS at 3 years was 86% and at 5 years was 79%, as good as historical controls with CSI to 35 Gy.
- COG ACNS0331 (*Michalski IJROBP* 2016 [abstract form only]). Average-risk patients age 3-7 randomized to low-dose CSI (18.0 Gy with posterior fossa boost to 23.4 Gy) vs standard-dose CSI (23.4 Gy). Second randomization for boost to posterior fossa vs tumor bed with margin to 54.0 Gy. Average-risk patients age 8-22 all received standard-dose CSI but underwent posterior fossa vs tumor bed with margin boost to 54.0 Gy. Preliminary data show that reducing the boost volume to the tumor bed with margin is acceptable, but there is increased risk of recurrence with reduced dose (18.0 Gy) CSI, and this is therefore not recommended.
- Proton therapy for CSI (*Howell Radiat Oncol* 2012). Evaluation of passive scatter proton vs photon radiotherapy for CSI at MDACC. Proton CSI reduced dose to the esophagus, heart, liver, thyroid, kidneys, and lungs.

Deferment of radiation for infants <3 years old

- Baby POG I (*Duffner NEJM* 1993; *Duffner Neuro-oncology* 1999). Postoperative chemotherapy and delayed radiation in children <3 years of age with malignant brain tumors. 198 patients with biopsy-proven malignant brain tumor (medulloblastoma, ependymoma, PNET, brainstem glioma, malignant glioma, choroid plexus carcinoma, other gliomas) received two 28-day cycles of cyclophosphamide plus vincristine followed by one 28-day cycle of cisplatin plus etoposide; repeated until disease progression or for 2 years in patients <24 months at age of diagnosis or for 1 year in patients ≥24-36 months of age at diagnosis. High response rate in patients with medulloblastoma, malignant gliomas, and ependymomas. Minimal response in brainstem glioma and PNET. Update for medulloblastoma showed 5-year PFS 32% and OS 40% with no difference if RT delayed by 1 or 2 years.

EPENDYMOMA

COURTNEY POLLARD III • ARNOLD C. PAULINO

BACKGROUND

- **Incidence/prevalence:** The third most common childhood brain tumor. Bimodal distribution with peaks at 4 and 35 years old. Approximately 200 cases per year in the United States
- **Outcomes:** Degree of resection most important predictor of outcomes. 5-Year overall survival ~75% with gross total resection (GTR) and ~35% with subtotal resection (STR)
- **Demographics:** Infratentorial lesions occur more commonly in younger children. Supratentorial lesions are more common in adolescents and adults. In children, 90% of tumors are intracranial.
- **Risk factors:** Spinal cord ependymomas are associated with neurofibromatosis type 2.

TUMOR BIOLOGY AND CHARACTERISTICS

- **Genetics:** Greater than 2/3 of supratentorial ependymomas have oncogenic fusions between *RELA* (which drives NF-κB) and *C11orf95*, leading to uncontrolled activation of NF-κB signaling pathway and driving tumorigenesis (Parker et al. *Nature* 2014). Among posterior fossa tumors, a poor prognostic subgroup is one which exhibits a CpG island methylator phenotype, which silences genes that prevent neuronal differentiation. This is prognostic of PFS and OS (Mack et al. *Nature* 2014).
- **Pathology:** Origin is the ependymal cells lining the ventricular system and spinal canal. Classic features are ependymal and perivascular pseudorosettes. GFAP, S100, and vimentin stain positive. Subependymomas are rare tumors that are found in adults in the 4th or lateral ventricles. These tumors appear benign histologically and grow slowly. Similarly, myxopapillary ependymomas are slow-growing and are found in adults almost exclusively within the conus and filum terminale of the spinal cord.
- **Imaging:** Classically hypointense on T1 MRI sequences and hyperintense on T2. Tumors enhance with gadolinium contrast. On CT, tumors will enhance with contrast and calcifications are commonly seen.

ANATOMY

Tumors can occur throughout the entire cranial spinal axis. If the tumor is in the posterior fossa, the most common site is the fourth ventricle and often involves the foramen of Luschka. Supratentorial tumors also arise in the ventricular system and spread through intraparenchymal extension. Direct extension through the foramen magnum into the upper cervical spinal canal is common. Subarachnoid seeding occurs in ~12% of children.

WORKUP

- **History and physical:** Common presenting symptoms include those resulting from increased ICP (headaches, nausea, vomiting) due to obstruction of CSF flow. For adults with myxopapillary ependymomas, chronic back pain is typically reported with or without neurologic deficits. Perform thorough neurologic exam.
- **Labs:** CBC, CMP
- **Procedure/biopsy:** CSF sampling with cytology (unless contraindicated due to obstructive hydrocephalus)
- **Imaging:** MRI of the brain and spine is essential. After resection, MRI should be obtained <24 hours to evaluate degree of resection. CSF cytology and MRI of the spine should be obtained ~2 weeks after surgery to avoid false-positive result.

EPENDYMOMA GRADE (*WHO 2016*)

WHO I	Subependymoma or myxopapillary ependymoma
WHO II	Classic ependymoma
WHO III	Anaplastic ependymoma

TREATMENT ALGORITHM

Localized ≥1 y old	Maximal safe surgical resection followed by postoperative radiation therapy (RT) for infratentorial lesions. For supratentorial tumors, postoperative RT is given if STR or anaplastic (grade III). Observation after a GTR is a valid option for supratentorial, grade II tumors.
Localized <1 y old	Maximal safe surgical resection followed by adjuvant chemotherapy until patient is at least 12 mo and then consider RT
Disseminated ≥3 y old	Maximal safe surgical resection of the primary tumor followed by craniospinal irradiation (CSI) and tumor bed boost
Disseminated <3 y old	Maximal safe resection of the primary tumor followed by chemotherapy
Recurrent ependymoma	No prior RT: Maximal safe surgical resection followed by adjuvant XRT Prior RT: Maximal safe surgical resection. Consider reirradiation.
Spinal/myxopapillary ependymoma	Maximal safe resection, if GTR can be observed. If STR or biopsy, follow with postoperative RT.

RADIATION TREATMENT DOSE/TARGET/TECHNIQUE

Infratentorial Tumor

- **SIM:** Supine, arms at side, aquaplast mask over head. For spinal tumor or CSI, use full body Vac-Lok. Sedation with general anesthesia may be required for children. Scan from the vertex of the skull through coccyx.
- **Dose:** 54-59.4 Gy in 30-33 fractions at 1.8 Gy/fx
- **Target:** CTV margin = preop GTV + 1 cm. Consider 3-5-mm CTV to PTV margin depending on IGRT and setup.
- **Technique:** Proton beam therapy or intensity-modulated radiation therapy for primary intracranial tumor. Treatment planning for CSI will require feathering of junctions to avoid potential hot spots at field borders (Fig. 17.1).

Supratentorial Tumor

- **Dose:** 54-59.4 Gy in 30-33 fractions at 1.8 Gy/fx for anaplastic tumors, if WHO grade I or II can be observed if completely resected.
- **Target:** Same as above
- **Technique:** Same as above

Spinal Tumor

- **Dose:** 45 Gy in 25 fractions at 1.8 Gy/fx, including two vertebral bodies/sacral nerve roots above and below tumor. Cone down to 50.4-54 Gy if safely below cord.
- **Target:** Same as above. May consider <3-mm PTV margins
- **Technique:** Same as above

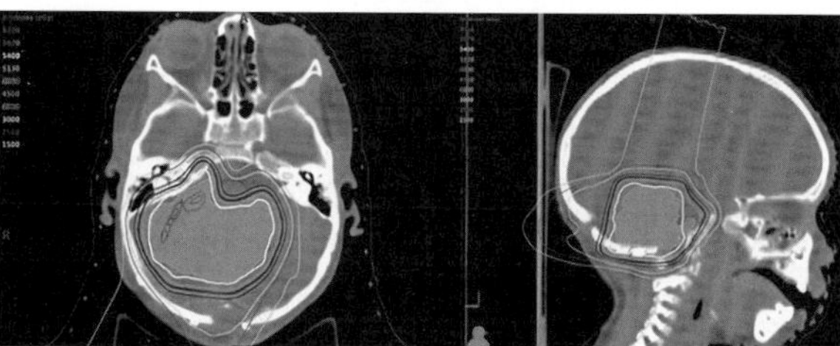

Figure 17.1 Representative proton beam plan for a posterior fossa ependymoma in a 3-year-old child. 54-Gy isodose line is represented by the *white line*.

PTV as per institutional standards and image guidance (we do 0.3-0.5 cm)
- **IGRT:** Daily kV imaging
- **Planning directive:**
  Spinal cord D_{max} < 50 Gy
  Brainstem D_{max} < 57 Gy, V54 Gy < 10%
  Chiasm D_{max} < 54 Gy
  Lt and Rt cochlea mean < 38 Gy, D_{max} < 45 Gy
  Lt and Rt eye D_{max} < 40 Gy
  Lt and Rt lens D_{max} < 5 Gy
  Lt and Rt parotid mean < 10 Gy
  Lt and Rt lacrimal gland mean < 26 Gy

SIDE EFFECT MANAGEMENT

- Nausea/vomiting: First line Zofran → second line Compazine
- Decline in IQ: More prominent in patients treated with CSI and in children <10 years old treated with localized fields, referral to neuropsychology and counsel parents
- Growth deficiency: Rule out growth hormone deficiency. Can occur with CSI secondary to irradiation of vertebral bodies and supporting musculature. Counsel parents.

FOLLOW-UP

- Follow-up period is long, ~10 years as ependymomas can recur very late following completion of treatment.
- History/physical with MRI: q3-4mo for year 1 → q4-6mo for year 2 → then q6-12mo thereafter
- If CSI, check growth hormone and TSH labs at least once per year.
- Consistent follow-up with neuropsychologist, especially with CSI

NOTABLE TRIALS

Adjuvant radiation

- St. Jude (*Merchant et al. JCO* 2004; *Merchant et al. Lancet Oncol* 2009): Prospective phase II trial evaluating whether the postoperative irradiated volume in patients with localized childhood ependymoma could be reduced to decrease late cognitive side effects without compromising disease control. All patients had maximal safe surgical resection followed by adjuvant RT. Patients ≥18 months (n = 73) received 59.4 Gy and patients <18 months (n = 15) received 54 Gy both to a margin of 1 cm. If patients had an STR, they were given chemo and then reevaluated for a second surgery and adjuvant RT. On preliminary analysis, 3-year PFS was 74% and IQ testing was stable after 2 years. Long-term analysis demonstrated that 7-year OS was 81%, 7-year LC was 87.3%, and 7-year EFS was 69.1%.
- Barrow Neurological Institute (*Rogers et al. J Neurosurg* 2005): Retrospective study evaluating if adjuvant RT is necessary for patients with posterior fossa ependymoma after GTR. 71% of patients had GTR. RT in 13/32 GTR and 12/13 STR. 10-Year LC: 50% for GTR alone, 100% for GTR + RT, and 36% for STR + RT. 10-Year OS: 67% for GTR alone, 83% for GTR + RT, and 43% for STR + RT
- ACNS0121 (ABSTRACT, *Merchant et al.* 2015): Prospective phase II trial observing WHO grade II with supratentorial ependymoma after microscopic GTR (stratum 1), chemotherapy with optional second surgery prior to RT for patients with STR at the time of protocol enrolment (stratum 2), immediate postoperative RT for patients after near-total resection (NTR) or GTR resection (stratum 3), and WHO grade III supratentorial or any grade infratentorial after GTR (stratum 4). 378 patients and 115 institutions participated. Median age was 5.3 years. There were 216 WHO grade II and 140 WHO grade III tumors.
  Stratum 1: 5-Year event-free survival (EFS) was 61.4%. Stratum 2: second surgery was performed in 25 of 64 patients; GTR was achieved in 14. There was no difference in EFS comparing the 25 patients that underwent the second surgery to 39 patients that did not (logrank test: P = .0790). Stratum 2: EFS was 39.2%. Stratum 3: EFS was 67.3%. Stratum 4: EFS was 69.5%. Among the 281 patients treated on stratum 3 and 4, EFS was 74.6% for WHO grade II and 60.7% for WHO grade III tumors according to central pathology review (P = .0047).

INTRACRANIAL GERM CELL TUMOR

ETHAN BERNARD LUDMIR • ARNOLD C. PAULINO

Background

- **Incidence/prevalence:** Intracranial germ cell tumor (GCT) accounts for 1%-2% of pediatric CNS tumors, higher in Asian/Pacific Islander populations, including those of Asian/Pacific Islander descent living in Western countries.
- **Outcomes:** Modern trials report 5-year PFS for pure germinoma >90%, for both localized and disseminated disease. Nongerminomatous GCT (NGGCT) 5-year PFS is poorer, ~70%-80% for localized NGGCT and ~50%-70% for disseminated NGGCT.
- **Demographics:** Median age of diagnosis 10-12 years old, male > female (2-3:1), as above Asians and those of Asian descent have 2-3× higher incidence of GCT.
- **Risk factors:** No major risk factors known

Tumor Biology and Characteristics

- **Genetics:** Aberrations in KIT/RAS and/or AKT/mTOR pathways in majority of intracranial GCTs
- **Pathology:** Histologic division of GCT into germinoma vs NGGCT. Germinomas are more RT sensitive and have better prognosis than NGGCT. Approximately 65% of intracranial GCTs are germinoma ("pure" germinoma). NGGCT includes embryonal carcinoma, yolk sac tumor (aka endodermal sinus tumor/endodermal sinus tumor), choriocarcinoma, teratoma, or mixed GCT. Mixed GCT may include germinoma components, but any NGGCT component makes tumor "mixed" and therefore treated as NGGCT (25% of NGGCT are mixed GCT). Helpful markers for GCT: B-hCG, alpha-fetoprotein (AFP), and placental alkaline phosphatase (PLAP). B-hCG and AFP can be examined on IHC, as well as in serum and CSF.

Serum/CSF B-hCG and AFP Differentiation of Tumor Histology		
Histology	**B-hCG**	**AFP**
Embryonal carcinoma	Wnl	Wnl
Yolk sac tumor	Wnl	Increased (can be marked)
Choriocarcinoma	Increased (can be marked)	Wnl
Teratoma	Wnl	Wnl
Germinoma	<50-100 IU/L	Wnl[a]

[a]Elevated AFP in serum (>10 ng/mL), in CSF, or on IHC **rules out** pure germinoma.
Intracranial GCT also classified as secreting vs nonsecreting depending on CSF AFP and B-hCG levels, w/ poorer prognosis for secreting tumors.

- Origin: Extragonadal GCT occurs intracranially, as well as in the sacrococcygeal region and the retroperitoneum, among other sites. Extragonadal GCT may arise from primordial germ cells that exhibit aberrant or incomplete migration during embryonal development.
- Location: Primary locations of intracranial GCT are the pineal gland and suprasellar region, pineal gland more common than suprasellar (2:1). Rare to occur at other intracranial sites. Approximately 5%-10% of cases have both pineal and suprasellar tumors, which are known as "bifocal" GCT.
- Imaging: GCT is usually iso-/hypointense on T1, and hyperintense on T2 (similar to MB), and like medulloblastoma shows postcontrast enhancement. No radiographic factors reliably differentiate germinomas from NGGCTs.

Workup

- **History and physical:** Recommend baseline evaluations by endocrinology, ophthalmology, audiology, and neuropsychology. Consideration should be made for baseline neurocognitive studies (for GCTs as well as other intracranial pediatric tumors). Clinical presentation varies by primary tumor site:
  - **Pineal tumors:** increased ICP (headaches, N/V, papilledema, lethargy/somnolence, due to obstructive hydrocephalus); ~40% of pineal GCTs present with increased ICP. Parinaud syndrome presents in 40%-50% of cases. This syndrome consists of upward gaze paralysis and sluggish pupillary reflex, as well as convergence nystagmus. This syndrome is thought to be due to compression of superior colliculus.

- **Suprasellar tumors:** neuroendocrinopathies/hypothalamus axis disruption, especially diabetes insipidus, precocious/delayed puberty, and bitemporal hemianopia (chiasm compression). Complete a neurologic exam including cranial nerve exam + funduscopy to evaluate papilledema.
- **Historical note:** Decades prior, germinoma was empirically diagnosed w/ initiation of RT. If response after ~20 Gy considered empirical diagnosis (w/out histologic/pathologic confirmation) of germinoma and RT continued. Not recommended in the modern era
- **Differential diagnosis:** Pineal tumor differential diagnosis includes GCT (germinoma/NGGCT), glioma, pineoblastoma, pineocytoma, PNET, ependymoma, lymphoma, and hamartoma. Suprasellar tumor differential diagnosis includes craniopharyngioma, Langerhans cell histiocytosis, glioma, GCT (germinoma/NGGCT), pituitary adenoma, meningioma, and aneurysm.

- **Procedures/biopsy:** LP and CSF analysis, including CSF AFP and B-hCG levels, as well as CSF cytology. CSF AFP and B-hCG are more sensitive than serum markers. Prefer LP for markers + cytology rather than ventricular CSF (ie, if shunt already placed for hydrocephalus). LP for CSF analyses 10-14 days after procedure (shunt placement, surgery). Biopsy mandatory for patients w/ normal serum and CSF markers (AFP and B-hCG). Biopsy is only needed for germinoma (no role for extent of resection), whereas data suggest possible role for maximal safe resection in NGGCT.
- **Labs:** CBC, CMP (including BUN/Cr and LFTs), serum AFP, serum B-hCG
- **Imaging:** MRI brain + entire spine w/ gadolinium contrast. MR spine critical as ~10% of patients will have spinal/leptomeningeal seeding at diagnosis.

Staging

M staging per modified Chang system as below used for intracranial GCTs as well as medulloblastoma (see Medulloblastoma).

Modified Chang Staging	
M0	No metastases (bifocal GCT [pineal + suprasellar tumors] w/out evidence of other metastasis = treated as localized/M0)
M1	Microscopic tumor cells in the CSF/positive CSF cytology
M2	Gross intracranial seeding
M3	Gross spinal seeding
M4	Metastases outside neuroaxis

Treatment Algorithm

- **Germinoma:** RT alone or neoadjuvant chemotherapy → RT. Chemotherapy-only approaches for germinomas have yielded inferior outcomes, with >50% rates of relapse, even after CR from chemotherapy (*Balmaceda et al. JCO* 1996).
- **NGGCT:** Several approaches, but in general, maximal safe resection → chemotherapy (6 cycles) → possible second-look surgery (if restaging after chemotherapy demonstrates sufficient residual tumor to warrant second-look surgery before CSI) → consolidative RT (including CSI)

Radiation Treatment Technique

- **SIM:** Supine (on foam board if CSI), thermoplastic mask. Sedation (anesthesia) may be required for younger patients.
- **Dose:**
  - Generally, treat at 1.5 Gy/fx for germinoma, and 1.8 Gy/fx for NGGCT, unless otherwise specified.
  - Localized germinoma: If RT alone, whole ventricle RT (WVRT) to 24 Gy → boost gross disease to 40-45 Gy.
  - Localized germinoma: If RT after chemotherapy, then treat per COG ACNS1123 RT dose depending on tumor response on repeat imaging after chemotherapy.
    - ACNS1123: If PR/SD after chemotherapy: 24 Gy WVRT → 12 Gy boost to primary site
    - ACNS1123: If CR after chemotherapy: 18 Gy WVRT → 12 Gy boost to primary site
    - Off protocol RT after induction chemotherapy: 21 Gy WVRT (rather than 18 Gy) → 15 Gy boost to primary site

- Bifocal germinoma: Treat as above for localized germinoma, but boost both primaries (suprasellar and pineal). Cannot have other tumors beyond these two sites to be classified as bifocal
- Disseminated (M+) germinoma: CSI to 24-30 Gy → boost to primary to total dose ~40-45 Gy
- NGGCT: Off protocol, current standard of care is CSI to 36 Gy and boost primary to 54 Gy. ACNS1123 is attempting to reduce field size from CSI to WVRT, pending results.

- **Target:**
  - Whole ventricular RT (WVRT): Outlined in ACNS1123 atlas online.
    - WVRT includes targets: Lateral, 3rd, and 4th ventricles, as well as suprasellar and pineal cisterns. Cover prepontine cistern if history of 3rd ventriculostomy (ie, done previously for obstructive hydrocephalus from tumor) or large suprasellar tumor. WVRT target well defined using T2 MRI fusion (or MRI simulation, if available)
    - Contour WV-CTV = ventricles/ventricular space, and then expand 5 mm (depending on IGRT) to generate WV-PTV.
  - Tumor bed boost:
    - Collapsed tumor bed and gross residual disease if present
    - 1-cm expansion from tumor bed for tumor CTV, then expand 5 mm for PTV (dependent on IGRT)
  - CSI:
    - Ensure coverage of cribriform plates, middle cranial fossae, and thecal sac.
- **Technique:** Similar to medulloblastoma, especially with regard to CSI. IMRT and proton beam therapy reasonable options. See **Medulloblastoma** chapter for CSI—considerations if CSI indicated.
- **IGRT:** Daily kV
- **Planning directive:** See **Medulloblastoma** chapter (Fig. 18.1).

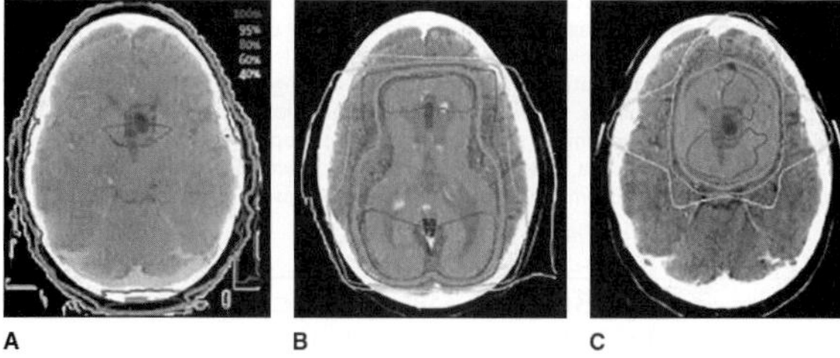

Figure 18.1 Axial imaging showing dose distribution with whole brain radiation **(A)** as part of CSI. WVRT **(B)** and focused radiation of a primary target, as would be conducted in a sequential boost **(C)** (*Rogers Lancet Oncol* 2005).

Chemotherapy

- Carboplatin/etoposide ×4 cycles typical for induction chemotherapy for germinoma (ACNS1123). Platinum-based chemotherapy ×6 cycles for NGGCT. Other regimens may include bleomycin and cisplatin for intracranial GCTs.

Notable Trials/Papers

Radiation for localized intracranial germinomas

- Patterns of failure review (*Rogers Lancet Oncol* 2005). Review of publications assessing radiation for localized intracranial germinomas from 1989 to 2004. Analysis demonstrated higher rates of failures (both local and spinal failures) if focal/involved field RT used for localized germinoma rather than WVRT or WBRT.
- SFOP Involved Field RT experience (*Alapetite Neuro Oncol* 2010). Review of SFOP experience treating localized germinoma w/ involved field RT. Among 10 patients with relapse after local therapy, predominate failure patterns were periventricular (8 of 10). This retrospective review supports the use of WVRT for germinoma pts.

- SIOP CNS GCT96 (*Calaminus Neuro Oncol* 2013). Prospective study with 190 pts w/ localized germinoma receiving CSI w/ tumor bed boost vs carbo/etop ×2 cycles alternating w/ ifos/etop followed by local RT. Study was nonrandomized. Chemotherapy and RT arm failures were all within the ventricular system, supporting WVRT at least; failures even w/ CR after chemotherapy. No difference in 5-year OS but improved FPS with CSI (97% vs 88%, $P = .04$). Suggests need at least WVRT even w/ CR

Treatment strategy of NGGCT

- COG Phase II Trial (*Goldman J Clin Oncol* 2015). Nonrandomized phase II trial of 102 pts with NGGCT treated with 6 cycles of induction chemotherapy +/– second look surgery followed by CSI with tumor/tumor bed boost. The 5-year EFS was 84% and OS was 93%. Currently this strategy is the backbone for treatment of these tumors in North America.

WILMS TUMOR

ETHAN BERNARD LUDMIR • ARNOLD C. PAULINO

Background

- **Incidence/prevalence:** Approximately 600 cases per year in the United States, about 7% of childhood malignancies (SEER)
- **Outcomes:** Markedly improved survival with the addition of radiation therapy (RT) and chemotherapy (CHT) over the last century; all-comers Wilms tumor (WT) overall survival (OS) ~10% in the 1920s to >90% by 2000. 4-Year OS for favorable histology (~90% of total) pts ≥90% for Stages I-III, and 85%-90% for Stages IV-V. Worse outcomes if unfavorable histology (UH) (Stage IV UH 4-year OS ~40%).
- **Demographics:** Median age at diagnosis is 44 months for unilateral cases and 31 months for bilateral cases. Sex predilection higher in girls (F:M = 1.1:1 for unilateral WT)
- **Risk factors:** Approximately 10% WT cases have a congenital syndrome, including WAGR (**W**T, **A**niridia, **G**U malformations, **R**etardation [mental]; deletion 11p13), Beckwith-Wiedemann syndrome (hemihypertrophy, visceromegaly, macroglossia, macrosomia, anterior abdominal wall defects; duplication 11p15), and Denys-Drash syndrome (nephrotic syndrome, XY pseudohermaphroditism; mutation 11p13).

Tumor Biology and Characteristics

- **Pathology/genetics:** Intrinsic renal tumor derived from nephrogenic blastemal cells, also known as nephroblastoma. 90% of WT are favorable histology (FH), classically "triphasic" including epithelial, blastemal, and stromal components. 10% of WT are unfavorable histology (UH), including tumors w/ focal anaplasia (FA) or diffuse anaplasia. UH tumors have higher rates of nodal and distant metastasis. LOH 1p16q is poor prognostic indicator (*Grundy et al. JCO* 2005). Other pediatric renal tumors (not WT family members) include clear cell sarcoma of the kidney (CCSK) and rhabdoid tumor of the kidney (RTK). RTK histologically not discernable from AT/RT of the brain (both show loss of nuclear INI1 staining).
- **Imaging:** Radiographic differentiation of WT vs NB: WT arises within the kidney (claw sign); rare calcifications in WT (~10%); WT rarely crosses midline (WT occasionally "overhang" onto contralateral side)

Workup

- **History and physical:** Pts typically present with painless abdominal mass, without constitutional symptoms. Approximately 33% of WT pts have abdominal pain, weight loss, or N/V. 25% have secondary HTN (elevated renin). 30% present with hematuria and 10% coagulopathy. Evaluate family history and assess for congenital syndromes, including GU malformations, macroglossia, hemihypertrophy, aniridia, and mental retardation.
- **Labs:** CBC, CMP, UA, and urine catecholamines (HMA/VMA)

- **Procedures/biopsy:** No biopsy unless unresectable or Stage V (bilateral). North American approach is staging after surgical resection, w/ surgical resection as first step in treatment paradigm for most patients.
- **Imaging:** Abdominal US w/ Doppler (assess vessel patency), usually followed by CT chest/abdomen/pelvis, w/ contrast, as well as CXR. Additional workup for uncommon histologies: CCSK = bone scan, BMBx, and MRI brain (assess for brain mets); RTK = MRI brain (assess for synchronous AT/RT)

Staging

- **Surgery:** In North America, up-front radical nephrectomy and LN sampling via transabdominal or thoracoabdominal incision, with en bloc removal of the kidney. Inspect contralateral kidney and assess for preoperative and intraoperative spill. Discussion between the surgeon and radiation oncologist is crucial for site(s) of intraop spill in particular.

Staging—WT	
I	Tumor confined to kidney, completed resected (R0)
II	Tumor completely resected (R0), with extension beyond the kidney through vessel involvement and/or penetration of renal capsule/sinus
III	R1 or R2 resection (+margins or STR), preop or intraop tumor spill, tumor biopsy, piecemeal resection (not en bloc), peritoneal implants, LN involvement in abd/pelvis, tumor penetration of peritoneal surface
IV	Hematogenous mets (lung, liver, bone, etc.), or LN outside abd/pelvis
V	Bilateral renal involvement

Treatment Algorithm

For FH patients

Stage I and II	Surgery → chemotherapy (omit RT for FH pts)
Stage III	Surgery → RT[a] → chemotherapy
Stage IV	Surgery → RT[b] → chemotherapy
Stage V	Neoadjuvant chemotherapy → surgery

[a]Flank RT for all "local" Stage III FH pts; whole abdomen irradiation (WAI) indicated if preoperative spill or diffuse intraoperative spill. Discuss with surgical team if intraoperative spill occurred to better delineate extent/location of spill, which will inform adjuvant treatment with flank RT vs WAI.

[b]Whole lung irradiation (WLI) for WT pts w/ lung mets if no radiographic complete response on CT after 6 weeks of VAAdr (regimen DD4A; *Dix et al. JCO* 2018). Generally recommend flank/abdominal RT w/in 14 days postop after nephrectomy. However, for sequencing, can delay flank/abdominal RT for Stage IV WT pts w/ lung mets until after 6 weeks of CHT; importance of early RT for WT pts appears to matter in the nonmetastatic setting (*Stokes et al. IJROBP* 2018). This allows flank RT/WAI to be delivered concurrently w/ WLI if needed for Stage IV pts.

For unfavorable histology and RTK patients: At least flank RT regardless of stage (I-IV)
For CCSK: At least flank RT for Stages II-IV. No RT for Stage I if adequate nodal sampling

Radiation Treatment Technique

- **SIM:** Supine, Vac-Lok, most will require sedation (anesthesia)
- **Dose (for FH):**
  - Flank (hemi-abdomen) RT to 10.8 Gy in 6 fx (1.8 Gy/fx).
    - If PA nodes involved, include PA chain in flank field from T11-L4.
    - If gross residual disease >3 cm, boost additional 10.8 Gy (in 6 fx).
  - WAI to 10.5 Gy in 7 fx (1.5 Gy/fx).
  - WLI to 12 Gy in 8 fx (1.5 Gy/fx); if pt <12 mo drop 1 fx (10.5 Gy in 7 fx).
  - Additional dosing specifications:
    - Undissected (gross) LNs—19.8 Gy/11 fx
    - Flank RT for Stage III diffuse anaplasia or RTK I-III—19.8 Gy/11 fx
    - Boost gross residual lung dz 2 weeks after WLI—7.5 Gy/5 fx
    - Bone mets: 25.2 Gy/14 fx (30.6 Gy/17 fx if age >16 years old)
    - Liver mets: Sx if local, whole liver if diffuse mets (19.8-21.6 Gy)
    - Brain mets: 21.6 Gy/12 fx WBRT or 30.6 Gy/17 fx if >16 years old

- **Target/technique (Flank RT, Fig. 19.1 below):**
  CTV: Preop tumor + kidney + 1 cm + entire vertebral body if block edge touches VB w/ AP/PA technique
  Technique: Generally AP/PA: Sup/Inf = 1 cm expansion off disease/kidney. Med = 1 cm lateral to whole VB (include whole VB in field, generally). Lat = body wall (no flash)

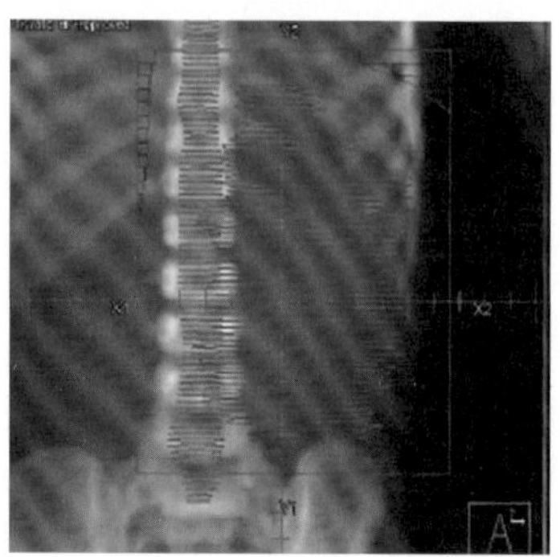

Figure 19.1

- **Target/technique (WAI, Fig. 19.2 below):**
  CTV: As above
  Technique: Generally AP/PA: Sup = 1 cm above diaphragm. Inf = bottom of obturator foramen (therefore, more accurately this is whole "abdominopelvic" RT, not just the abdomen). Lat = body wall (no flash)

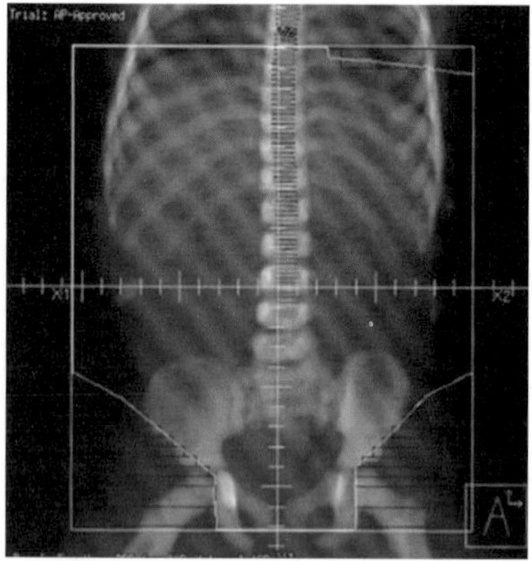

Figure 19.2

- **Target/technique (WLI, Fig. 19.3):**
  CTV: Includes bilateral lungs, mediastinum, and pleural recesses
  Technique: AP/PA or IMRT (cardiac-sparing IMRT warrants 4D-CT simulation; see *Kalapurakal et al. IJROBP* 2012). If AP/PA: Sup = 1 cm above clavicle/lung apex (flash SCV fossa). Inf = below diaphragm. Lat = chest wall

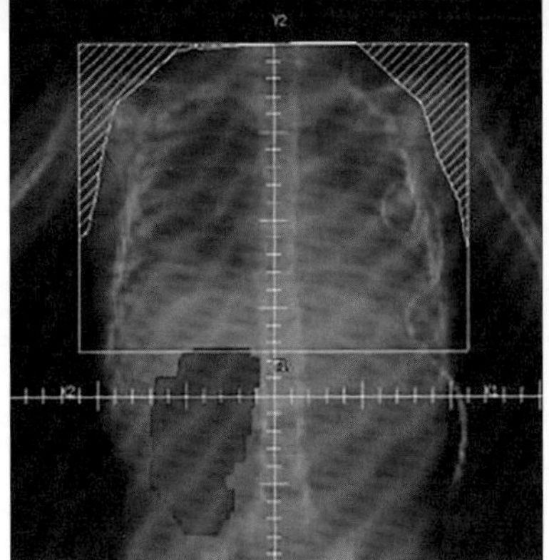

Figure 19.3

- **Planning directive:**
  Contralateral kidney: V14.4 < 33%
  Liver: V19.8 < 50%

Chemotherapy

- Generally, vincristine/actinomycin D/Adriamycin (VAA; regimen DD4A); with addition of cyclophosphamide/etoposide (with VAA; regimen M) for higher-risk Stage III/IV

Side Effect Management

Acute: Skin reaction, nausea/vomiting, indigestion, diarrhea, esophagitis, pneumonitis

Late (varies by treatment field, age, among others): Height loss, kyphosis/lordosis/scoliosis, chronic renal insufficiency (rare <1%, unless bilateral Wilms tumor), muscular hypoplasia, pneumonitis (4% with whole lung irradiation), pulmonary fibrosis, infertility, malabsorption, SBO, VOD, increased risk of cardiac morbidity, second malignancy (1%-2% at 15 years)

Follow-up

- Follow-up with imaging recommended q3mo for 2 years, then q6mo for 2 further years. Imaging recommend alternating between CXR + abdominal US and CT C/A/P. Most relapses occur w/in first 2 years; some question regarding role of further imaging beyond 2 years (*Brok et al. Lancet Oncol* 2018).
- Long-term monitoring for late effects, which may include echocardiography, height/growth abnormalities/bone density, hypogonadism, chronic renal insufficiency, pulmonary function testing, screening for second malignancies (breast, colon).

Notable Trials

NWTS 3 (*D'Angio Cancer* 1989). Randomized trial including 1439 patients, treatment adaptive by stage and histology. Stage II FH pts had no difference in outcomes with no RT vs 20 Gy RT. Stage III FH pts randomized 10 vs 20 Gy flank RT, with no difference in outcomes. Established use of 10 Gy for flank RT

COG AREN0533 (*Dix JCO* 2018). Prospective trial in which 292 Stage IV FH patients w/ CT-identified isolated lung metastases were treated w/ 6 weeks of DD4A and assessed w/ repeat CT. Those without LOH 1p/16q with complete response on repeat CT (total 133 patients) continued DD4A without WLI and had 4-year EFS of 79.5% and OS of 96.1%. Patients with incomplete response or LOH 1p/16q received IWLI and four cycles of cyclophosphamide in addition to DD4A. These patients had a 4-year EFS of 88.5% and OS of 95.4%. Overall, there was an excellent OS observed after omission of lung RT in select stage IV patients, although there were more events than was expected. Additional cycles of chemo + lung RT improved survival in high-risk stage IV patients when compared to historical control arm (data from the prior NWTS-5 study).

NEUROBLASTOMA

AHSAN FAROOQI • ETHAN BERNARD LUDMIR • ARNOLD C. PAULINO

BACKGROUND

- **Incidence/prevalence:** Accounts for ~8% of all childhood cancers in the United States. Approximately 650 new cases per year diagnosed in the United States, overall 10 cases per million children (SEER data)
- **Outcomes:** 5-Year OS for low- and intermediate-risk patients is >90%. For high-risk neuroblastoma, the 5-year OS is between 40% and 50%. Neuroblastoma is a rare cancer that has the potential to spontaneously regress without any treatment.
- **Demographics:** Most common extracranial tumor of childhood. Median age at diagnosis is ~17 months. Most common malignancy of infants (~50%). No sex predilection, M:F is 1.2:1
- **Risk factors:** Majority of cases (>98%) sporadic due to chance mutations. However, in 1%-2% of cases, neuroblastoma develops due to a hereditary mutation in either the *ALK* or *PHOX2B* genes (Mosse et al. *Nature* 2008).

TUMOR BIOLOGY AND CHARACTERISTICS

- **Genetics:** *MYCN* is a DNA binding transcription factor, which can cause malignant transformation due to downstream effects. It is found to be amplified in 25% of all neuroblastoma and is associated with rapid progression and poor prognosis (Seeger et al. *NEJM* 1985; Chan et al. *Clin Can Res* 1997). *ATRX* mutations were recently identified in adolescents and young adults with neuroblastoma and are associated with an indolent disease course (Cheung et al. *JAMA* 2012).
- **Pathology:** Arise from primitive neural crest sympathetic ganglion cells. Small, round, blue cell tumor of childhood (like Ewing's, medulloblastoma, rhabdomyosarcoma, and PNET). Shimada pathologic classification dependent on degree of differentiation, mitosis-karyorrhexis index, stromal component, and nodularity (Shimada et al. *Cancer* 1999). Classically stains positive for synaptophysin, chromogranin A, and neurofilaments
- **Imaging:** X-rays may demonstrate calcifications in ~80% of neuroblastomas (in comparison with Wilms tumors, which classically do not have calcifications). CT of the abdomen with contrast is typically performed, which can help identify extent of tumor and presence or absence of regional or distant metastatic disease. Importantly, nuclear medicine meta-iodobenzylguanidine (MIBG) radionuclide scans can be used to identify distant sites of disease and response to systemic therapy (Fig. 20.1).

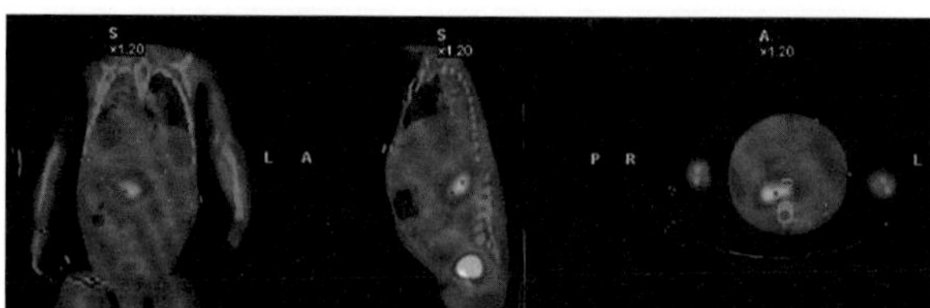

Figure 20.1 Representative coronal, sagittal, and axial (*left* to *right*) MIBG scans in a patient presenting with a right adrenal neuroblastoma. The avidity can be seen in his right suprarenal area, consistent with the primary malignancy. There were no additional MIBG-avid sites, suggesting absence of distant metastases.

ANATOMY

- May arise from any site in the sympathetic nervous system. Most common sites are adrenal gland in the abdomen, paraspinal ganglia along the abdomen, thorax, and head and neck.

WORKUP

- **History and physical:** Patients typically present with an abdominal mass with additional symptoms such as malaise, irritability, and pain. Evaluate for Horner syndrome (meiosis, ptosis, anhidrosis) due to involvement of the sympathetic chain on the ipsilateral affected side. Evaluate for back pain due to possible bony involvement. Important to do careful skin examination as metastatic disease can present with a bluish tinge ("blueberry muffin" sign) and may be indicative of stage 4S disease. Opsoclonus-myoclonus syndrome—presenting as truncal ataxia and/or cerebellar encephalopathy—may be seen.

- **Labs:** CBC, CMP. Include measurement of urinary catecholamines HVA and VMA, which are found to be elevated in >90% of patients with stage IV disease
- **Procedures/biopsy:** Can obtain tissue from primary site or from gross lymph nodes. **Bone marrow aspirate and biopsy are required for appropriate staging of neuroblastoma.**
- **Imaging:** Abdominal x-rays may show calcification in up to 80%-85% of neuroblastomas. Obtain CT of the abdomen with contrast and MIBG nuclear medicine scan at diagnosis to determine extent of metastatic disease. Consider MRI of the abdomen w/ and w/o contrast if equivocal findings on CT scan.

STAGING/GRADING

International Neuroblastoma Staging System (INSS) (*Brodeur et al. JCO* 1998)

Stage 1: Tumor removed completely during surgery, without microscopic residual disease. Ipsilateral lymph nodes excised during surgery negative for tumor (but nodes attached to primary tumor may be positive)

Stage 2A: Localized tumor with incomplete gross excision. Ipsilateral lymph nodes do not contain cancer.

Stage 2B: Localized tumor with or without gross excision. Ipsilateral lymph nodes do contain cancer.

Stage 3: Unresectable unilateral tumor extending past midline, which has or has not spread to regional lymph nodes or other areas near the tumor but not to other parts of the body

Stage 4: The original tumor has disseminated to distant lymph nodes, bones, bone marrow, liver, skin, and/or other organs, except for those listed in stage 4S, below.

Stage 4S: The original tumor is located only where it started (as in Stages 1, 2A, or 2B), and it has spread **only** to the skin, liver, and/or bone marrow, in infants younger than 1 year. The spread to the bone marrow is minimal; usually <10% of cells examined show cancer.

TREATMENT ALGORITHM

Low-risk	Surgery → omit adjuvant chemo or RT if favorable biology If unresectable: preoperative chemo → surgery
Intermediate-risk	If <1 y: Surgery → chemotherapy If >1 y: Surgery → chemotherapy → adjuvant RT to primary and regional lymph node basin
High-risk	Induction chemotherapy → Surgery → myeloablative therapy and ABMT → consolidative RT to tumor bed and residual MIBG-avid sites → maintenance therapy with isotretinoin and immunotherapy
Stage IVS	Clinical diagnosis. Omit therapy and observe for probable spontaneous regression

RADIATION TREATMENT TECHNIQUE

- **SIM:** Supine, Vac-Lok, nearly all will require anesthesia.
- **Dose:** 21.6 Gy in 12 fractions
- **Target:**

  GTV: Define tumor bed using postinduction and chemotherapy preoperative CT or MRI. Treat postinduction residual MIBG sites as well (*Mazloom et al. IJROBP* 2014).

  CTV: Tumor bed + 1-1.5-cm margin, limiting to anatomic barriers of spread (bone, etc.).

  PTV: 0.5-1 cm depending on institutional standards and image guidance

  Considerations: Different than other pediatric tumors, the GTV is not based upon the initial tumor volume. Consider shorter RT course. Consider 4.5 Gy/3 fx regimen for palliation of liver metastases.

- **Technique:** IMRT typically used, especially if tumor extended past midline. Consider AP/PA techniques if well-lateralized tumor (may spare dose to contralateral kidney). Proton therapy can be considered if dosimetric advantage.
- **IGRT:** daily kV imaging
- **Planning directive:**
  Kidneys—D_{mean} < 14.4 Gy

Chemotherapy

Commonly used induction and myeloablative chemotherapy regimens include cyclophosphamide or ifosfamide, cisplatin/carboplatin, vincristine, doxorubicin, etoposide, topotecan, and busulfan or melphalan (for stem cell transplant).

Side Effect Management

Acute: Skin reactions, mucositis, diarrhea, and fatigue are commonly seen. Prescribe Aquaphor for mild skin reactions; consider Silvadene if worse.

Late: Spinal deformities are commonly seen due to RT to the bony structures. Children may be shorter than their peers. Chronic renal insufficiency rarely seen in survivors. Risk of secondary malignancies about 1%-2% per decade of life

Follow-up

Typically will resume care with medical oncologist following completion of RT for maintenance therapy (for Stage IV patients). Follow-up with abdominal and whole body imaging is recommended q3mo for 1 year, q6mo for 2-4 years, and then every year.

Notable Trials

COG 3891 (*Matthay et al. NEJM* 1999). Randomized 539 high-risk Stage IV or III with MYCN amplification patients to myeloablative therapy and autologous bone marrow transplant (ABMT) with TBI vs intensive nonmyeloablative chemotherapy. Patients underwent a second randomization to either receive 6 cycles of adjuvant therapy with 13-cisretinoic acid or no further therapy. 3-Year EFS are 34% (ABMT) vs 22% (no ABMT) (P = .034) and 46% (retinoic acid) vs 29% (no retinoic acid) (P = .027).

COG ANBL0032 (*Yu et al. NEJM* 2011). 226 high-risk neuroblastoma patients who had a response to induction therapy and stem cell transplantation were assigned to (1) standard maintenance therapy consisting of 6 cycles of isotretinoin or (2) immunotherapy (Ch14.18 with GM-CSF and IL-2) + 6 cycles of isotretinoin. EFS superior with immunotherapy (66% vs 46% at 2 years, P = .01). OS superior with immunotherapy (86% vs 75% at 2 years, P = .02).

EWING SARCOMA

ETHAN BERNARD LUDMIR • ARNOLD C. PAULINO

Background

- **History:** Described in 1921 by James Ewing as a bone tumor sensitive to radiation. Ewing family of tumors (EFT) includes Ewing sarcoma (EWS) (both osseous and extraosseous), as well as malignant small cell tumor of the chest well (Askin tumor), and primitive neuroectodermal tumor (PNET). Osseous EWS accounts for ~85% of EFT; 8% of EFT are extraosseous EWS.
- **Incidence/prevalence:** Approximately 200 cases per year dx in the United States of EFT including EWS ~3% of adolescent malignancies. Second most common pediatric malignant bone tumor after osteosarcoma
- **Outcomes:** 5-Year OS for localized EWS ~70% (~60% for pelvic primaries, 80% for extremity primaries). 5-Year OS for metastatic EWS ~30% (~40% for lung mets only).
- **Demographics:** Median age at diagnosis is 14 years. 20%-30% of EFT occur in ptts <10 years old, and another 20%-30% occur in pts >20 years old. Higher incidence in M (M:F = 1.5:1 for EFT) and in Caucasians (very uncommon among African Americans)

- **Risk factors:** No known/established congenital syndrome associated w/ EFT. Rare reports of EWS as a second malignancy after treatment with chemotherapy
- **Prognostic factors:** Better prognosis w/ extremity tumors vs axial tumors. Larger size has worse prognosis (both those treated definitively with surgery and RT). Also prognostic: extent of viable tumor after neoadjuvant chemotherapy (≥5% residual viable tumor is a poor prognostic marker) and older age. Better prognosis for fusion of exon 7 of *EWS* to exon 6 of *FLI*

Tumor Biology and Characteristics

- **Pathology/genetics:** Proposed neuroectodermal origin of EFT, though other hypotheses exist. Histologically, EFT are small round blue cell tumors, differentiated by expression of vimentin, c-myc, and CD99 (CD99 being sensitive for EWS, but not specific as it is also expressed in rhabdomyosarcoma). Most cases involve breakpoints clustered within *EWSR1* gene on chromosome 22. 80%-90% of EFT have t(11;22), generating an *EWS-FLI* fusion protein, which has been shown to function as a transcription regulator. An additional 5%-10% of EFT have other translocations involving *EWSR1*, including t(21;22) and t(7;22) and less commonly t(17;22) and t(2;22).

Anatomy

For osseous EWS, pooled data from European Intergroup Cooperative Ewing Sarcoma Studies (EI-CESS) trials demonstrated that 54% of tumors had primary axial skeletal sites and 42% had primary appendicular skeletal sites (*Cotterill et al. JCO* 2000). Pelvic primary tumors = 25% of osseous EWS, and femoral primary tumors = 16% of osseous EWS. Primary location is typically diaphyseal.

Workup

- **History and physical:** Patients typically present with pain and swelling at the primary tumor site; often, minor trauma can precipitate pain/swelling at the site, which worsens over weeks. Pain associated with primary tumor is often worse at night and w/ exercise. Pts can present with pathologic fracture as well. Constitutional symptoms, including fevers and weight loss, occur in ~10%-20% of EWS pts at presentation and can portend metastatic dz + poorer prognosis.
- **Imaging:** Plain x-ray of primary site ("onion skin" appearance in EWS vs "sunburst" in osteosarcoma). Contrasted MR or CT of primary site (MRI preferred due to soft tissue delineation and involvement of neurovascular structures, surgical planning/considerations). Metastatic workup outlined per guidelines (*Meyer Pediatr Blood Cancer* 2008) generally includes PET/CT and radionuclide bone scintigraphy (bone scan). Also, note that repeat imaging prior to local therapy is recommended (usually MRI of primary site) to guide surgical planning and/or RT volumes.
- **Labs:** CBC, CMP (including BUN/Cr and LFTs), LDH, ESR.
- **Procedures/biopsy:** Core needle biopsy (often CT-guided) or incisional biopsy. Ensure surgeon is involved before biopsy, especially for cases where limb salvage is being considered (extremity EWS cases). At least unilateral bone marrow biopsy is recommended due to a significant risk of bone marrow metastases from EFT as well.

Staging

- No commonly used staging systems are present for EFT; rather the primary categorization of EWS (osseous and extraosseous) is localized or metastatic.
- Notably, 25% of EWS pts p/w metastatic disease, most commonly in the lungs (50%), bones (30%), and bone marrow (25%). Rare spread (<10%) to LNs, brain, and liver. If mets to other bones, vertebral column most often involved. Patterns of relapse mirror de novo sites of metastatic disease, w/ lung as most common site of relapse.

Treatment Algorithm

Conceptually, even localized EWS pts should be regarded as having occult systemic disease.

- **General treatment algorithm:** VDC/IE × 12 weeks → local therapy → VDC/IE through week 48 (~14-17 total cycles of VDC/IE)
- **Local therapy:** Surgery (+adj RT if needed) vs definitive RT
- **Surgery:** Favored if possible, to decrease risk of second malignancy and often less morbidity of resection in developing child than RT. Often, surgery is favored if limb reconstruction/sparing approach is possible. Resectable/dispensable bones (generally amenable to surgery): fibula (proximal), ribs, portions of hands/feet (esp small

tumors), and distal clavicle, among others. In an effort to avoid exposing pts to both surgery and adjuvant RT, definitive surgery should generally be pursued if complete resection is feasible.

- **Radiation:** Concurrent non–doxorubicin-containing chemotherapy is often delivered with RT during local therapy. Common indications for adjuvant RT include +margin/incomplete resection (R1 or R2), >10% viable tumor after induction chemotherapy (12 weeks of VDC/IE), or tumor spill. Per COG AEWS0031, adequate surgical margins are >1 cm for bone and >5 mm for soft tissue. Also, for bulky tumors in challenging sites, preop or postop RT can be utilized in conjunction with surgery. Similarly, adjuvant hemithoracic RT can be indicated in high-risk chest wall primary tumors (especially those w/ pleural infiltration or intraop contamination of pleural space). Whole lung irradiation (WLI) is generally recommended for pulmonary metastases, especially for those with good response to initial chemotherapy.

Radiation Treatment Technique

- **SIM:** Dependent on primary tumor site; some pediatric patients may require sedation (anesthesia)
- **Dose (primary EWS site):**
  - Definitive RT: 55.8 Gy (lower if paraspinal EWS w/ respect to cord tolerance)
  - Adjuvant RT: 55.8 Gy for gross residual, 50.4 Gy for microscopic residual
  - Doses in 1.8 Gy fractions (55.8 Gy in 31 fractions, for instance)
- **Target (primary EWS site):**
  - Definitive:
    - GTV1 = Pre-CHT bone and pre-CHT soft tissue involved
    - GTV2 = Pre-CHT bone and post-CHT soft tissue involved
    - GTV1 + 1.5 cm = CTV1
    - GTV2 + 1.5 cm = CTV2
    - CTV1 + 5 mm (generally) = PTV1 → treat to 45 Gy in 25 fractions
    - CTV2 + 5 mm (generally) = PTV2 → treat to additional 10.8 Gy in 6 fractions (total to 55.8 Gy/31 fx).
  - Adjuvant:
    - As per definitive, but GTV2 = postop residual/site of positive margins
    - CTV2 = GTV2 + 1.5 cm
    - CTV2 + 5 mm (generally) = PTV2 → treat to additional 5.4 Gy if microscopic residual or additional 10.8 Gy if macroscopic residual
  - Paraspinal EWS considerations:
    - Challenge with respect to cord tolerance. Often dose limited to 45 Gy or 50.4 Gy for those tumors w/ proximity to cord
- **Technique (primary EWS site):**
  Proton beam therapy and intensity-modulated radiation therapy (IMRT) are reasonable options. For certain pelvic tumors, consideration can be given to bladder filling, if full bladder displaces bowel from the treatment field. Daily bladder scanning may be helpful if this is the case. For hands/feet, use bolus/compensators. Consider bolus to scar/drain sites if adjuvant RT.
- **WLI/Hemithorax RT:**
  Dose: 15 Gy/10 fx
  CTV: Includes the bilateral lungs, mediastinum, and pleural recesses for WLI. For hemithorax RT (ie, due to pleural effusion), includes the ipsilateral lung + pleural recess
  Technique: AP/PA or IMRT (cardiac-sparing IMRT warrants 4D-CT simulation; see *Kalapurakal IJROBP* 2012). If AP/PA borders are as follows: Superior = above the clavicle/lung apex (flash SCV fossa). Inferior = below the diaphragm. Lateral = chest wall. See **Wilms Tumor** chapter for representative fields.
- **Planning directive constraints:**
  Specific constraints are largely dependent on the primary site, but in general:
  - Cord D_{max} < 45 Gy (though consideration can be given to a D_{max} < 50.4 Gy, depending on circumstances)
  - Avoid circumferential limb irradiation (see "Soft Tissue Sarcoma" section for more information), sparing 1-2 cm strip of skin to reduce lymphedema risk.
  - Extra care should be given to avoid unnecessary bladder dose given cystitis associated w/ EWS CHT agents cyclophosphamide and ifosfamide, which are often given concurrent w/ RT.
  - Avoid premature epiphyseal closure by avoiding RT to uninvolved epiphyseal growth plates.

Chemotherapy

- VDC/IE = Vincristine + doxorubicin + cyclophosphamide (VDC) alternating with ifosfamide + etoposide (IE)

Side Effects

- Acute: Varies by treatment field/primary site
- Late: Varies by treatment field/primary site, but in general: height loss, premature epiphyseal closure/decreased bone growth (and therefore skeletal asymmetry in some cases), kyphosis/lordosis/scoliosis, fracture, cystitis, pneumonitis, pulmonary fibrosis, infertility, and second malignancy (SMN). Note the relatively high rate of SMN for EWS survivors, w/ CCSS report of 24% cumulative SMN risk at 35 years (*Marina et al. Cancer* 2017).

Follow-up

- End-treatment imaging with PET/CT at completion of chemotherapy and MRI of primary site ~3-4 months after definitive local treatment (*Meyer Pediatr Blood Cancer* 2008)
- Follow-up q3mo for first 2 years, then q6mo for years 2-5, then annually for another 5 years, and likely longer than that. Includes H&P, labs, as well as primary + chest imaging, generally plain films unless concerning/focal sxs present, or abnormality detected on XR
- Late relapses not uncommon w/ EWS, per CCSS occurring in 13% of 5-year EWS survivors by 20 years. Site-specific monitoring for late effects should also be pursued (relevant site-specific guidelines available from COG).

Notable Trials

POG 8346 (*Donaldson IJROBP* 1998). Randomized trial including 178 children w/ EWS, 79% with localized disease. Patients who achieved a CR/PR after induction VDC + dactinomycin and with primary tumors involving nonexpendable bone randomized to whole-bone RT field vs involved field RT (GTV + 2 cm). 53% LC in both RT arms, establishing involved field RT for EWS, compared to whole-bone RT

INT-0091 (*Grier NEJM* 2003). Randomized trial in which 518 EFT pts were randomized to induction VDC + dactinomycin vs VDC + dactinomycin alternating with IE. For pts with localized EFT, alternating VDC + dactinomycin with IE resulted in a significant improvement in 5-year OS (72% vs 61%, $P = .01$) and LC (95% vs 85%, $P < .001$).

RHABDOMYOSARCOMA

ETHAN BERNARD LUDMIR • ARNOLD C. PAULINO

Background

- **Incidence/prevalence:** Rhabdomyosarcoma (RMS) is the most common pediatric soft tissue sarcoma, with ~350-400 cases per year in the United States. Accounts for ~3%-4% of pediatric malignancies
- **Outcomes:** Varies by primary tumor site, histology, translocation status, and risk stratification, among others. The 5-year overall survival (OS) by COG risk stratification: low risk = 92%, intermediate risk = 65%, and high risk = 14%
- **Demographics:** Male predominance; M:F = ~1.4:1. Slight racial trends in RMS incidence: African Americans > Caucasians > Asians. Incidence peaks at 2-6 years old (embryonal histology) and 10-14 (alveolar histology). However, 7% of RMS is in infants (<1 year old), and 13% of RMS is in pts 15+ years old, including cases in adults.
- **Risk factors:** Limited knowledge, w/ most RMS cases being sporadic. RMS has been associated w/ some genetic syndromes including Li-Fraumeni, NF-1, and Beckwith-Wiedemann.

Tumor Biology and Characteristics

- **Pathology:** Small round blue cell tumor. IHC helpful to distinguish from other small blue round cell tumors. RMS positive for muscle-specific proteins including myoglobin, Z-band protein, myogenic differentiation 1 (MyoD1), actin, myosin, and desmin.

- **Cell of origin:** Hypothesized to arise from primitive mesenchymal cells, though emerging data suggest nonmesenchymal origin may be possible for fusion-negative RMS (*Drummond et al. Cancer Cell* 2018).
- **Histology:** Multiple histologic subtypes with prognostic importance. From the best to the worst prognosis: botryoid, spindle cell, embryonal, alveolar, and pleomorphic/undifferentiated. Botryoid and spindle cells are variants of embryonal histology and confer excellent prognosis. Botryoid is common in infants and tumors of the GU tract (ie, vaginal RMS in infants, typically botryoid histology, which has "bunch of grapes" appearance on physical exam). Embryonal histology displays patchy myogenin staining, with appearance similar to embryonal skeletal muscle; RMS of head and neck enriched for embryonal histologies (especially orbital tumors). Alveolar histology, with a worse prognosis, occurs in older children (10+) and has diffuse myogenin staining. Furthermore, alveolar tumors occur in more unfavorable sites, especially the extremities, perineum, and trunk. Approximately 50%-55% of RMS are embryonal, and ~25% are alveolar.
- **Genetics:** Translocations involving *FOXO1* on chromosome 13 have been shown to be associated with alveolar RMS. Approximately 80% of alveolar RMS have either *PAX3-FOXO1* or *PAX7-FOXO1* fusion transcripts, corresponding to t(2;13) and t(1;13), respectively. Of those w/ fusion transcripts, majority are *PAX3-FOXO1* fusions. *PAX-FOXO1* is a negative prognostic indicator (*Sorenson et al. JCO* 2002). Moreover, fusion-negative alveolar RMS has comparable outcomes to embryonal RMS (*Williamson et al. JCO* 2010). Therefore, there is a trend toward fusion status for risk assignment and trial design (including ongoing COG trials).

Anatomy

Approximately 20% GU, ~15% H&N parameningeal, ~10% orbital, ~10% H&N nonparameningeal, ~20% extremity, and ~15% other (including trunk, retroperitoneum)

*Parameningeal H&N includes MMNNOOPP mnemonic = Middle ear, Mastoid, Nasal cavity, Nasopharynx, infratemporal fOssa, pterygopalatine fOssa, Paranasal sinuses, and Parapharyngeal space

Classify primary site into favorable and unfavorable prognostic categories:

- **Favorable sites:** Orbit, nonparameningeal H&N, biliary, nonprostate/nonbladder GU
- **Unfavorable sites:** All other sites

Diagnostic Evaluation

- **History and physical:** Clinical presentation varies by primary site. Orbital: proptosis, ophthalmoplegia. Parameningeal H&N: nasal/aural/sinus obstruction, CN deficits, and altered mental status (consider intracranial extension). Other H&N: painless enlarging mass. Extremities: mass (+/– pain associated with mass), swelling. GU: hematuria/urinary obstruction (bladder), discharge (vagina), scrotal/inguinal enlargement (paratesticular)

  Nodal metastasis rates, including at presentation, vary by primary site/histology; highest risks of LNs involved by site are prostate, paratesticular, and extremity tumors. H&N alveolar tumors may also have increased risk of LN mets.

  Distant mets in ~20% of RMS pts at diagnosis, usually the lung, bone marrow, and bone. Mets within the CNS can occur in parameningeal RMS pts w/ intracranial extension (seeding within CSF).
- **Imaging:** Assess primary site: MRI preferred. Assess for LN + distant mets: PET/CT; can omit chest CT and bone scan if PET/CT performed. Bone marrow biopsy recommended, though bilateral BMBx not required for embryonal RMS pts and clinically node-negative pts.
  - **Parameningeal RMS:** These tumors have high risk of extension into the CNS (intracranial extension, as well as cranial bone erosion and CN deficits). Therefore, for parameningeal RMS, CSF cytology (LP) as well as MRI of the brain is needed.
- **Labs:** CBC, CMP (including BUN/Cr and LFTs), uric acid
- **Procedures/biopsy:** Core needle or incisional Bx. As above, for parameningeal RMS, LP is needed for CSF cytologic analysis.
  - **Nodal evaluation:** Biopsy any suspicious LNs to confirm nodal status. Sentinel LN biopsy indicated for extremity tumors. Males >10 years old w/ paratesticular RMS are recommended for ipsilateral nerve-sparing retroperitoneal LN dissection.
- **Miscellaneous:** Sperm banking/fertility consult, as indicated

RISK STRATIFICATION/STAGING

- Risk stratification guides treatment; 4-step process
  1. **Site: favorable vs unfavorable:** See above re: dividing primary sites into favorable vs unfavorable categories.
  2. **Stage:** Start by site, and then determine the stage (I-IV) as below:

Stage	Site	Size	L Nodes	Mets
I	Favorable	Any	Any	M0
II	Unfavorable	≤5 cm	N0	M0
III	Unfavorable	>5 cm OR N1 (any size)		M0
IV	Any	Any	Any	M1

Favorable site: Orbit, non-PM H&N, nonbladder/prostate GU, biliary tract
Unfavorable site: PM, everything else

3. **Group (extent of surgery):** IRS grouping based on the extent of surgery

Group	Definition
1	R0 (complete) resection
2	R1 resection and/or LN+ (with R0-1)
3	R2 resection or unresectable/Bx only
4	Metastatic disease

4. **Risk stratification:** Combination of stage + group, as well as histology (now fusion status; *Pappo et al. JCO* 2017). See above for OS rates for each risk category.
   - **Low risk:** Fusion-negative: Stage 1 Group 2, Stage 2 Groups 1 and 2, and orbital Stage 1 Group 3
   - **High risk:** All Stage 4 Group 4 except fusion-negative pts <10 years old
   - **Intermediate risk:** All others

TREATMENT ALGORITHM

- Overarching Tx paradigm: maximal safe resection (or biopsy) → chemotherapy, start RT as indicated during chemotherapy, timing noted below
- RT used as definitive local therapy for sites w/ limited options for primary resection w/o significant morbidity, including orbital as well as other H&N (esp parameningeal).
- RT dosing, timing, and indications vary by stage/group/risk stratification as above.

RADIATION TREATMENT TECHNIQUE

- **SIM:** Primary site dependent; sedation (anesthesia) may be required in children <8 years old, for both sim and treatment.
- **Dose:** All in 1.8 Gy fractions, generally
  - Group I embryonal = no RT
  - Group I alveolar = 36 Gy to prechemo site
  - Group II N0 (microscopic residual after surgery) = 36 Gy to prechemo site
  - Group II N1 (resected LN involvement) = 41.4 Gy to prechemo site and nodal region
  - Group III nonorbital = 50.4 Gy
  - Group III orbital = 45 Gy (if CR after induction chemo) and 50.4 Gy (if non-CR after induction chemo)
  - No RT indicated for additional settings (including nonembryonal RMS): N0 extremity RMS s/p amputation; paratesticular s/p R0 resection
- **RT timing:** Relative to start of chemotherapy, generally by risk stratification
  - Low risk = week 13 (per ARST0331)
  - Intermediate risk = previously week 4 (ARST0531) though current COG ARST1431 moving this to week 13
  - High risk = week 20
  - Emergent RT should be initiated as soon as indicated, regardless of the above.
  - Parameningeal RMS w/ intracranial extension conventionally treated weeks 0-2. ARST1431 delaying RT start to week 13.
- **Target:**
  - In general: GTV = prechemotherapy volume and CTV = GTV + 1 cm
  - PTV margin depends on site(s) being treated, IGRT utilized, etc.

- **Technique:** Varies by treatment site, but in general proton beam therapy and IMRT are reasonable options, w/ multiple series utilizing both techniques across primary sites.
- **IGRT:** Primary site dependent, usually at least daily kV-IGRT
- **Planning directive dose constraints:** Primary site dependent

Chemotherapy

- Commonly utilized: VAC (vincristine/dactinomycin/cyclophosphamide), VI (vincristine/irinotecan), and IE (ifosfamide/etoposide)

Side Effects

- **Acute:** Varies by treatment field/primary site
- **Late:** Varies by treatment field/primary site. For orbital tumors, for instance, xerophthalmia, cataracts, decreased visual acuity H&N RT leads to dentofacial abnormalities, facial asymmetry/hypoplasia, endocrinopathies, and neurocognitive deficits. Other late risk factors include premature epiphyseal closure and decreased bone growth (and therefore skeletal asymmetry), fracture, cystitis, urinary incontinence, infertility (especially w/ cyclophosphamide), and second malignancy (SMN).

Notable Trials/Papers

- IRS I (*Maurer Cancer* 1988). Group I favorable histology pts: VAC vs VAC-RT, with no difference in OS (93% vs 81%, respectively, $P = .67$); therefore no RT for Group I favorable histology. Also showed that for Group II/III pts, RT coverage of whole muscle vs involved fields resulted in no difference in LC (therefore no need for whole muscle coverage). For pts >6 years old, LR 32% for RT < 40 Gy and LR 12% for RT > 40 Gy ($P > .4$); no dose response demonstrated.
- IRS IV (*Crist JCO* 2001). Group III pts randomized to 50.4 Gy in 1.8 Gy daily fx vs hyperfractionated 59.4 Gy in 1.1 Gy BID fx. No difference in failure-free survival or LC ($P = .85$ and .9, respectively), w/ increased mucositis in hyperfractionated arm. Therefore, conventional daily fractionation remains standard.

OSTEOSARCOMA/RETINOBLASTOMA/ BRAINSTEM GLIOMA

ETHAN BERNARD LUDMIR • ARNOLD C. PAULINO

Osteosarcoma

- **Background:**
  - Most common pediatric bone tumor (2nd most is Ewing sarcoma [EWS]), w/ ~400 pediatric cases per year. Bimodal distribution w/ peak in teenage years and another peak >65 years old. M > F and African American > Caucasian
  - Increased risk of osteosarcoma in pts w/ history of germline *RB* mutation as well as h/o RT for retinoblastoma (irrespective of germline *RB* mutation presence)
  - Presents with local symptoms including pain, swelling, palpable mass, and fracture. Less common for systemic symptoms at presentation than EWS. "Sunburst" pattern on films vs "onion skin" appearance in EWS
  - 80% of cases in appendicular skeleton, majority of which originate in metaphysis (distal femur > tibia)
  - 90% of osteosarcoma pts have radiographically localized disease at dx, but w/ symptoms alone, ~80% of pts will develop lung mets within 12 months. Therefore, like w/ EWS, osteosarcoma is an "occult systemic" disease.
- **Treatment paradigm:**
  Neoadjuvant chemotherapy → surgery* → adjuvant chemotherapy (usually double doxorubicin/cisplatin)
  *Pathologic response to neoadjuvant chemotherapy on surgical specimen is prognostic, with >90% necrosis resulting in ~80% relapse-free survival.

- **Role of RT:**
  - Unlike EWS, osteosarcoma is generally considered radioresistant (variant histologies of osteosarcoma are to some extent more radiosensitive).
  - Beyond palliative indications, RT may be used in the definitive setting for inoperable pts (inoperable due to pt and/or disease factors) or in the adjuvant setting for those with close or positive margins.
  - Definitive RT, or RT after R2 resection (gross residual dz), is thought to require high doses of RT (60-70 Gy, usually at least 66 Gy in 2 Gy fractions).
  - Data suggest no role for prophylactic WLI despite high risk of lung metastases.

RETINOBLASTOMA (RB)

- **Background:**
  - Most common primary intraocular pediatric malignancy, with ~300 cases per year. Occurs usually in infants/toddlers (~2 years median age at dx). 95% of cases in those <5 years old
  - 60% of Rb cases are sporadic, and 40% are heritable (germline *RB* mutation). Most heritable *RB* mutation is via de novo germline mutations, since <10% of *RB* patients have family history of *RB* mutation.
  - Approximately 1/3 of Rb cases are bilateral, generally suggestive of germline *RB* mutation. However, 15% of unilateral Rb pts have germline mutation, so genetic testing should be considered even in unilateral cases. Trilateral retinoblastoma cases refer to bilateral retinoblastoma with a concordant pineoblastoma. Occurs in 5% of patients with *RB* mutation
  - Earlier age of presentation (~1-1.5 years old) for bilateral Rb pts and pts w/ germline *RB* mutation
  - Usually p/w leukocoria, although can p/w strabismus, nystagmus, and others
  - Multiple classification systems; COG currently using the International Classification of Intraocular Retinoblastoma system, where the eyes are risk stratified from A through E.
    A: Small tumors (3 mm), limited to the retina and not near important structures
    B: All other tumors, limited to the retina
    C: Well-defined tumors with small amount of spread under the retina or vitreous seeding
    D: Large or poorly defined tumors with widespread vitreous or subretinal seeding
    E: Large tumor, extending near the front of the eye. Bleeding, causing glaucoma, or have almost no chance the eye can be served
- **Treatment paradigm:**
  - Variable but includes both systemic therapy (usually VCE = vincristine/carboplatin/etoposide) and focal therapies w/ the goal of sparing the eye from enucleation if possible
  - Array of local treatment options available, including intra-arterial chemotherapy, intravitreous chemotherapy, cryotherapy, laser photocoagulation, external beam RT, and plaque brachytherapy
  - EBRT may be indicated in adjuvant setting after enucleation as well, if positive margin or nodal involvement is identified; enucleation is often indicated for advanced (very high risk = group E) tumors, among others.
- **Role of EBRT and brachytherapy:**
  - EBRT was developed as the first technique to allow globe sparing. However, it is used less now due to concerns for second malignancy. Roarty et al. examined bilateral Rb pts; 35% had second malignant neoplasm after EBRT vs 6% for those who didn't have EBRT (*Roarty et al. Ophthalmology* 1988). Data support field and dose dependence of second malignant neoplasm incidence after RT for Rb. Second malignant neoplasm after RT for Rb includes osteosarcoma of bones within the treatment field around the orbit.
  - EBRT (usually with concurrent chemotherapy) is often indicated in adjuvant setting after enucleation w/ +margin or +LN. Doses 36-45 Gy.
  - Plaque brachytherapy provides a custom-design shielded source that decreases RT dose to bones and therefore reduces risk for developing secondary malignant neoplasms.
  - Usually I-125 or Ru-106 sources for plaques, **prescribing** 45 Gy to 1 mm beyond the apex of the tumor
  - Logistically challenging, as plaques remain in place for ~2 days in these young children before returning to the operating room for plaque removal. Similarly, technically challenging; therefore not used often in the frontline setting, but rather considered in the setting of persistent dz after other local therapies exhausted

Brainstem Glioma

- **Background:**
  - 80% of pediatric brainstem gliomas arise from pons. Most pontine tumors are diffuse intrinsic pontine gliomas (DIPGs). Approximately 20% of pediatric brainstem gliomas = focal, predominantly at cervicomedullary jxn (low medulla) and tectum (upper midbrain). Usually present with CN palsies, especially CNs VI and VII, as well as ataxia, incr ICP (H/A, N/V, lethargy/somnolence). Pontine gliomas are primarily infiltrative, high-grade, and aggressive and portend poor prognosis.
  - Nondiffuse nonpontine lesions include dorsally exophytic lesions, usually low-grade gliomas including JPA (WHO grade I tumors).
  - Incidence: DIPGs usually present at 4-9 years old, ~300 cases per year. No gender predilection for DIPG
  - Pathology: Emerging understanding of molecular pathogenesis of DIPG, including high incidence of mutations in *H3F3A* (histone H3 gene). Approximately 80% of DIPG in one study found to have *H3F3A* mutation (*Wu et al. Nat Genet* 2012). These *H3 K27M* mutations have been identified as portending poor prognosis. 2016 WHO classification includes "H3 K27M-mutant diffuse midline glioma" as a diagnostic entity.
  - DIPG on MRI demonstrates characteristic T1-hypointense and T2-hyperintense expansile infiltrative pattern within the pons, w/ variable rates of Gd contrast enhancement.
- **Treatment paradigm:**
  - Management of peritumoral edema (steroids) and management of hydrocephalus (shunt) as indicated. Biopsy of tumor only indicated if atypical appearance on imaging questioning DIPG dx. Emerging studies/protocols are demonstrating safety of biopsy of DIPG, but outside of protocol, do not biopsy due to risks of injury to the brainstem.
  - The only standard antitumor therapy is RT. Despite this, median survival ~1 year, w/ minimal (<5%) survival at 5 years. Of note, non-DIPG brainstem gliomas, such as dorsal exophytic brainstem gliomas, have better prognosis (~75% 10-year OS)
  - Limited role for conventional chemotherapeutics, though increasingly HDAC inhibitors/inhibitors of histone demethylation are being utilized on the protocol.
- **Role of RT:**
  - Dose: RT for DIPG involves treatment to 54 Gy in 30 fractions (1.8 Gy/fx)
  - Target: Tumor volume (MRI fusion helpful) + 1-1.5 cm for CTV. Additionally, 5 mm PTV w/ daily kV-IGRT
  - Technique: Photon-based RT (IMRT/VMAT) rather than proton beam therapy, owing to theoretical considerations regarding higher risk of brainstem injury w/ protons.
  - Alternative RT dose via hypofractionation, using 39 Gy at 3 Gy/fx (13 daily fractions) or 44.8 Gy at 2.8 Gy/fx (16 daily fractions). Matched cohort analysis (*Janssens et al. IJROBP* 2013) suggested comparable outcomes with shorter treatment time/burden. However, RCT from Egypt randomized DIPG pts to 54 Gy/30 fx vs 39 Gy/13 fx found similar results between 2 arms, but w/ PFS differences exceeding prespecified noninferiority assumption (PFS favoring conventional arm).
  - Therefore, we continue to utilize conventional fractionation at MDACC at present.
  - RT usually results in response and symptom improvement in majority (~65%-75%) of pts, but virtually all will recur 1 year after RT.

LATE EFFECTS

ETHAN BERNARD LUDMIR • ARNOLD C. PAULINO

Background

- **Overview:**
  - Late toxicity from radiotherapy, especially in pediatric pts, informs treatment choices and risks.
  - Increasing concern regarding late toxicity given improved survival of pediatric pts across disease sites over the last 50 years.

- Top causes of mortality in 5-year survivors of childhood cancers are recurrent disease (57%), secondary malignancies (SMNs; 15%), and cardiac toxicities (7%) (*Mertens et al. JCO* 2001).
- **Factors affecting late effects:**
  - Factors may affect risk of late toxicity to different organ systems/sites.
  - Host factors, including age, gender, comorbidities, ethnicity/race, and genetic predisposition, may affect late toxicity.
  - Age of patient is particularly important for OARs, given differential rates of maturation. For example, early development of brain vs teenage development of reproductive system; conceptually, brain more sensitive to RT during development in early childhood, whereas gonads more sensitive to RT during puberty
  - Genetic effects are also important: NF1 pts after RT for optic pathway gliomas had ~50% risk of second malignancy (*Sharif et al. JCO* 2006). Similarly, increased risk for moyamoya syndrome for NF1 pts after RT and also increased risk of cutaneous basal cell carcinomas in field after RT in pts w/ Gorlin syndrome (see *Happle JAAD* 1999). Secondary neoplasm risk in Rb pts markedly increased if hereditary Rb vs nonhereditary after RT (33% vs 13%; *Marees et al. JNCI* 2008)
  - Gender is also critical, as discussed below; there is evidence for increased sensitivity for RT toxicity in females, including neurocognitive deficits and height impairments after cranial RT for leukemia, hypothyroidism, and secondary malignancies after mediastinal RT for Hodgkin lymphoma (specifically breast).
  - Treatment parameters also influence toxicity: radiation dose, fraction size, volume treated, concurrent chemotherapy, as well as timing of chemotherapy and radiation; also important are other oncotherapeutics employed, including surgery and chemotherapy. Multiple modalities may synergize to increase the risk of toxicity.

Late Effects by Organ Site

- **CNS:**
  - Neurocognitive effects due to brain radiation; most sensitive in utero and then for the first few years of life. Synaptogenesis, axonal growth, dendritic arborization, and maturation of neural networks over these early years are thought to be central to RT neurotoxicity in the very young.
  - Neurocognitive changes affected by age of RT; IQ scores for pediatric low-grade glioma pts show more significant long-term IQ deficits w/ younger age at RT (*Merchant et al. JCO* 2009).
  - CSI + posterior fossa boost for medulloblastoma pts is shown to affect both verbal and nonverbal IQ (*Ris et al. JCO* 2001).
  - The above study suggested female pts are more likely to have verbal IQ deficits after RT; possible gender sensitivity to IQ changes in females in study w/ ALL pts s/p CSI: 50% of girls vs 14% of boys had IQ < 90 on follow-up (*Waber et al. JCO* 1992).
  - Cranial RT may also cause leukoencephalopathy, though unlikely (<1%) in the absence of methotrexate (IV or intrathecal).
- **Musculoskeletal:**
  - RT injury to bone is dependent on portion of bone treated; for example, epiphyseal RT arrests chondrogenesis.
  - Skeletal effects are observed across multiple series, including scoliosis, kyphosis/lordosis, and iliac wing hypoplasia, among others. The most common of these (dependent on RT fields) is scoliosis.
  - Height deficits after RT are also noted, dependent on both dose and age at RT. Example is Wilms tumor pts treated w/ RT: 8-year-old pts s/p 10 Gy had only 0.8 cm height loss, whereas 2-year-old pts s/p 30 Gy had 7.2 cm height loss (*Hogeboom et al. Med Pediatr Oncol* 2001).
  - Prior to puberty, if a vertebral column or growth plate cannot avoid radiation, then it is better to treat the entire column or growth plate to avoid asymmetric growth.
  - Similarly thought to have gender bias w/ female more sensitive to RT-related height loss
  - Growth abnormalities d/t both direct RT to developing bones and cranial RT (GH deficits). Short stature risk for pts s/p cranial RT > 20 Gy for ALL pts (*Chow et al. J Pediatr* 2007).
- **Second malignancy:**
  - Secondary breast cancer ~9%-10% incidence after RT for Hodgkin's
  - Increased sensitivity for secondary breast cancer if patient is pubescent (~12-16 years old) at RT vs younger (<12 years old; *Constine IJROBP* 2008).
  - After RT for Hodgkin lymphoma, secondary thyroid cancer is also observed with comparable frequency to SBC (*O'Brien JCO* 2010).

- Secondary malignancy is risk linked closely to RT use, among other factors (including certain chemotherapeutics such as procarbazine, anthracycline, and etoposide); secondary sarcoma is largely related to prior RT, and secondary GI malignancies are similarly related to prior abdominal RT.
- Differential secondary malignancy rates by primary tumor histology (see **Ewing Sarcoma** chapter; high secondary malignancy incidence for EWS). Other reports describe low secondary malignancy risk for other lesions, including ~1%-2% at 10-15 years for Wilms tumor, ALL, and rhabdomyosarcoma.
- SMN studies are challenging due to time lapse between RT, treatment, and tumor-causing events; modeling suggests modern techniques have decreased risk of RT-related secondary malignancies. Emerging data suggest trend toward decreased secondary malignancies with progressive era of treatment (*Turcotte et al. JAMA* 2017).

Strategies to Reduce Late Toxicity

- **Delaying/omitting RT**
  - Utilized in young children, especially <3-year-old pts w/ brain tumors. CSI delayed to >3 years old for MB and other CNS pts. Approach of deferring/delaying RT supported infants w/ ependymoma (*Merchant et al. JCO* 2004).
- **Hyperfractionated RT**
  - Relying on radiobiological principles, hyperfractionation is thought to decrease late effects, supported by a few series. Examples include decreased fracture and muscle atrophy in Ewing sarcoma pts w/ hyperfractionation and decreased hypothyroidism with RT for medulloblastoma w/ hyperfractionation.
  - Trials across multiple disease sites, however, have found limited to no difference w/ fractionation (IRS-IV, EWS CESS-86, MB HIT-SIOP PNET 4).
- **Decreasing RT dose and volume**
  - Decreased RT dose is successfully applied in NWTS-3, the results of which decreased adjuvant RT dose for Stage III favorable histology Wilms tumor pts from 20 to 10 Gy w/ addition of doxorubicin to chemo regimen. Used additional chemotherapy to offset decreased RT dose.
  - In medulloblastoma patients, ACNS0031 demonstrated that involved field boost is equivalent to posterior fossa boost, which translated into a significant reduction in total brain doses.
  - Significant RT dose reductions for Hodgkin lymphoma, previously total nodal/subtotal nodal/mantle field RT to 36-44 Gy, now involved field/site/nodal RT to much lower doses (20-30 Gy generally).
  - May also attempt to eliminate RT for favorable subsets of pts: for example, in COG AREN0533, elimination of WLI for Wilms tumor pts w/ lung metastases w/ favorable chemo response. Also, see multiple Hodgkin lymphoma trials recommending RT for pts w/ PR after chemo vs observation for pts w/ CR after chemo.
- **Advanced RT technologies**
  - IMRT Example: Decreased ototoxicity in MB pts w/ IMRT vs 3DCRT (*Huang et al. IJROBP* 2002)
  - Proton beam therapy: see **Proton therapy** chapter, minimal exit dose via Bragg peak particularly advantageous for certain disease sites. Among the most notable examples, CSI, sparked 2013 debate in *IJROBP* whether proton beam therapy "only ethical" approach for pediatric pts needing CSI
  - Despite a concern for secondary neutron production/contamination w/ proton beam therapy, clinical data are not suggestive of increased risk of secondary malignancies with protons (*Sethi et al. Cancer* 2013).
  - PENTEC group, pediatric analog of the QUANTEC effort, developing quantitative, evidence-based guidelines for RT treatment planning and dose constraints, among others

ORAL CAVITY

GARY WALKER • ADAM SETH GARDEN

BACKGROUND

- **Incidence/prevalence:** ~30 000 cases diagnosed annually in the United States
- **Outcomes:** 5-Year survival across all stages estimated at 67% (SEER data)
- **Demographics:** M > F, older age
- **Risk factors:** Smoking, smokeless tobacco, alcohol, betel nut, and premalignant lesions (leukoplakia 5% risk of developing cancer, erythroplakia 50% risk)

TUMOR BIOLOGY AND CHARACTERISTICS

- **Genetics:** Majority associated with genetic alterations from external factors
- **Pathology:** Vast majority are SCC. Rare histologies include adenoid cystic, adenocarcinoma, sarcoma, and melanoma.

ANATOMY

- **Subsites:** Oral tongue, mucosal lip, buccal mucosa, alveolar ridge, retromolar trigone, floor of the mouth, hard palate
- **Extrinsic muscles of the tongue:** Genioglossus, hyoglossus, styloglossus, palatoglossus
- **Lymph node drainage** (35% are cN+):
  - Primary drainage to Ib and IIA.
  - The upper lip can drain to preauricular.
  - The lower lip and FOM can drain to IA.
  - About 15% bypass II and go directly to level III-IV.
  - Level IV-V can be involved with advanced nodal disease.

HEAD AND NECK LYMPH NODE LEVELS

The neck is divided into six LN levels (Fig. 25.1). For all the remaining chapters in this section, please refer to the following definitions:

Level I: Inferior to mylohyoid muscle and above the caudal border of the hyoid bone/carotid bifurcation:

- **Ia (submetal):** Between anterior bellies of the bilateral digastric muscles
- **Ib (submandibular):** Posterolateral to the anterior belly of the digastric muscle and anterior to the posterior border of the submandibular gland

Level II (internal jugular chain): Base of the skull to caudal border of hyoid bone/carotid bifurcation. Anterior to the posterior border of SCM. Posterior to the posterior border of the submandibular gland:

- **IIa:** Anterior or immediately adjacent to (eg, inseparable from) the internal jugular vein
- **IIb:** Posterior to internal jugular vein with a fat plane separating node from vein (otherwise considered level IIa)

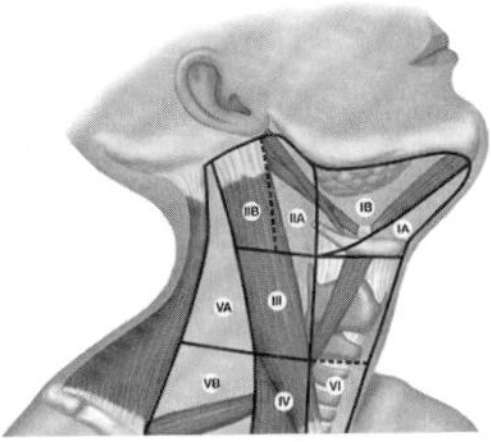

Figure 25.1 Diagram of LN stations of the neck. (Adapted from Edge SB, Byrd DR, Compton CC, Fritz AG, Greene FL, Trotti A III. eds. *AJCC cancer staging manual*. 7th ed. New York, NY: Springer; 2010. Copyright c 2010 American Joint Committee on Cancer. Reproduced with permission of Springer in the format Book via Copyright Clearance Center.)

Level III (internal jugular chain): Caudal border of hyoid to caudal border of cricoid. Anterior to posterior border of SCM. Lateral to medial margin of the common/internal carotid artery

Level IV (internal jugular chain): Caudal border of cricoid to clavicle. Anterior to posterior border of SCM. Lateral to the medial margin of common carotid artery

Level V (posterior triangle/spinal accessory): Posterior to SCM and anterior to trapezius muscle:

- **Va:** Superior half, posterior to level II and III LN levels
- **Vb:** Inferior half, posterior to level IV LN levels

Level VI (Prelaryngeal/pretracheal/delphian node): Caudal edge of hyoid bone to the manubrium, anterior to levels III and IV and visceral space (Fig. 25.2)

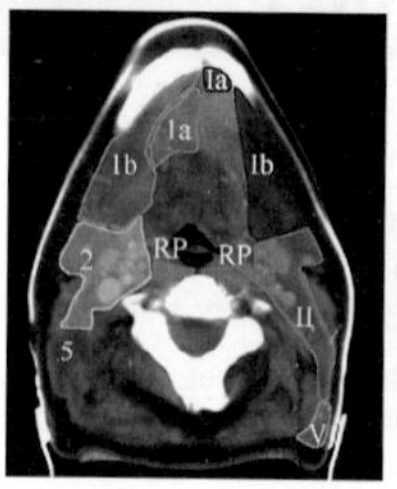

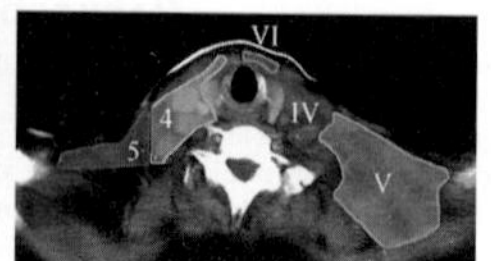

Figure 25.2 Axial CT images showing LN levels at the lower edge of the mandible **(left panel)** and low neck **(right panel)**. **See color insert**. (Reprinted from Grégoire V, Levendag P, Ang KK, et al. CT-based delineation of lymph node levels and related CTVs in the node-negative neck: DAHANCA, EORTC, GORTEC, NCIC, RTOG consensus guidelines. *Radiother Oncol.* 2003;69(3): 227-236. Copyright © 2003 Elsevier Ireland Ltd. With permission.)

Workup

- **History and physical:** Assess presenting symptoms including oral cavity function, cranial nerve deficits, otalgia, and trismus. Direct palpation and visualization of tumor and adjacent subsites with nasolaryngoscope and/or mirror exam useful to assess disease spread
- **Labs:** CBC, CMP
- **Procedures/Biopsy:** Biopsy of primary and FNA of enlarged LNs as clinically indicated
- **Imaging:** CT or MRI with contrast of head and neck. Consider CT of the chest. FDG-PET/CT recommended for Stage III/IV disease
- **Additional consultations:** Multidisciplinary evaluation with head and neck surgical oncology, radiation oncology, medical oncology, speech, nutrition, and dental (fluoride/extractions)

Oral Cavity Cancer Staging *(AJCC 8th Edition)*

T Stage		**N Stage**	
Tis	Carcinoma in situ	N1	1 ipsi LN, ≤3 cm without ENE
T1	Tumor ≤2 cm, ≤5 mm depth of invasion (DOI)	N2a	1 ipsi/contra LN ≤ 3 cm with ENE, 1 ipsi LN > 3 cm ≤ 6 cm without ENE
T2	Tumor ≤2 cm, DOI > 5 mm and ≤10 mm **Or** Tumor >2 cm and ≤4 cm and DOI ≤ 10 mm	N2b	>1 ipsi LN ≤ 6 cm without ENE
T3	Tumor >4 cm or any tumor DOI > 10 mm	N2c	>1 ipsi/contra LN > 6 cm without ENE
		N3a	1 + LN > 6 cm without ENE
		N3b	1 ipsi LN, >3 cm with ENE, 1 + ipsi/contra LN with ENE
		M Stage	
T4a	Moderately advanced local disease: (lip) tumor invades through cortical bone or involves the inferior alveolar nerve, floor of the mouth, or skin of the face (ie, chin or nose); (oral cavity) tumor invades adjacent structures only (eg, through the cortical bone of the mandible or maxilla, or involves the maxillary sinus or skin of the face); note that superficial erosion of the bone/tooth socket (alone) by a gingival primary is not sufficient to classify a tumor as T4	M1	Metastatic disease
T4b	Very advanced local disease; tumor invades masticator space, pterygoid plates, or skull base and/or encases the internal carotid artery		

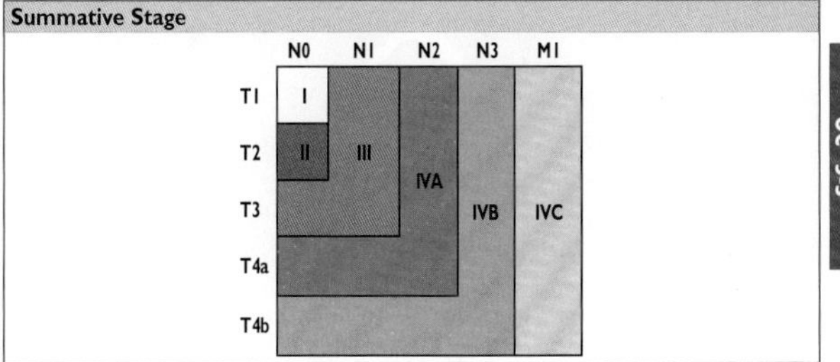

Treatment Algorithm

	Surgery
T1-2, N0	Resection of primary ± ipsi neck dissection (>4 mm DOI) or SNL Bx
T3N0, T1-4 N+	Resection of primary + ipsi or bilateral neck dissection
	Adjuvant Radiation
Positive margins	Adjuvant chemoRT (cisplatin Category I) if can't be reresected
ECE	Adjuvant chemoRT
Other risk factors[a]	RT or consider chemoRT

[a]pT3/T4, N2/N3, PNI, level IV/V, LVSI.

Radiation Treatment Technique

- **Timing:** Should be started within 4-6 weeks of surgery
- **Dose:** Highest risk (close/positive margins/ECE)—63-66 Gy in 30-33 fractions
  High risk (tumor bed)—60 Gy in 30 fractions
  Intermediate risk (operative bed and dissected neck)—57 Gy in 30 fractions
  Low risk (elective nodal coverage)—54 Gy in 30 fractions
- **Target:** Tumor bed, operative bed, and draining lymphatics (levels I-IV, level V if node positive). Consider unilateral treatment for a well-lateralized retromolar trigone, buccal mucosa, or alveolar ridge without nodal disease.
- **Technique:** VMAT, IMPT, and IMRT with half-beam block and matched AP low-neck field
- **SIM:** Supine, consider mouth opening with the tongue forward (oral tongue), tongue lateralizing (buccal/alveolar/retromolar trigone) or ramp (FOM) dental stent, and aquaplast mask. Wire scar. 3-mm bolus 2 cm around the scar (Fig. 25.3)
- **IGRT:** Daily kV with weekly CBCT or daily CBCT.
- **Planning directive (for conventional fractionation):**

PTV	>95% coverage
Spinal cord	Max < 45 Gy
Brainstem	Max < 54 Gy
Optic nerve	Max < 54 Gy
Mandible	Max less than prescription dose to CTV_{HD}
Total lung	V20 < 40%
Cochlea	Max < 35 Gy
Lens	Max < 5 Gy
Parotids	Mean < 26 Gy, lower for contralateral
Larynx	Mean < 30 Gy
Cervical esophagus	Mean < 30 Gy

Surgery

- WLE and partial, hemi-, or total glossectomy
  - Close margin is <5 mm.
  - Advanced resections may need flap/graft reconstruction.

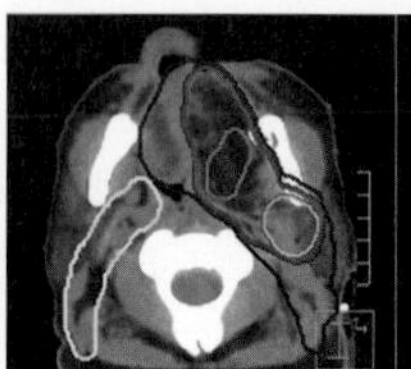
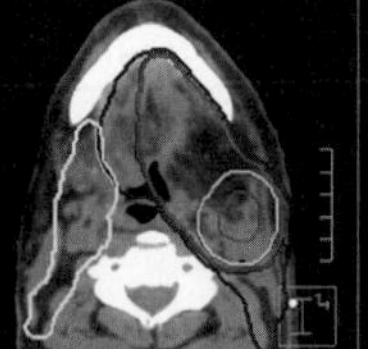
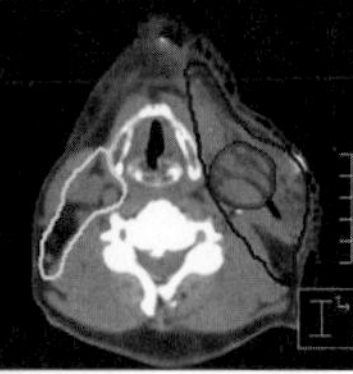

Figure 25.3 A 64-year-old with a resected pT2N2a (4.5 cm LN with ECE) SCC of the oral tongue reconstructed with a pectoralis flap treated with chemoRT. GTV (*green*), GTV-N (*forest green*), CTV63 (*aqua*), CTV60 (*red*), CTV57 (*blue*), and CTV54 (*yellow*) in 30 fractions. **See color insert.**

- Neck dissection for node positive or DOI > 4 mm. Consider neck dissection if is DOI 2-4 mm.
  - Rad neck dissection = I-V, CN XI, IJV, SCM
  - Mod rad neck dissection = I-V, preserve one of the following (CN XI, IJV, SCM)
  - Supraomohyoid = I-III
  - Lateral = II-IV
  - Selective neck dissection = LNs based on site

Chemotherapy

- **Concurrent:** High-dose cisplatin (100 mg/m^2), weekly cisplatin (40 mg/m^2), weekly carboplatin.
- **Induction:** TPF (docetaxel/cisplatin/5-FU); should not be done off protocol

Side Effect Management

- Nausea/vomiting: First-line Zofran (4-8 mg q8h prn) → second-line Compazine (5-10 mg q6h prn) → ABH (lorazepam 0.34 mg, diphenhydramine 25 mg, and haloperidol 1.5 mg) 1 capsule q6h
- Anxiety: Aquaplast mask can cause anxiety; lorazepam 1 mg 30 minutes to 1 hour before simulation or treatment
- Oral infection: Candidiasis; if superficial—nystatin 500000 units tid; if significant—diflucan 100 mg tablet once daily. Bacterial superinfection: tongue VERY red, send to dental for oral cultures.
- Pain: Hydrocodone/acetaminophen (7.5/325) mg q6h prn and hydromorphone 2 mg q3-6h prn (can increase frequency). If refractory, fentanyl 12.5-25 mcg transdermal patch q72h with prn breakthrough narcotics. If pain is recalcitrant to the above, consider a pain management specialist.
- Skin: Dermatitis: Routine moisturizer use (ie, Aquaphor, coconut oil, Egyptian magic, NutriShield). Pruritus: Hypoallergenic soap and lotion and hydrocortisone 1% ointment. Moist desquamation: Mepilex dressing, Biafine cream. Crusting: consider Domeboro soaks. Infectious dermatitis: Most likely MSSA, can be treated with Bactroban 2% ointment 3× daily for 7-10 days. If infection does not clear, consider consult to infectious disease specialists.
- Thick secretions: Baking soda rinses, diet ginger ale gargles, papaya juice gargles, Mucinex, Robitussin, portable suction device. Scopolamine patches and Hycodan can be tried for refractory cases.
- Xerostomia: Acupuncture and Biotene spray; encourage hydration

Follow-up

- History/physical exam and CT neck: Every 3 months for 1 year → every 4 months for the 2nd year → every 6 months for the 3rd year → yearly to 5 years
  Assess compliance with fluoride trays and neck range of motion/lymphedema exercises.

Notable Trials

Adjuvant chemoRT vs RT

- RTOG 95-01 (*Cooper et al. NEJM* 2004; *Cooper et al. IJROBP* 2012)—Phase III randomized study enrolling 459 patients with oral cavity, oropharynx, larynx, and hypopharynx cancer after complete resection. Patients must have had the presence of high-risk features (two or more positive lymph nodes, ECE, or SM+). Patients were randomized to RT alone vs RT with concurrent cisplatin (100 mg/m^2 given every 3 weeks). RT 60/30 plus optional boost to 66/33 high-risk areas. At initial report, DFS was significantly longer with concurrent chemotherapy (HR = 0.78, *P* = .04). At updated follow-up, 10-year DFS was not significantly different (19.1% vs 20.1%).

- EORTC 22931 (*Bernier NEJM* 2004)—Phase II randomized study enrolling 334 patients with oral cavity, oropharynx, hypopharynx, or larynx cancer after complete resection. Patients must have been high risk by being in one of the following risk groups: T3-4 any N with negative margins, T1-2 N2-3, T1-2 N0-1 with high-risk features (ECE, SM+, PNI, LVI), or oral cavity/oropharynx with LN+ at level IV or V. Patients were randomized to adjuvant RT alone vs RT + concurrent cisplatin (100 mg/m^2 given every 3 weeks). RT dose 54/27 + boost to 66 Gy high-risk areas. At first analysis, combination chemoradiation was associated with improved PFS (HR = 0.75, *P* = .04) and OS (HR = 0.7, *P* = .02).
- EORTC 22931/RTOG 95-01 (*Bernier et al. Head Neck* 2005): Combined analysis showed ECE or SM+ had an overall survival benefit with treatment utilizing RT and concurrent cisplatin.

OROPHARYNX

JAY PAUL REDDY • ADAM SETH GARDEN

Background

- **Incidence/prevalence:** Approximately 12 000 cases annually in the United States
- **Outcomes:** 5-Year survival across all stages estimated at ~80% for HPV-positive and 50% for HPV-negative
- **Demographics:** Current incidence in men is greater than women, 3:1 for HPV-negative and 8:1 for HPV-positive.
- **Risk factors:** Historically linked with tobacco and alcohol abuse, but now dramatic rise in HPV-associated OPC. Increased by 225% from 1988 to 2004 (SEER data)

Tumor Biology and Characteristics

- **Pathology:** Majority are squamous cell carcinomas (>95%). Majority of cases are HPV positive, which are associated with better prognosis. p16/HPV testing should be performed for all OPC. Common serotypes are 16, 18, 31, and 33.
- **Symptoms:** The most common presentation in HPV-associated OPC is enlarging, painless neck mass. Otalgia, dysphagia, or odynophagia is possible. HPV-associated OPC tends to present with smaller primary disease and advanced nodal, often cystic, disease.

Anatomy

- Sites: Base of the tongue, tonsil (subsites: anterior and posterior tonsillar pillars and tonsillar fossa), soft palate, and posterior/lateral pharyngeal wall
- Borders: Circumvallate papillae (anterior), pharyngeal wall (posterior), tonsillar fossa (lateral), soft palate (superior), vallecula (inferior)
- Lymph node drainage: 80%-90% of patients are cN+:
  - The tonsil primarily drains to ipsilateral level IIA.
  - BOT drains to levels II and III bilaterally.
  - Bilateral RP and levels II-IV should be covered in all cases.
  - See **Oral Cavity** chapter for neck LN description (Fig. 26.1).

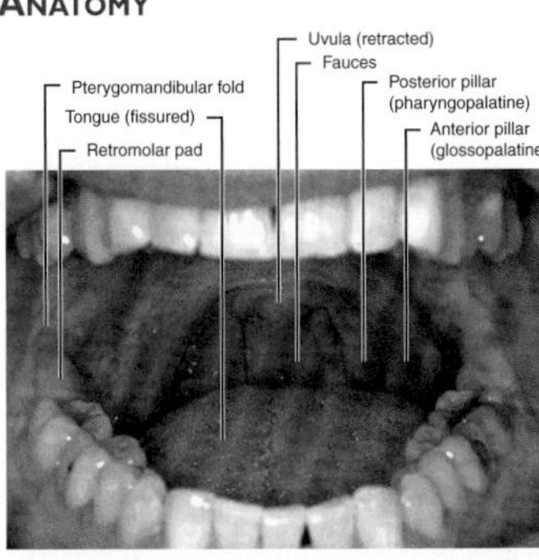

Figure 26.1 Sites of the oropharynx.

WORKUP

- **History and physical:** Assess presenting symptoms including oral function, cranial nerve deficits, speech quality, otalgia, and trismus. Direct palpation and visualization of tumor and adjacent subsites with nasolaryngoscope and/or mirror exam to assess disease spread
- **Labs:** CBC, CMP
- **Procedures/biopsy:** Biopsy of primary and FNA of enlarged LNs as clinically indicated
- **Imaging:** CT or MRI with contrast of the head and neck. Consider CT chest or chest x-ray. FDG-PET/CT recommended for Stage III/IV disease
- **Additional consultations:** Multidisciplinary evaluation with head and neck surgical oncology, radiation oncology, medical oncology, speech, nutrition, dental (fluoride/extractions)

OROPHARYNX STAGING (*AJCC 8TH EDITION*, 2018)

Staging now depends on HPV status.

HPV-associated (p16+) OPC

T Stage	
T1	Tumor ≤2 cm
T2	Tumor >2 cm but ≤4 cm
T3	Tumor >4 cm or extension to lingual surface of the epiglottis
T4	Tumor invades any of the following: larynx, deep/extrinsic muscles of the tongue, medial pterygoid, hard palate, mandible, or beyond

N Stage (Clinical)	
N0	No regional LN metastasis
N1	≥1 ipsilateral LN(s), ≤6 cm
N2	Contralateral or bilateral LN(s) ≤ 6 cm
N3	LN(s) >6 cm

N Stage (Pathologic)	
pN0	No regional LN metastasis
pN1	≤4 LN(s)
pN2	>4 LN(s)

Summative Stage (Clinical)

	N0	N1	N2	N3	M1
T1	I	I	II	III	IV
T2	I	I	II	III	
T3	II	II	II	III	
T4	III	III	III	III	

Summative Stage (Pathologic)

	N0	N1	N2	M1
T1	I	I	II	IV
T2	I	I	II	
T3	II	II	III	
T4	II	II	III	

Non–HPV-associated (p16–) OPC

T Stage	
T1	Tumor ≤2 cm
T2	Tumor >2 cm but ≤4 cm
T3	Tumor >4 cm or extension to lingual surface of the epiglottis
T4a	Tumor invades any of the following: larynx, deep/extrinsic muscles of tongue, medial pterygoid, hard palate, or mandible
T4b	Tumor invades lateral pterygoid, pterygoid plates, lateral nasopharynx, and skull base or encases carotid artery

N Stage	
N0	No regional LN metastasis
N1	1 ipsilateral LN, ≤3 cm, and ENE-negative
N2a	1 ipsilateral LN, >3 cm but ≤6 cm, and ENE-negative
N2b	>1 ipsilateral LN(s), ≤6 cm, and ENE-negative
N2c	Contralateral or bilateral LN(s) ≤6 cm, and ENE-negative
N3a	LN(s) >6 cm, and ENE-negative
N3b	Clinically overt ENE-positive LN

Summative Stage

	N0	N1	N2	N3	M1
T1	I	III	IVA	IVB	IVC
T2	II	III	IVA		
T3	III	III	IVA		
T4a	IVA	IVA	IVA		
T4b	IVB	IVB	IVB		

TREATMENT ALGORITHM

(T Stage has historically determined RT alone vs chemoRT)

Definitive RT	
T1/2	RT alone (consider ipsilateral RT,[a] concurrent cetuximab or accelerated fx for bulky T2)
T3/4	Concurrent chemoradiation with cisplatin
Bulky/low LN	Consider induction chemo[b] → RT or chemoRT
Postoperative RT	
+Margins or ECE	Adjuvant chemoRT
Other risk factors[c]	RT or consider chemoRT

[a]Criteria for ipsilateral RT: tonsil primary, <1 cm soft palate involvement, no BOT involvement, ipsilateral nodal disease. Risk of contralateral neck failure 0%-3%

[b]Given recent data from randomized trials, there is little evidence to support the use of induction chemotherapy.

[c]Risk factors include pT3/T4, N2/N3, PNI, level IV/V, and LVSI.

RADIATION TREATMENT TECHNIQUE

Definitive radiation therapy

- **Dose:**

	CTV_{HD}	CTV_{ID}	CTV_{ED}	Fx #
T1/2	66	60	54	30
Bulky T2 (Acc. fx)	70	63	57	33 or 35[a]
T3/4 (chemoRT)	70	63	57	33
PORT	60	57	54	30

[a]Finish in 6 weeks (DAHANCA, eg, 6 fx/wk).

- **Target:**
  - **General:** CTV_{HD} includes GTV + 8-mm margin, CTV_{ID} includes high-risk mucosal and nodal volumes, and CTV_{ED} includes uninvolved regions at risk for microscopic spread.
  - **Tonsil:** CTV_{HD} includes the entire tonsillar fossa from maxillary tuberosity to superior to hyoid. CTV_{ED} typically begins at pterygoid plates. Typically includes GP sulcus and parapharyngeal space
  - **BOT:** CTV_{HD} inferior from soft palate to vallecula (if involved) with coverage of the entire hyoid. Anterior extent typically includes posterior 2 cm of tongue.
  - **Nodal:** CTV_{ED} routinely covers RP nodes (from the jugular foramen to C2) and levels II-IV on uninvolved side of the neck. Cover ipsilateral Ib and V on involved side of the neck
- **Technique:** VMAT, IMRT with half-beam block and matched AP low-neck field, or IMPT in experienced centers.

- **SIM:** Supine, aquaplast mask covering the head and shoulders, mouth-opening, tongue-depressing stent (for BOT/soft palate), isocenter at or below the cricoid. Pull straps for shoulder retraction. If the patient had neck dissection, wire scars and place 3-mm bolus on top of wired scars. Patient should be reminded not to swallow during simulation as this distorts anatomy.

Post-op

- **Target/Dose: Region of resected gross disease:** 60 Gy in 2 Gy fractions (high dose) and 66 Gy in 2 Gy fractions for positive margins
  Operative bed: 57 Gy (intermediate dose)
  Nondissected at risk regions including nondissected at risk nodal levels: 54 Gy (low dose)
- **Technique:** IMRT or VMAT. Scanning beam proton therapy can be used in capable centers.
- **SIM:** See Oral Cavity section.

IGRT

- Daily kV imaging with weekly CBCT or daily CBCT

Planning directive

See **Oral Cavity** chapter.

Special circumstances

- **Indications for boosting stoma with post-op XRT:** (1) Emergency tracheostomy was performed, (2) subglottic extension of disease, and (3) anterior soft tissue extension.
- **Indications for neck dissection after definitive XRT or chemoRT:** Persistent neck disease.
- **Transoral robotic surgery (TORS):** Increasingly common minimally invasive surgical technique utilizing robot arms controlled remotely to remove lesions in the tonsil, BOT, and soft palate. Neck dissection may also be performed during the same procedure.
  - **PORT indications:** Positive margin, ECE, pT3/4, PNI, multiple nodes, N3, and LVI
  - However, the above factors do not necessarily account for the overall good prognosis of HPV+ patients. This area is evolving.
- **Ipsilateral treatment:** Consider for T1-2 tumors limited to the tonsillar fossa with N0-1 (N2b per AJCC 7) ipsilateral neck involvement.

Chemotherapy, side effect management, and follow-up

See **Larynx** chapter.

NOTABLE TRIALS

HPV status as a positive prognostic marker in oropharynx patients

- RTOG 0129 (*Ang et al. NEJM* 2010): Phase III randomized study of 743 patients with stage III/IV oral cavity, oropharynx, hypopharynx, or larynx cancer randomized to two arms: Arm 1, accelerated fractionation (72 Gy/42 fx in 6 weeks), vs Arm 2, standard fractionation (70 Gy/35 fx). Both arms were given with concurrent high-dose cisplatin. No difference in overall survival and toxicity between arms. Post hoc analysis of this trial found that among oropharynx patients, 3-year OS was 82.4% in HPV+ vs 57.1% in HPV–. RPA was used to risk-stratify patients (with 3-year OS as endpoint) into low (p16+ and <10-year PY, 94%), intermediate (p16+ and >10 PY, or p16– and <10 PY, 67%), and high (p16– and >10 PY, 42%) risk groups based on HPV status, pack-year smoking history, T stage, and N stage.

Accelerated fractionation

- RTOG 00-22 (*Eisbruch et al. IJROBP* 2010): Single-arm study assessing feasibility of modest acceleration in early-stage OPC (T1/2 N0/1) by treating to 66 Gy/30 fx. 2-Year LRF 9%. Acceptable toxicity, frequent grade ≥2 toxicities were salivary (67%), mucosa (24%), esophagus (19%), skin (12%), and osteoradionecrosis (6%).
- RTOG 90-03 (*Fu et al. IJROBP* 2000; *Beitler IJROBP* 2014): A randomized four-arm randomized clinical trial of 1113 stage III-IV OPC, oral cavity, hypopharynx, and larynx cancer. Arms were Arm 1, standard fx (70 Gy/35 fx); Arm 2, hyperfractionated (81.6 Gy/68 fx [1.2 Gy bid]); Arm 3, accelerated fractionation with split course (67.2 Gy/42 fx [1.6 Gy bid]) with a 2-week break; and Arm 4, accelerated fx with concomitant boost (54 Gy/30 fx + 18 Gy/12 fx bid boost to a total of 72 Gy).

All arms did not receive concurrent chemotherapy. 2-Year LRC: Arm 1 46% vs Arm 2 54% vs Arm 3 47% vs Arm 4 54%. At 5 years, only the comparison of Arm 1 vs Arm 2 was significant for locoregional control (HR = 0.79, *P* = .05) and OS (HR = 0.81, *P* = .05).

- DAHANCA 6/7 (*Overgaard et al. Lancet* 2003): Two randomized trials enrolling 1485 patients. DAHANCA 6 randomized patients with glottic tumors and DAHANCA 7 randomized patients with OC and pharynx cancer. In both studies, patients were randomized to either 5 or 6 fx/wk. All patients received concurrent nimorazole. Six fractions a week improved local control (5-year LRC: 60% vs 70%, *P* = .0005) and disease-specific survival (5-year DSS: 73% vs 66%, *P* = .01). No OS difference

Concurrent cetuximab

- Bonner trial (*Bonner et al., Lancet Oncology* 2010; *Bonner et al., NEJM* 2006): A randomized two-arm study enrolling 424 patients with stage III/IV OPC, hypopharynx, or larynx cancer. Patients were randomized to radiation + cetuximab vs radiation alone. Patients were randomized to RT + cetuximab exhibit significantly better OS (5 years: 46% vs 36%, *P* = .018). Benefit associated with development of grade 2 cetuximab-associated rash (HR = 0.49, *P* = .002)

SINONASAL AND NASOPHARYNX

SHANE MESKO • ADAM SETH GARDEN

BACKGROUND

Nasopharynx

- **Incidence/prevalence:** 86 000 cases, with 55 000 deaths annually worldwide. Marked geographic variation: incidence 0.5-2 per 100 000 in the United States and Western Europe vs endemic regions at 25 per 100 000. Estimated 3000-4000 cases per year in the United States annually
- **Outcomes:** 5-Year survival estimated 38%-72% (Stage I-IV) (SEER data)
- **Demographics:** Median age 55, endemic to Southern China, common in N. Africa and Middle East
- **Risk factors:** Endemic regions: Male sex (RR 2-3), EBV, and preserved and smoked foods; nonendemic: smoking and alcohol

Sinonasal

- **Incidence/prevalence:** Incidence 0.56 per 100 000, estimated 2000 cases per year in the US annually, nasal cavity and maxillary sinus most common
- **Outcomes:** 5-Year survival estimated 35%-63% (Stage I-IV) (SEER data)
- **Demographics:** Median age 50-60; higher frequency of cases in Japan and South Africa
- **Risk factors:** Male sex, environmental/occupational exposures (eg, wood dusts, glues, adhesives), smoking, HPV, retinoblastoma

TUMOR BIOLOGY AND CHARACTERISTICS

Nasopharynx

- **Pathology:**
  - Keratinizing (WHO I): most common sporadic form (25% US, 2% endemic)
  - Nonkeratinizing differentiated (WHO II): (12% US, 3% endemic)
  - Nonkeratinizing undifferentiated (WHO III): commonly associated with endemic disease and has favorable prognosis (63% US, 95% endemic)

Sinonasal

- **Pathology:** Squamous cell (36%-58%) is most common, but adenocarcinoma (12%-15%), melanoma (6%-8%), adenoid cystic carcinoma (6%), olfactory neuroblastoma (3%-6%), and sinonasal undifferentiated carcinoma (SNUC) (3%) are also seen.

Anatomy

Nasopharynx

- Anterior border: Nasal cavity posterior to choana
- Lateral border: Torus tubarius, pharyngeal recess (fossa of Rosenmüller)
- Superior border: Clivus
- Posterior border: Clivus/occipital bone, C1/C2 vertebral bodies
- Inferior border: soft palate
- Lymph node drainage:
  - RP nodes
  - Jugular chain (levels II-IV)
  - Spinal accessory nodes (level V)
  - See **Oral Cavity** chapter for neck LN description.
- Local invasion:
  - Lateral tumors can occlude the eustachian tube (causing hearing loss). Tumors that extend beyond the nasopharynx laterally can invade the masticator space.
  - Inferior extension can invade the oropharynx.
  - Anterior extension can invade the nasal cavity.
  - Superior extension can invade the base of the skull (clivus). Further extension can invade the sphenoid sinus. Intracranial extension can occur through either the clivus or adjacent foramina. Foramen lacerum provides easy access to intracranial invasion. Foramen ovale and rotundum can lead to V3 and V2 deficits and are a conduit to the cavernous sinus where the abducens nerve (VI) and less commonly III can be involved. Very advanced cases can either push or invade the temporal lobe.
  - Posterior extension can invade the prevertebral muscles and eventually adjacent bones (inferior clivus, C1). Further extension through the bone can impinge on the brainstem, or the adjacent posterior cranial nerves (IX-XII) that emerge from the lateral aspects of the brainstem.

Sinonasal

- Includes the nasal cavity and the paranasal sinuses (maxillary, ethmoid, sphenoid, and frontal)
- The nasal cavity:
  - Anterior border: Limen nasi and nasal vestibule
  - Posterior border: Choana
  - Lateral border: Maxillary sinus
  - Inferior border: Hard palate of the oral cavity
  - Superior: Frontal sinus and cribriform plate
  - The borders of the sinuses are complex. The main point is that they all abut the orbit and also are in close proximity to the brain.
- Lymph node drainage:
  - Nasal vestibule: Submandibular, facial, preauricular, can be bilateral
  - Nasal cavity and ethmoid sinuses: Retropharyngeal and levels I-II
  - Maxillary sinus drains to levels I-II; tumors with premaxillary space or skin involvement can drain to buccal and facial nodes.
  - See **Oral Cavity** chapter for neck LN description.
- Local invasion:
  - Orbital structures, bones of the hard palate, nasal meatus, cribriform plate, dura, brain, clivus, and middle cranial fossa

Workup

- **History and physical:** Assess presenting symptoms including cranial nerve dysfunction. Direct visualization of tumor and adjacent subsites with nasolaryngoscope.
- **Labs:** CBC and CMP; consider EBV virus titers pre and post therapy.
- **Procedures/biopsy:** Biopsy of primary and FNA of enlarged LNs as clinically indicated
- **Imaging:** CT with contrast of the head and neck/skull base to evaluate bony invasion and LN involvement. MRI with contrast of the head and neck/skull base to evaluate soft tissue component and cranial nerve involvement. Consider CT of the chest. FDG-PET/CT is recommended for Stage III/IV disease.
- **Additional consultations:** Multidisciplinary evaluation with head and neck surgical oncology, radiation oncology, medical oncology, nutrition, and dental (fluoride/extractions). Consider ophthalmologic and endocrine evaluation.

Nasopharyngeal Cancer Staging *(AJCC 8th Edition)*

T Stage		N Stage	
T0	No tumor identified, but EBV-positive cervical node(s)	N1	Unilateral cervical lymph node, or unilateral/ bilateral retropharyngeal node(s), <6 cm in greatest dimension and above the caudal border of the cricoid cartilage
Tis	Carcinoma in situ	N2	Bilateral cervical lymph nodes, <6 cm in greatest dimension and above the caudal border of the cricoid cartilage
T1	Confined to nasopharynx or extends to oropharynx and/or nasal cavity without parapharyngeal involvement	N3	Unilateral or bilateral cervical lymph nodes, larger than 6 cm in the greatest dimension and above the caudal border of the cricoid cartilage
T2	Extends to parapharyngeal space and/or adjacent soft tissue (eg, medial/lateral pterygoid, prevertebral muscles)	**M Stage**	
		M0	No distant metastasis
		M1	Distant metastasis
T3	Infiltrates bony structures of skull base, cervical vertebra, pterygoid structures, and/or paranasal sinuses		
T4	Intracranial extension; involvement of cranial nerves, hypopharynx, orbit, and parotid gland and/or soft tissue involvement beyond the lateral surface of lateral pterygoid		

Summative Stage

	N0	N1	N2	N3	M1
T1	I	II	III	IVA	IVB
T2	II	II	III	IVA	IVB
T3	III	III	III	IVA	IVB
T4	IVA	IVA	IVA	IVA	IVB

Treatment Algorithm

Nasopharynx

Stage I	Definitive RT alone
Stage II-IVa	Concurrent chemoRT ± adjuvant chemotherapy *OR* induction chemotherapy followed by concurrent chemoRT
Stage IVb	Chemotherapy alone or concurrent chemoRT

Sinonasal Cancer Staging *(AJCC 8th Edition)*

Maxillary Sinus T Stage		Nasal Cavity and Ethmoid Sinus	
Tis	Carcinoma in situ		
T1	Tumor limited to maxillary sinus mucosa without erosion or destruction of the bone; except extension to posterior wall of maxillary sinus and pterygoid plates	T1	Tumor restricted to any one subsite, with or without bony invasion
T2	Tumor with bony erosion or destruction, including extension into the hard palate or middle nasal meatus	T2	Tumor invading two subsites in a single region or extending to involve adjacent region within the nasoethmoidal complex, with or without bony invasion
T3	Tumor invades any of the following: The bone of the posterior wall of maxillary sinus, subcutaneous tissues, floor or medial wall of the orbit, pterygoid fossa, and ethmoid sinuses	T3	Tumor extends to invade the medial wall or floor of the orbit, maxillary sinus, palate, or cribriform plate

T4a	Moderately advanced local disease: Tumor invades anterior orbital contents, skin of the cheek, pterygoid plates, infratemporal fossa, cribriform plate, sphenoid or frontal sinuses
T4b	Very advanced local disease: Tumor invades any of the following: orbital apex, dura, brain, middle cranial fossa, cranial nerves other than maxillary division of trigeminal verve (V2), nasopharynx, or clivus
N Stage *(All Sinonasal)*	
N0	No regional lymph node metastasis
N1	Metastasis in a single ipsilateral lymph node, 3 cm or smaller in greatest dimension and extranodal extension negative (ENE–)
N2a	Metastasis in a single ipsilateral node larger than 3 cm but not larger than 6 cm in greatest dimension and ENE(–)
N2b	Metastasis in multiple ipsilateral nodes, none larger than 6 cm in greatest dimension and ENE(–)
N2c	Metastasis in bilateral or contralateral lymph nodes, none larger than 6 cm in greatest dimension and ENE(–)
N3a	Metastasis in a lymph node larger than 6 cm in greatest dimension and ENE(–)
N3b	Metastasis in any node(s) with ENE
M Stage *(All Sinonasal)*	
M0	No distance metastasis
M1	Distant metastasis
Summative Stage *(All Sinonasal)*	

	N0	N1	N2	N3	M1
T1	I	III	IVA	IVB	IVC
T2	II	III	IVA	IVB	IVC
T3	III	III	IVA	IVB	IVC
T4a	IVA	IVA	IVA	IVB	IVC
T4b	IVB	IVB	IVB	IVB	IVC

Treatment Algorithm

Sinonasal: ethmoid sinus and nasal cavity

T1-2	Definitive RT alone or surgical resection followed by (RT ± chemo[a]) or (observation[b])
T3-4a	ChemoRT or surgical resection followed by RT ± chemo
T4b	ChemoRT or RT alone

[a]Indications for post-op chemoRT: positive margins, intracranial extension, ENE
[b]For select T1N0 tumors centrally located, low grade, and with negative margins

Consider systemic therapy for all patients with sinonasal undifferentiated carcinoma (SNUC), small cell neuroendocrine carcinoma (SNEC), or small cell tumors.

Sinonasal-Maxillary Sinus

T1-2, N0	Surgical resection followed by (RT ± chemo[a]) or (observation) or (reresection[b])
T3-4a	Surgical resection[c] followed by RT ± chemo
T4b, any N	ChemoRT or RT alone

[a]Indications for post-op RT: PNI, positive margins, intracranial extension, adenoid cystic histology, ENE, T3/4 disease
[b]For positive margins, if feasible. Follow with RT ± chemo
[c]Add neck dissection for any node-positive disease

Consider systemic therapy for all patients with sinonasal undifferentiated carcinoma (SNUC), small cell neuroendocrine carcinoma (SNEC), or small cell tumors.

RADIATION TREATMENT TECHNIQUE

- **Dose/target:**
  - **Nasopharynx (Definitive, Fig. 27.1)**
  - *Gross disease (CTV_{HD}):*
    - *Dose:* 70 Gy in 33-35 fractions, daily
    - *Target:* GTV (tumor + involved nodes) + 5-8 mm margin (margins may be tighter if GTV abuts critical neural structures)
  - *Intermediate risk (CTV_{ID}):*
    - *Dose:* 59.4-63 Gy in 33-35 fractions
    - *Target nasopharynx*: Entire nasopharynx, RP nodes, clivus (anterior 1/2 if uninvolved, entire clivus if involved), pterygoid fossa, parapharyngeal space, sphenoid sinus (inferior 1/2 if uninvolved, entire if involved or cavernous sinus disease), posterior 1/3 of maxillary sinus and nasal cavity, cavernous sinus in locally advanced disease, and skull base (rotundum, ovale, lacerum).
    - *Target neck (excludes neck covered by CTV_{HD})*: In the positive neck, cover the remaining neck level in the axial plane not covered in CTV_{HD} and 2 cm cranially and caudally.
  - *Low risk (CTV_{ED}):*
    - *Dose*: 54-56 Gy in 33-35 fractions
    - *Target (excludes neck covered by CTV_{HD} and CTV_{ID})*: In the N0, neck levels II-IV should be covered. In the involved neck levels Ib-V; the bilateral RPs should be covered.
  - *PTV expansion*: 3-5 mm depending on the setup and IGRT
  - **Sinonasal**

Definitive:

High-risk or gross disease (CTV_{HD}):
- *Dose:* 66-70 Gy in 33-35 fractions
- *Target:* GTV (gross tumor + involved LNs) + 5-8 mm margin unless constrained by critical normal tissues

Intermediate risk (CTV_{ID}):
- *Dose:* 60 Gy in 30 fractions, 63 Gy in 33-35 fractions
- *Target:* entire disease subsite, include nerves to skull base if PNI or adenoid cystic histology, ipsilateral involved nodal levels if N+, cribriform plate if esthesioneuroblastoma or ethmoid sinus involvement

Low risk (CTV_{ED}):
- *Dose:* 54 Gy in 30 fractions, 56 Gy in 33-35 fractions
- *Target:* Uninvolved neck nodal levels (see Anatomy section)

Post-op:

High risk (CTV_{HD}):
- *Dose:* 60 Gy in 30 fractions to preoperative tumor bed with 1-2 cm margins
- *Consider 3-6 Gy boost target:* Positive margins and gross nodal disease + 5-8 mm margin

Intermediate risk (CTV_{ID}):
- *Dose:* 57 Gy in 30 fractions
- *Target:* operative bed including primary and LN operative areas. Include the entire flap if utilized

Low risk (CTV_{ED}):
- *Dose:* 54 Gy in 30 fractions
- *Target:* Uninvolved neck nodal levels (if at risk, dependent on site and histology); cover nerve pathways to base of skull (or beyond) dependent on histology and extent of PNI

  - *PTV expansion:* 3-5 mm depending on setup
- **Technique:** IMRT with 6-MV photons is preferred; option to consider matched low-neck field of 40 Gy in 20 fractions with larynx block, followed by 10 Gy in 5 fractions with full midline block, however IMRT/VMAT plans with larynx avoidance may achieve excellent dosimetric results. Start post-op cases within 6 weeks of surgery.
- **SIM:** Supine, thermoplastic mask, shoulder pull straps. Mouth-opening tongue-depressing stent (with space to fill cavities in maxillary sinus cancers, may optimize position to displace tissues that don't need treatment, posterior head cradle, isocenter at arytenoids). Consider adding MR simulation, and/or fuse previous MRI imaging.
- **IGRT:** Daily kV imaging, cone beam CT
- **Planning directive (for conventional fractionation)**

  Brainstem: General goal <45 Gy; proximity of targets may require higher dose and constraint can be set at 54 Gy
  Spinal cord: Max 45 Gy
  Parotids: Mean < 26 Gy
  Mandible: Less than prescribed dose to CTV_{HD}
  Brachial plexus: <66 Gy if treating adjacent disease; otherwise max < 60 max
  Larynx: Mean < 30 Gy or ALARA
  Esophagus: Mean < 30 Gy
  Oral cavity: <40 Gy
  Optic nerves/chiasm: <54 Gy

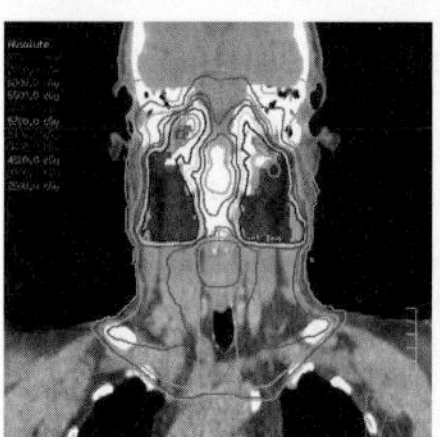
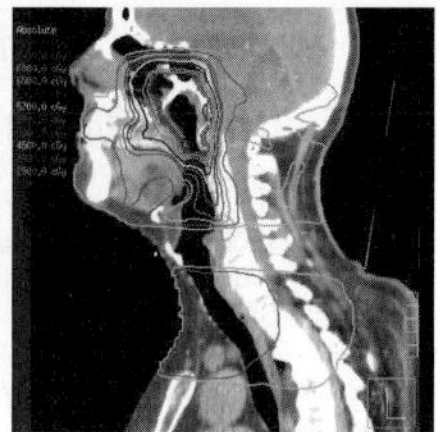

Figure 27.1 Definitive chemoradiation planning showing treatment IMRT treating to 70 Gy to CTV_{HD} and 59.4 Gy to CTV_{ID}. A 3D conformal field is treating 45 Gy to the low neck.

Chemotherapy

Nasopharynx

- **Concurrent:** Cisplatin 30-40 mg/m^2 weekly or 100 mg/m^2 on days 1, 22, and 43 (cumulative cisplatin dose goal 200 mg/m^2); carboplatin can be used in patients who cannot tolerate or have contraindication to cisplatin.
- **Adjuvant:** Cisplatin 80 mg/m^2 weekly + 5-FU 1000 mg/m^2 q4wk × three cycles
- **Induction:** No defined standard of care; possible regimens include
  Docetaxel + cisplatin ± 5-FU
  Cisplatin + 5-FU
  Cisplatin + epirubicin + paclitaxel

Sinonasal

- **Concurrent:** Cisplatin 30-40 mg/m^2 weekly or 100 mg/m^2 on days 1, 22, and 43 (cumulative cisplatin dose goal 200 mg/m^2); carboplatin can be used in patients who cannot tolerate or have contraindication to cisplatin. Can consider cetuximab

Side Effect Management

See **Oral Cavity** chapter.

Follow-up

- First posttreatment follow-up at 8 weeks with MRI and/or CT imaging.
- Consider PET/CT at 12 weeks if suspicion for persistent disease or lack of response.
- Consider neck dissection for PET-positive lymph nodes with >1 cm of residual primary disease.
- History/physical with nasopharyngoscopy: Every 3-4 months for years 1-3 → every 6 months for years 4-5
- Thyroid function tests every 6 months
- Can consider EBV titer monitoring if initially positive pretreatment for nasopharyngeal
- Consider longer-term follow-up for esthesioneuroblastoma as recurrence can occur >15 years after primary treatment.

Notable Trials

Nasopharynx

Benefit of chemoRT over RT alone

- Intergroup-0099 (*Al-Sarraf et al. JCO* 1998): Phase III randomized study of 147 stage III-IV nasopharyngeal cancer patients randomized to definitive RT vs concurrent cisplatin/RT+ adjuvant cisplatin. The total dose was 70 Gy in 1.8-2 Gy/fx, 66 Gy for involved nodes, and 50 Gy for elective nodes. 3-Year PFS of 24% vs 69% (P < .001) and OS of 46% vs 78% (P = .005) in favor of chemoRT
- Singapore phase II (*Wee et al. JCO* 2005): Phase II randomized study randomizing 221 stage III-IV nasopharyngeal cancer patients to definitive RT vs concurrent cisplatin/RT+ adjuvant cisplatin. Found improved 2-year OS (78% vs 85%; HR = 0.51, P = .0061) and DFS and DM favoring chemoRT arm. Confirmed the results of Intergroup-0099 in an endemic (Asian) population
- MAC-NPC meta-analysis (*Blanchard et al. Lancet Oncol* 2015): 19 trials and 4806 patients. Found improved overall survival and progression-free survival with addition of

concomitant chemotherapy over RT alone—10-year OS benefit of 9.9% and 10-year PFS benefit of 9.5%. There was no OS benefit observed for induction or adjuvant chemotherapy alone.

Benefit of IMRT for nasopharynx cancer

- *Kam et al. JCO* 2007: Randomized 60 patients with T1-2bN0-1M0 nasopharynx cancer to either IMRT or 2DCRT. Patients were treated to 66 Gy in 33 fractions to gross tumor and 60-54 Gy to the node-negative regions. At 1 year after RT, patients in the IMRT arm had lower rates of xerostomia (39.3% vs 82.1%, $P = .001$).
- *Pow et al. IJROBP* 2006: Randomized 51 patients with T2N0-1M0 nasopharynx cancer to IMRT vs conventional RT. IMRT significantly improves quality of life ($P < .001$). Most significant improvement in xerostomia-related symptoms at 12 months for IMRT group.

Induction chemotherapy

- GORTEC NPC 2006 (*Huang et al. Eur J Cancer* 2015): 10-Year outcome of 408 patients with locoregionally advanced nasopharyngeal carcinoma randomized to induction chemotherapy (carboplatin + floxuridine) followed by either chemoRT (carboplatin) or RT alone. No significant differences in OS (induction chemo 50.4% vs no induction chemo 48.8%, $P = .71$), locoregional failure (induction chemo 79% vs no induction chemo 82.5%, $P = .41$), or distant failure-free survival (induction chemo 67.7% vs no induction chemo 66.1%, $P = .90$).
- *Sun et al. Lancet Oncol* 2016: Phase III multicenter trial randomized 480 patients with locally advanced nasopharyngeal cancer to induction TPF (cisplatin, fluorouracil, docetaxel) + chemoRT (cisplatin) vs chemoRT alone. 3-Year failure-free survival favored the induction group (80% vs 72% $P = .034$).
- *Cao et al. Eur J Cancer* 2017: Phase III multicenter trial randomized 476 patients with locoregionally advanced NPC to induction (cisplatin, fluorouracil) + chemoRT (cisplatin) vs chemoRT alone. 3-Year DFS (82% vs 74%, $P = .028$) and DMFS (86% vs 82%, $P = .056$) favored the induction arm. However, OS (88.2% vs 88.5%, $P = .815$) and locoregional relapse-free survival (94.3% vs 90.8%, $P = .430$) showed no difference. There was a significant ($P < .001$) increase in grade 3-4 toxicity in the induction arm.

Adjuvant chemotherapy

- *Chen et al. Eur J Cancer* 2017: Long-term update of phase III multicenter randomized trial with 251 patients with locoregional advanced NPC. Patients were randomized to chemoRT (cisplatin) vs chemoRT + adjuvant chemo (cisplatin, fluorouracil). There was no significant difference in 5-year failure-free survival (adjuvant 75% vs no adjuvant 71%, $P = .45$) or late grade 3 or 4 toxicity (adjuvant 27% vs no adjuvant 21%, $P = .14$).

LARYNX AND HYPOPHARYNX

COURTNEY POLLARD III • JACK PHAN

Background

- **Incidence/prevalence:** Approximately 13 400 laryngeal cancers and ~2500 hypopharyngeal cancers annually in the United States
- **Outcomes:** 5-Year survival across all stages estimated at ~60% for larynx and 30% for hypopharynx (SEER data).
- **Demographics:** Majority of patients are male and associated with advanced age (>60).
- **Risk factors:** Larynx cancer—smoking is associated with the vast majority of cases; in nonsmokers, GERD is associated with larynx cancer. Hypopharyngeal cancer—in addition to smoking, alcohol abuse, chronic voice strain, vitamin C and iron deficiencies (Plummer-Vinson syndrome), and prior head and neck malignancy particularly if the patient received prior head and neck radiation.

Tumor Biology and Characteristics

- **Pathology:** Majority are squamous cell carcinomas (>95%). Minority of cases are HPV positive but clinical implications are not established. p16/HPV testing should be considered for all supraglottic cancers and hypopharyngeal cancers, particularly those arising in nonsmokers. In larynx cancer, invasive cancer can progress from leukoplakia or erythroplakia (premalignant lesions).

- **Symptoms:** Hoarseness, sore throat, dysphagia, odynophagia, globus sensation in the throat, referred otalgia from branch of cranial nerve X (Arnold nerve), and asymptomatic neck mass

Anatomy

- The larynx consists of three sites each with multiple subsites (Fig. 28.1):
  - *Supraglottis* (suprahyoid and infrahyoid epiglottis, aryepiglottic folds, arytenoids, false vocal folds, and ventricles)
  - *Glottis* (true vocal cords including anterior/posterior commissures, 5 mm inferior to free margin of true cords)
  - *Subglottis* (lower boundary of the glottis to the inferior aspect of the cricoid cartilage). Site incidence: Glottis (65%-70%) > supraglottis (25%-30%) > subglottis (1%)
- The hypopharynx consists of the pyriform sinuses, the postcricoid area, and the posterior pharyngeal wall (3 Ps). Site incidence: Pyriform sinus (75%) > posterior pharyngeal wall (20%) > postcricoid (5%) (Fig. 28.1)

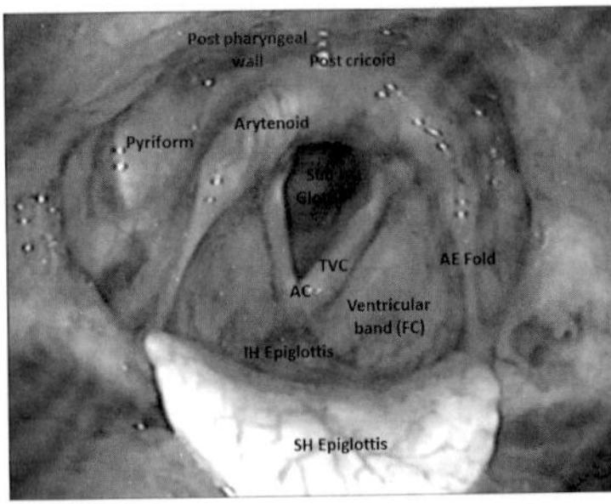

Figure 28.1 Larynx and hypopharynx structures. AC, anterior commissure; AE, aryepiglottic; FC, false cord; IH, infrahyoid; PC, posterior commissure; SH, suprahyoid; TVC, true vocal cord. (Adapted from http://www.laryngologysurgery.com/examinationendoscopy.html. Reprinted by permission from Dr. Rahmat Omar.)

Workup

- **History and physical:** Assess presenting symptoms; assess including voice quality, swallow function, breathing, and ability to protect airway. Visualization of tumor and adjacent subsites with nasolaryngoscope and/or mirror exam to assess disease spread. Consider videostroboscopy. Palpate the thyroid to evaluate for pain as it may be indicative of cartilage invasion.
- **Labs:** CBC, CMP
- **Procedures/biopsy:** Biopsy of primary and FNA of enlarged LNs as clinically indicated
- **Imaging:** MRI with contrast or CT with contrast and thin-angled cuts through the larynx. Evaluation of cartilage invasion and infiltration of adjacent subsites. Consider CT of the chest. FDG-PET/CT recommended for stage III/IV disease
- **Additional consultations:** Multidisciplinary evaluation with head and neck surgical oncology, radiation oncology, medical oncology, speech/swallow (swallowing exercise regime), nutrition, and dental (fluoride/extractions)

Larynx and Hypopharynx Staging (*AJCC 8th Edition*, 2018)

The different sites of the larynx have different T staging.

Glottis

T Stage	
Tis	Carcinoma in situ
T1	Tumor limited to the true vocal cords with normal mobility (T1a, 1 vocal cord; T1b, both vocal cords)
T2	Tumor extends to the supra- or subglottis, and/or with impaired vocal cord mobility
T3	Tumor is limited to the larynx with vocal cord fixation and/or invasion into the paraglottic space and/or partial invasion of the inner cortex of thyroid cartilage

T4a	Tumor invades through the outer cortex of the thyroid cartilage and/or invades tissues beyond the larynx (trachea, soft tissues of neck, deep extrinsic muscles of tongue, strap muscles, thyroid, esophagus)
T4b	Tumor invades prevertebral space, encases carotid artery, or invades mediastinal structures

Supraglottis

T Stage	
Tis	Same as glottis, see above
T1	Tumor limited to 1 subsite of the supraglottis, with normal vocal cord mobility
T2	Tumor invades mucosa of more than 1 adjacent subsite of the supraglottis or glottis or regions outside the supraglottis (mucosa of BOT, medial wall of piriform sinus, vallecula), no fixation of the larynx
T3	Tumor limited to the larynx, with vocal cord fixation; and/or invasion of the postcricoid area, pre-epiglottic space, and paraglottic space; and partial invasion through the inner cortex of thyroid cartilage
T4a	Same as glottis, see above
T4b	Same as glottis, see above

Subglottis

T Stage	
Tis	Same as glottis, see above
T1	Tumor limited to the subglottis
T2	Tumor extends to the vocal cord(s) with normal or impaired mobility
T3	Tumor limited to the larynx, with vocal cord fixation and/or paraglottic space extension, and/or invasion of inner cortex of thyroid cartilage
T4a	Tumor invades outer portion of the thyroid or any portion of cricoid cartilage and/or invades tissues beyond the larynx (trachea, soft tissues of the neck, deep extrinsic muscles of the tongue, strap muscles, thyroid, esophagus)
T4b	Same as glottis, see above

Hypopharynx

T Stage	
Tis	Same as glottis, see above
T1	Tumor limited to 1 subsite and/or ≤2 cm
T2	Tumor involves >1 subsite and/or an adjacent site or measures >2 cm but not more than 4 cm, no fixation of the hemilarynx
T3	Tumor >4 cm and/or with fixation of the hemilarynx or extension to the esophagus
T4a	Tumor invades thyroid or cricoid cartilage, hyoid bone, thyroid gland, or central compartment soft tissue (prelaryngeal strap muscles, subcutaneous fat)
T4b	Same as glottis, see above

Larynx/Hypopharynx NM Staging

N Stage	
N1	Single, ipsi, ≤3 cm, ENE(−)
N2a	Single, ipsi, >3 cm, ≤6 cm, ENE(−)
N2b	Multiple, ipsi, ≤6 cm, ENE(−)
N2c	Bilateral or contralateral, ≤6 cm, ENE(−)
N3a	>6 cm, ENE(−)
N3b	Any clinically overt ENE(+)
M Stage	
M0	No distant metastasis
M1	≥1 site of distant metastasis

Larynx/Hypopharynx Group Staging

Summative Stage	N0	N1	N2a	N2b	N2c	N3	M1
T1	I	III	IVA	IVA	IVA	IVB	IVC
T2	II	III	IVA	IVA	IVA	IVB	IVC
T3	III	III	IVA	IVA	IVA	IVB	IVC
T4a	IVA	IVA	IVA	IVA	IVA	IVB	IVC
T4b	IVB	IVB	IVB	IVB	IVB	IVB	IVC

Note: TisN0M0 is group stage 0.

Larynx Treatment Algorithm

Stage I-II	Definitive XRT, laser cordectomy, partial laryngectomy
Stage III-V	Total laryngectomy w/ thyroidectomy → adv XRT or CRT for + margin or + ENE; definitive CRT alone; or definitive XRT (altered fractionation). It is important that definitive CRT or XRT is not offered to patients who have impaired larynx function.

Hypopharynx Treatment Algorithm

T1-2	Partial pharyngectomy or definitive XRT. Add concurrent chemotherapy if bulky T2.
T3 and/or N+	• Good glottis function (eg, no dysphagia or other symptoms): Induction chemotherapy → concurrent CRT or surgery depending on response to concurrent CRT • Poor glottis function (eg, dysphagia and other symptoms): Consider total laryngectomy or partial pharyngectomy.
T4	Total laryngectomy w/ thyroidectomy/partial pharyngoesophagectomy → post-op XRT or chemoRT for + margin or + ENE.

Radiation Treatment Technique

Early stage glottic

- **Dose: T1:** 63 Gy in 28 fractions at 2.25 Gy/fx.
  T2: 70 Gy in 35 fractions at 2 Gy/fx or 65.25 in 2.25 Gy/fx; consider hyperfractionation (79 Gy at 1.2 bid) or mild acceleration (bid once per week to complete treatment in 6 weeks)
  Factors that influence local control (especially T2): (1) fraction size 2.25 Gy > 2 >> 1.8 Gy (*Le et al. IJROBP* 1997), (2) overall treatment time $\leq$43 days (*Le et al. IJROBP* 1997), and (3) altered fractionation increases local control ~10% in T2N0 disease (*Trotti et al. IJROBP* 2014; DAHANCA—*Overgaard et al. Lancet* 2003).
- **Target: T1:** Entire glottic larynx, anteriorly flash 1 cm, posteriorly cover to anterior edge of vertebral bodies, superiorly cover to top of thyroid cartilage, and inferiorly cover to bottom of cricoid cartilage (Fig. 28.2)
  T2: Same as T1 with adjustments superiorly and/or inferiorly if T2 based on supraglottic or subglottic extension. Typically with conventional techniques field border 2 cm above or below GTV
- **Technique:** 3DCRT: right and left opposed laterals, **can consider 3 beam (0, 70, 290 degrees) IMRT for carotid sparing in experienced centers** (*Rosenthal et al. IJROBP* 2010).
- **SIM:** Supine w/ neck hyperextended, aquaplast mask covering the head and shoulders, isocenter in midlarynx. Pull straps for shoulder retraction. Consider thin bolus for patients with anterior disease. Patient should be reminded not to swallow during simulation or treatment as this can cause distortion of anatomy.

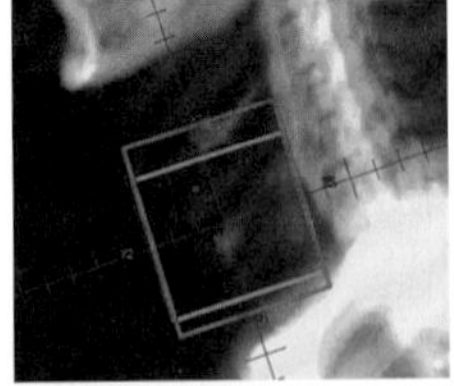

Figure 28.2 Classic early-stage glottic fields. *Smaller box* represents T1 lateral field. *Larger box* represents T2 lateral field.

Advanced Stage Glottic, Supraglottic, Subglottic, and Hypopharyngeal

- **Dose:**
  Primary tumor and involved nodes: 70 Gy in 33-35 fractions (high dose, CTV_{HD}) (Fig. 28.4)
  High-risk regions (involved nodal level and disease adjacent mucosa): 60-63 Gy (intermediate dose, CTV_{ID})
  Subclinical disease (at-risk nodal levels): 50 Gy in 25 fractions, 54 Gy in 30 fractions, or 57 Gy in 33 fractions (low dose, CTV_{ED})
- **Target:** Primary tumor with 8 mm to 1 cm CTV margin and involved nodes receive high dose (CTV_{HD}). Adjacent at-risk tissue, involved nodal levels, and 1 nodal level above and below involved nodal levels receive intermediate-risk subclinical dose (CTV_{ID}). Uninvolved at-risk nodal levels receive low-risk subclinical dose (CTV_{ED}).
- **Technique:** IMRT or VMAT. Scanning beam proton therapy can be used in experienced centers.
- **SIM:** Same as for early larynx

Lymph Node Drainage

- Supraglottic cancers most commonly spread to levels II, III, and IV LNs. Glottic cancers have almost no LN drainage, so LNs are not covered for stage I disease and rarely in stage II disease. Subglottic cancers can involve level VI nodes (Fig. 28.3).

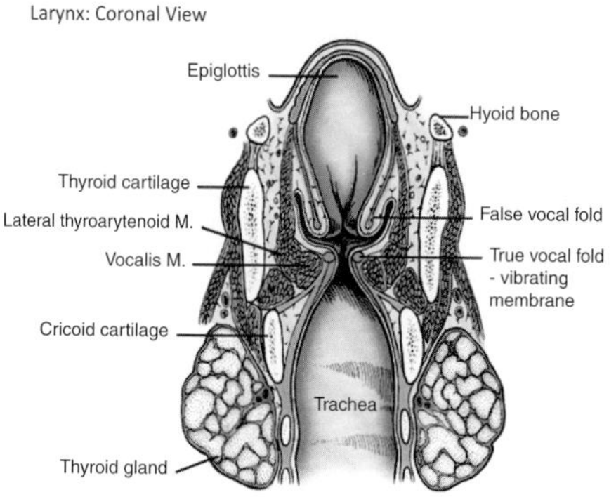

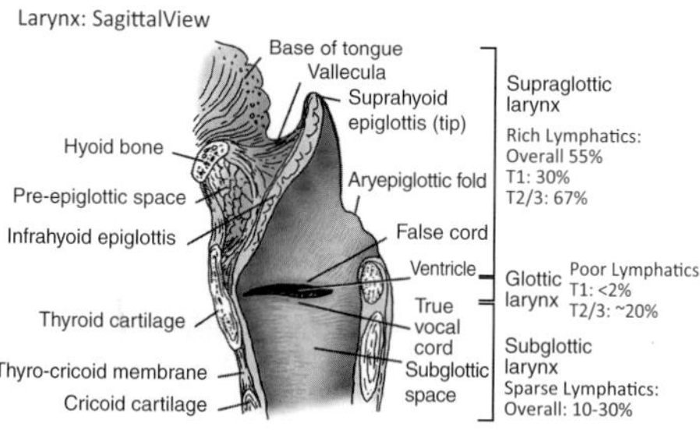

Figure 28.3 Lymph node involvement of laryngeal cancer based on site. (Top: Reprinted from Garrett CG, Ossoff RH. Hoarseness. *Med Clin N Am*. 1999;83(1):115-123. Copyright © 1999 Elsevier. With permission. Bottom: Reproduced with permission from Koch WM, Machtay M, Best S. Treatment of early (stage I and II) head and neck cancer: The larynx. In: UpToDate, Post TW (Ed), UpToDate, Waltham, MA. (Accessed on [Date].) Copyright © 2019 UpToDate, Inc. For more information visit www.uptodate.com.)

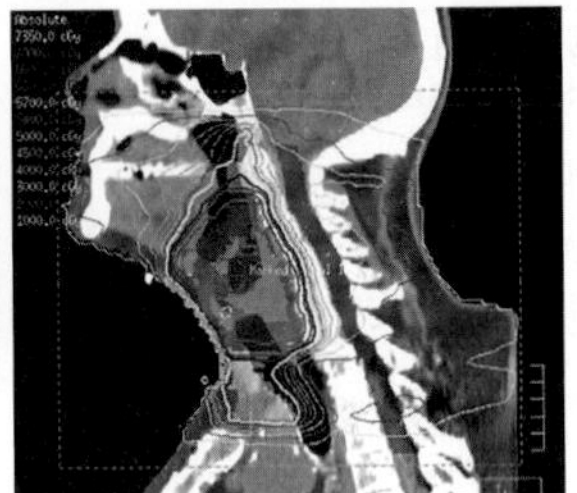

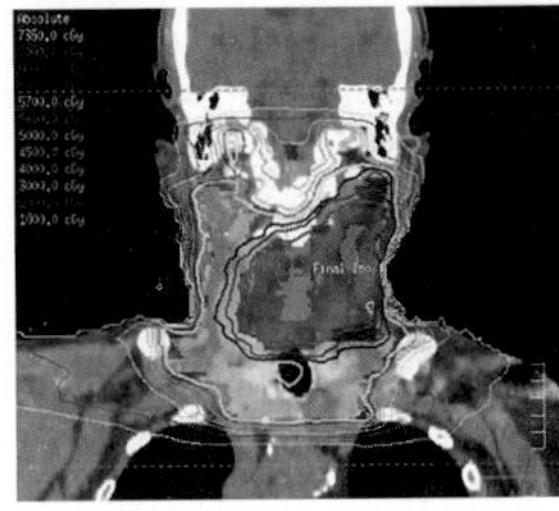

Figure 28.4 Representative VMAT treatment plan of patient with hypopharyngeal cancer involving structures of the larynx including epiglottis. Note extensive elective LN coverage. Inner RT field shows high-risk dose (CTV_{HD}) treated to 70 Gy and intermediate-dose CTV (CTV_{ID}) treated to 63 Gy. The outer RT field shows low-dose CTV treated to 57 Gy.

- Hypopharyngeal cancers are richly drained by lymphatics and ~75% have nodal involvement at diagnosis. Levels II, III, VI, and V and RP LNs are most commonly involved and should be covered when planning XRT. Will often cover level IV as well.
- See **Oral Cavity** chapter for neck LN description.

Post-Op

- **Target/dose: Region of resected gross disease:** 60 Gy in 2 Gy fractions (high dose, CTV_{HD}), 66 Gy in 2 Gy fractions for positive margins
  Operative bed of primary and LNs: 57 Gy (intermediate dose, CTV_{ID})
  Nondissected at-risk regions including nondissected at-risk nodal levels: 54 Gy (low dose, CTV_{ED}). The stoma is typically included in this volume.
  Note: if stoma or tracheostomy is made emergently through tumor, then this is included in the CTV_{HD}.
- **Technique:** IMRT or VMAT. Scanning beam proton therapy can be used in capable centers.
- **SIM:** Same as above. Wiring scars helps define the operative bed. Especially if there was neck disease with ECE, consider bolus for scars, and also consider bolus for stoma if at increased risk due to disease proximity.
- **IGRT**: Daily kV Imaging
- **Planning directive (for conventional fractionation):**

PTV	>95% coverage
Parotid gland	bilateral mean < 26 Gy
Submandibular gland	bilateral mean < 30 Gy
Spinal cord	D_{max} < 45 Gy
Brainstem	D_{max} < 45 Gy
Mandible	D_{max} < 70 Gy
Cochlea Lt and Rt	D_{max} < 35 Gy
Brachial plexus	D_{max} < 66 Gy
Total lung	V20 < 20%
Cervical esophagus	Mean < 30 Gy
Brachial plexus	D_{max} < 66 Gy

Special Circumstances

- **Indications for neck dissection after definitive XRT or CRT:** Persistent neck disease. Avoid treatment of brachial plexus to doses >66 Gy. If nodal disease is adjacent to brachial plexus, consider treating disease to 60-64 Gy with a planned nodal dissection.

Surgery

- Endoscopic resection: For early-stage tumors—done either via a transoral laser microsurgery (TLM) technique or transoral robotic surgery (TORS) technique. Preserves the larynx. Compared to RT, results in equivalent oncologic outcomes but voice outcomes may not be as good as RT (controversial)

- Total Laryngectomy: Resection of the entire larynx including all three substructures (supraglottis, glottis, subglottis) and creation of a stoma to provide a method for the patient to breathe. Requires total thyroidectomy. Typically can receive primary closure
- Pharyngolaryngectomy: Resection of the entire larynx including all three substructures (supraglottis, glottis, subglottis) and partial resection of the soft tissues of the pharynx. Performed for bulky hypopharyngeal cancers, used sparingly secondary to morbidity. Requires creation of a stoma, total thyroidectomy, and typically requires a flap resection of pharyngeal structures

CHEMOTHERAPY

- **Concurrent:** IV cisplatin 100 mg/m^2 every 3 weeks (days 1, 22, and 43) of RT OR weekly IV cisplatin at a dose of 40 mg/m^2. If the patient cannot tolerate cisplatin secondary to toxicity, weekly carboplatin or cetuximab can be considered.
- **Neoadjuvant:** Most common regimen is TPF (docetaxel, cisplatin, 5-flourauracil). Consists of docetaxel at a dose of 75 mg/m^2, administered as a 1-hour infusion on day 1; followed by cisplatin at a dose of 75 mg/m^2, administered as a 1-hour infusion on day 1; and fluorouracil at a dose of 750 mg/m^2, administered by continuous infusion on days 1 to 5 (*Vermorken et al. NEJM* 2007). Can give up to 4 cycles every 3 weeks. Primarily used for downstaging, *NO* survival advantages.
- **Adjuvant:** No role.

SIDE EFFECT MANAGEMENT

See **Oral Cavity** chapter.

FOLLOW-UP

- General—History/physical with nasolaryngoscopy, TSH, T4, BUN, Cr, CT, or MRI (use the same imaging as pretreatment): q3mo at year 1 → q4mo at year 2 → q6mo at years 3-5 → annually after year 5. PET/CT as baseline posttherapy evaluation ~12 weeks posttreatment, particularly in the node-positive patient treated definitively
- Can consider stopping imaging after year 2 as this is the highest-risk time period for recurrence; imaging can be saved for clinical symptoms or suspicious PE findings. Annual CXR—screening for metastases and second primary.
- For early-stage glottic cancers, imaging is not needed; just use videostroboscopy and regular follow-up with MD.
- If PEG tube is placed, follow up with speech pathology and nutrition.

NOTABLE TRIALS

Feasibility of larynx preservation with induction chemotherapy followed by RT

- VA Larynx Trial (*Wolf et al. NEJM* 1991; *Hong et al. Cancer Res* 1993): Phase III randomized controlled trial randomizing 332 ≥ stage III laryngeal cancer patients to total laryngectomy + post-op RT vs sequential RT: Induction chemo (cis/5-FU) followed by RT. At 2 years, OS was the same (68%) with overall larynx preservation rate of 64% in the chemoRT arm. Decreased DM in the chemoRT arm (11% vs 17%, $P = .016$) but with higher rates of local recurrence at the primary site (12% vs 2%, $P = .0005$). 5-year follow-up showed no OS difference and persistent larynx preservation benefits.

Larynx preservation superior with chemoRT

- RTOG 91-11 (*Forastiere et al. NEJM* 2003; updates *JCO* 2006 and 2013): Phase III randomized of 547 patients with stage III cancers of the glottis and supraglottis. Patients were randomized to 3 arms: Arm (1) Induction chemo (cis/5-FU) followed by XRT (or laryngectomy if poor response plus adjuvant RT to 50-70 Gy depending on surgical margin status), Arm (2) concurrent cisplatin and RT, and Arm (3) RT alone (70 Gy in 35 fractions). Elective neck and SCV received 50 Gy in 25 fractions. Both induction and concurrent chemoRT regimens improved laryngectomy-free survival over XRT alone, HR 0.75, $P = .02$ and .78, $P = .03$, respectively. No OS difference between the three arms. Larynx preservation rate was improved with concurrent chemoRT arm vs the induction arm (HR 0.58, $P = .005$). Larynx preservation was similar between the induction chemoRT arm and XRT alone arm.

SALIVARY GLAND NEOPLASMS

CHRISTOPHER WILKE • BRIAN J. DEEGAN

BACKGROUND

- **Incidence/Prevalence:** Malignant salivary gland tumors account for ~5% of all H&N malignancies. Annual incidence is ~1 per 100 000 (SEER). Peak incidence occurs during the sixth decade of life.
- **Outcomes:** 5-Year survival across all stages and sites is estimated at 70%.
- **Risk factors:** Prior radiation, smoking (Warthin tumor), male sex, solvent exposure

TUMOR BIOLOGY AND CHARACTERISTICS

- **Genetics:** t(11;19)(q21;p13) translocation creates a fusion oncogene (*CRTC1-MAML2*), which is associated with the development of mucoepidermoid carcinomas (*Tonon et al. Nat Genet* 2003). t(6;9) translocations produce the *MYB-NFIB* fusion protein commonly observed in many adenoid cystic carcinomas (*Persson et al. Proc Natl Acad Sci USA* 2009).
- **Pathology:** Most tumors (~70%) arise in the parotid gland; however, a majority (70%-80%) of all parotid tumors are benign. In contrast, tumors of the minor salivary glands are most likely malignant. Mucoepidermoid carcinoma (MEC) is the most common malignant histology followed by adenoid cystic (ACC), acinic cell and adenocarcinomas. MEC varies from low to high grade. Although ACC exhibit different grades, histologic subtypes substitute for grade with cribriform and tubular being low grade while solid type is considered high grade. Acinic cell carcinoma is almost always low grade. Adenocarcinoma is often a catchall descriptor and includes low-grade polymorphous adenocarcinoma and salivary duct carcinoma. The latter is a very aggressive high-grade tumor and in recent years is identified separately. Mixed malignant tumors (MMT) most commonly have components resembling benign pleomorphic adenomas but despite this are often high grade.

ANATOMY

- The parotid gland abuts the posterior mandibular ramus and is separated into the superficial and deep lobes by the plane of the facial nerve.
- The facial nerve arises from the base of the pons, traverses through the temporal bone, and exits the skull base at the stylomastoid foramen.
- The submandibular gland is located within the submandibular triangle and is bounded superiorly by the lower border of the mandible and inferiorly by the anterior belly of the digastric muscle. The hypoglossal nerve traverses inferior to the gland, and the lingual nerve (a branch of V3) traverses over the gland. Either can be involved by cancer, particularly if the cancer is neurotropic.
- Lymph node involvement is less common compared with other H&N sites, particularly for well-differentiated cancers. Primary drainage is to the periparotid nodes (for parotid primaries) and ipsilateral neck (primarily levels I and II). See **Oral Cavity** chapter for neck LN description.

WORKUP

- **History and physical:** Head and neck evaluation with special attention to cranial nerve deficits. Direct palpation and visualization of tumor and possibly with nasolaryngoscope and/or mirror exam to assess disease spread. Major salivary gland masses may represent a lymph node metastasis from a separate primary site, specifically cutaneous squamous cell carcinoma of the skin; thus, consider a skin examination of the head and neck.
- **Labs:** CBC, CMP
- **Procedures/biopsy:** Biopsy of primary and FNA of enlarged LNs as clinically indicated
- **Imaging:** CT or MRI with contrast of the head/neck. MRI useful for evaluation of nerve invasion and soft tissue component. CT useful for evaluation of bone invasion. Consider CT of the chest. Ultrasound can also be of value for superficial tumors of the parotid or submandibular glands.
- **Additional consultations:** Multidisciplinary evaluation with head and neck surgical oncology, radiation oncology, medical oncology, nutrition, and dental (fluoride/extractions).

Major Salivary Gland Staging *(AJCC 8th edition)*

Major salivary gland defined as parotid, submandibular, or sublingual gland

T Stage		N Stage	
T1	Tumor ≤2 cm without extraparenchymal extension	**N1**	Single ipsilateral LN ≤ 3 cm and ENE(−)
T2	Tumor >2 but ≤4 cm without extraparenchymal extension	**N2a**	• Single ipsilateral LN ≤ 3 cm and ENE(+) **or**
T3	Tumor >4 cm or with extraparenchymal extension		• Single ipsilateral LN > 3 cm but ≤6 cm and ENE(−)
T4a	Involves the skin, mandible, ear canal, or facial nerve	**N2b**	Multiple ipsilateral LNs all <6 cm and ENE(−)
T4b	Involves the skull base or pterygoid plates or encases carotid artery	**N2c**	Bilateral or contralateral LN(s) all <6 cm and ENE(−)
		N3a	LN > 6 cm and ENE(−)
		N3b	• Single ipsilateral LN > 3 cm and ENE(+) **or** • Multiple ipsilateral, contralateral or bilateral LN any with ENE(+) **or** • Single contralateral LN ≤ 3 cm and ENE(+)

Group Staging

	N0	N1	N2	N3	M1
T1	I				
T2	II				
T3	III				IVC
T4a	IVA				
T4b	IVB				

Minor Salivary Gland Staging *(AJCC 8th edition)*

Tumors arising in minor salivary glands are staged the same as a head and neck squamous cell carcinoma arising from the same anatomical location. For example, a minor salivary gland cancer arising from the tonsil region would be staged as an oropharynx cancer.

Surgery

- Surgical management is preferred with definitive radiotherapy reserved for patients who are not operative candidates or those with unresectable tumors.
- Patients with cN+ typically are treated with a planned neck dissection. While there is no consensus regarding the role of an elective neck dissection in all clinically N0 patients, it is generally recommended for those with high-grade histologies felt to be at highest risk of occult nodal disease.

Chemotherapy

- While the use of platinum agents is often extrapolated from other H&N sites, there is a lack of prospective data for use in salivary gland tumors (currently under investigation on RTOG 1008).
- Retrospective series have failed to demonstrate a survival benefit with adjuvant chemoradiotherapy vs radiotherapy alone in these patients *(Amini et al. JAMA Otolaryngol Head Neck Surg 2016)*.

Indications for Postoperative Radiotherapy

- Extraglandular extension
- High-grade histology
- Close or positive surgical margins
- Perineural invasion
- Lymph node metastases
- Recurrent disease

Conventional Borders for Postoperative Radiation Fields

As a general rule of thumb, it is useful to use the contralateral intact gland as a reference in all patients. All borders listed below are contingent on tumor extent.

Parotid	
Superior	Zygomatic arch
Inferior	Hyoid
Anterior	Anterior edge of the masseter muscle
Posterior	Just behind the mastoid process
Submandibular	
Superior	Line extending from oral commissure to mandibular ramus just inferior to temporomandibular joint
Inferior	Thyroid notch
Anterior	Determined by surgery. Shield oral commissure if possible
Posterior	Just behind the mastoid process

Modern Radiation Treatment Technique (Simultaneous Integrated Boost)

- **Dose: High risk** (CTV_{HD}): 60 Gy in 30 fractions at 2 Gy/fx (Fig. 29.1)
  **High-risk areas for residual disease (ECE, +margin) can be boosted to 66 Gy.*
  Intermediate risk (CTV_{ID}): 57 Gy (1.9 Gy/fx)
  Low risk/elective dose (CTV_{ED}): 54 Gy (1.8 Gy/fx)
- **Target:**
  CTV_{HD}: Primary and nodal tumor bed with 8- to 10-mm expansion
  CTV_{ID}: Remaining operative bed not included in CTV_{HD}
  CTV_{ED}: Ipsilateral neck levels II-IV in N0 patients with high-grade tumors, coverage of at-risk perineural tracks
- **Technique:** IMRT or IMPT
- **SIM:** Supine with head extended. Thermoplastic mask extending to the shoulders for immobilization. A tongue-lateralizing oral stent can help displace the tongue away from the target volume. Scan vertex to the carina.
- **IGRT:** Daily 2D kV orthogonal imaging or cone beam CT
- **Dose constraints (at 2 Gy/fx):**
  Contralateral parotid: Mean < 10 Gy
  Oral cavity: Mean < 30 Gy
  Larynx: Mean < 30 Gy
  Spinal cord: Max < 45 Gy
  Brainstem: Max < 45 Gy
  Brachial plexus: Max < 66 Gy
  Optic nerves and chiasm: Max < 54 Gy. Can go to Max < 60 Gy if necessary; (ex PNS salivary gland cancer abutting optic structure)
  Cochlea: Max < 35 Gy; soft constraint if have to cover facial nerve through temporal bone
  Mandible: Max less than prescription dose for CTV_{HD}

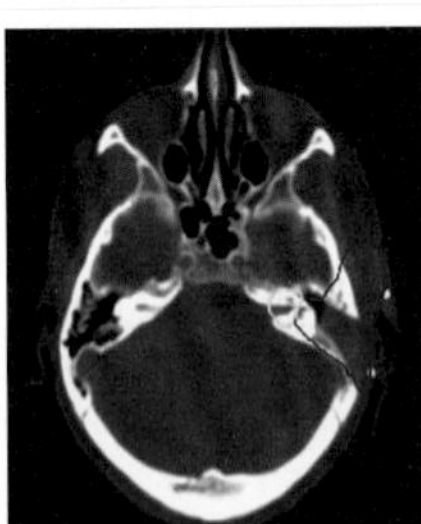
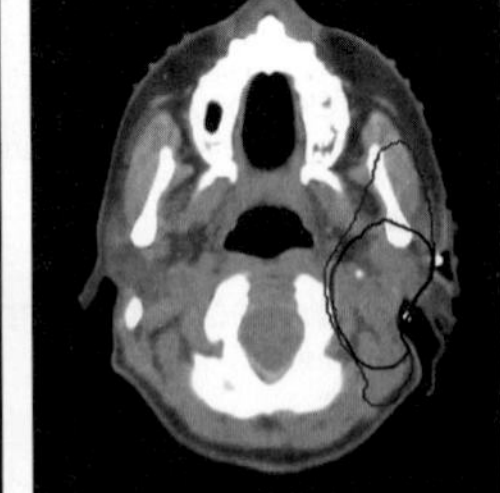

Figure 29.1 Adjuvant treatment for an early-stage adenoid cystic carcinoma of the left parotid gland with perineural invasion. *Maroon*, CTV_{HD} 60 Gy.

SIDE EFFECT MANAGEMENT

See **Oral Cavity** chapter.

FOLLOW-UP

- Posttreatment clinical assessment at 4-6 weeks → if response/no recurrence, then PET/CT at 3 months
- History/physical with imaging: Every 3 months for 2 years → then every 6 months for 3 years → annual clinical exam thereafter
- TSH every 6-12 months if the neck was treated
- Dental evaluation every 6-12 months
- Audiology and speech/swallow assessment as needed

NOTABLE TRIALS

Retrospective series assessing risk factors and radiation doses

- Dutch Cooperative Group (*Terhaard et al. IJROBP* 2005): Retrospective analysis of 498 patients with salivary gland tumors treated with surgery followed by adjuvant radiotherapy or observation. Radiotherapy improved 10-year local control for T3/T4 tumors (84% vs 18%, $P < .001$), close margins (95% vs 55%, $P = .003$), incomplete resection (82% vs 44%, $P < .001$), bone invasion (86% vs 54%, $P = .04$), and perineural invasion (88% vs 60%, $P = .01$). For pN+ patients, adjuvant radiotherapy improved 5-year locoregional control (83% vs 57%, $P = .04$).
- UCSF (*Chen et al. IJROBP* 2007): Retrospective study of 251 patients with cN0 carcinomas of the salivary gland treated with surgery and adjuvant radiotherapy. 52% received elective nodal irradiation. 10-Year nodal relapse-free survival was significantly improved with elective nodal irradiation (26% vs 0%, $P = .0001$). Histologies associated with the highest rate of nodal relapse included squamous cell carcinoma (67%), undifferentiated carcinoma (50%), adenocarcinoma (34%), and mucoepidermoid carcinoma (29%). No nodal failures occurred with omission of elective neck radiotherapy in adenoid cystic or acinic cell histologies.
- MD Anderson (*Garden et al. IJROBP* 1995): Retrospective analysis of 198 patients with adenoid cystic carcinomas of the head and neck who received adjuvant radiotherapy. 10-Year local control rates worse with positive margins vs close/negative margin (77% vs 93%, $P = .006$) and worse with named nerve involvement vs named nerve not involved (80% vs 88%, $P = .02$); both positive margins and named nerve involvement vs one feature vs none (70% vs 83% vs 93%, $P = .002$). Improved local control with doses ≥56 Gy in patients with positive margins (88% vs 40%, $P = .006$). Recommended doses of 60 Gy to the tumor bed with boost to 66 Gy for patients with positive margins.

Prospective trial demonstrating the benefit of neutron-based radiation

- **RTOG-MRC Neutron Trial** (*Laramore et al. IJROBP* 1993): Two-arm prospective randomized phase III trial comparing fast neutron radiotherapy to conventional photon and/or electron radiotherapy for inoperable or recurrent malignant salivary gland tumors. Neutron dose was 16.5-22 Gy in 12 fractions. Conventional RT dose was 55 Gy/4 weeks or 70 Gy/7.5 weeks. Trial stopped after accrual of 32 patients due to significantly improved local control in neutron arm. Significantly improved 10-year local control with neutrons (56% vs 17%, $P = .009$); however, no difference in OS (15% vs 25%, $P = .5$)

THYROID CANCER

GARY WALKER • JEENA VARGHESE • ADAM SETH GARDEN

BACKGROUND

- **Incidence/prevalence:** Approximately 56 000 cases diagnosed annually in the United States
- **Outcomes:** 5-Year survival for well differentiated across all stages estimated at 98% (SEER data). 5-Year survival for anaplastic histology is <5%.
- **Demographics:** F > M, 63% are age 35-65
- **Risk factors:** Family history, diet low in iodine, history of goiter, radiation exposure (diagnostic tests, previous cancer treatment, and nuclear fallouts), genetics (Cowden's, MEN2 for medullary), nodules (4% are malignant)

TUMOR BIOLOGY AND CHARACTERISTICS

- **Genetics:** Papillary and follicular thyroid cancer associated with defects in the gene PRKAR1A, familial adenomatous polyposis (FAP), Cowden disease, Carney complex, and familial nonmedullary thyroid carcinoma. Medullary thyroid cancer can be familial, either as part of the multiple endocrine neoplasia type 2 (MEN2) or isolated familial medullary thyroid cancer syndrome. Anaplastic thyroid cancers appear to arise from differentiated cancers.
- **Pathology:** Differentiated histologies: Papillary (85%) and follicular (11%)
  Derived from neuroendocrine C cells: Medullary (2%)
  Undifferentiated histology: Anaplastic (ATC) (1%)
  Other pathologies of the thyroid include primary thyroid lymphomas.

ANATOMY

- The thyroid is deep to sternohyoid muscle. Consists of two lobes and isthmus
- Lymph node drainage (35% are cN+)
  - Prelaryngeal (level VI, delphian)
  - Pretracheal/paratracheal nodes/mediastinal
  - Levels II-IV
  - See **Oral Cavity** chapter for neck LN description.

WORKUP

- **History and physical:** Assess presenting symptoms including symptoms of hyper/hypothyroidism. Direct palpation and visualization of the thyroid and vocal cords with nasolaryngoscope when advanced
- **Labs:** CBC, CMP, TSH, free T4/T3, T4/T3
- **Procedures/biopsy:** US-guided FNA of primary and enlarged LNs as clinically indicated
- **Imaging:** Ultrasound, ^{123}I thyroid uptake and scan, CT or MRI of the neck with contrast for locally advanced, PET/CT for anaplastic histology
- **Additional consultations:** Multidisciplinary evaluation with head and neck surgical oncology, endocrinology, nuclear medicine, radiation oncology, medical oncology, speech (evaluation of vocal cord mobility), nutrition, dental (fluoride/extractions)

THYROID CANCER STAGING *(AJCC 8TH EDITION)*

T Stage		**N Stage**	
T1a	≤1 cm limited to thyroid	N0a	≥1 cytologically or histologically confirmed benign LN
T1b	>1 cm but ≤2 cm limited to thyroid	N0b	No radiologic or clinical evidence of LN disease
T2	>2 cm but ≤4 cm limited to thyroid	N1a	Level VI or VII LNs either unilateral or bilateral
T3a	>4 cm limited to thyroid	N1b	Level I, II, III, IV, or V or retropharyngeal either unilateral or bilateral
T3b	Extrathyroid extension invading only strap muscles	**M Stage**	
T4a	Invades soft tissue, larynx, trachea, esophagus, or recurrent nerve	M1	Distant metastasis
T4b	Invades prevertebral fascia, incases carotid/mediastinal vessels		

Summative Stage (Depends on Patient's Age and Histology)

Age < 55 y

	N0	N1	M1
T1	I	I	II
T2	I	I	II
T3	I	I	II
T4	I	I	II

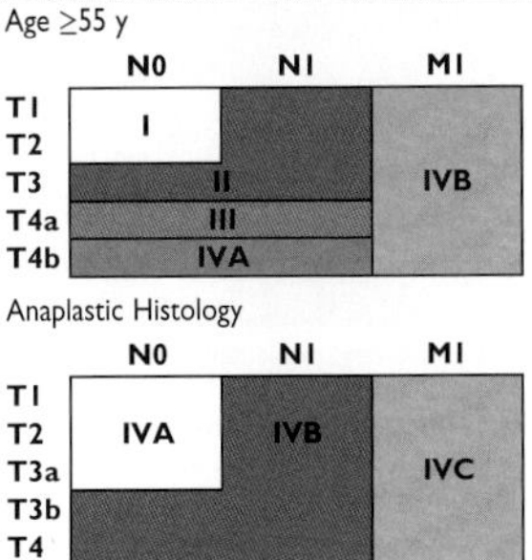

TREATMENT ALGORITHM

Indications for Postoperative Radioiodine (RAI) Decision-Making[a]		
ATA Risk Stratification[a]	**TNM Stage**	**RAI Indicated?**
Low risk	T1a N0 M0	No
Low risk	T1b N0 M0	Not routine
Low risk	T2 N0 M0	Not routine
Low to intermediate risk	T3 N0 M0	Consider if age > 55 and large size or in patients with ETE
Low to intermediate risk	Any T, N+ M0	Strongly consider, especially if advanced age or clinically evident lymph nodes
High risk	T4 any N/M	Yes
High risk	Any T/N, M+	Yes

[a]Ref: *Haugen et al. Thyroid* 2016.

ATC (M0)	**Consider Resection + Adjuvant EBRT ± Chemotherapy**			
Indications for Adjuvant External Beam Radiation for Differentiated Disease				
	ATA	**NCCN**	**BTA**	**ESMO**
Locally advanced	Yes		Yes	
>60 y with ETE	Consider			
Multiple reoperations	Consider	Yes	Yes	Yes
Residual gross disease		Consider	Yes	
No radioactive iodine uptake		Consider	Yes	Consider

NCCN, National Comprehensive Cancer Network; ATA, American Thyroid Association; BTA, British Thyroid Association; ESMO, European Society of Medical Oncology.

EXTERNAL RADIATION TREATMENT TECHNIQUE

- **Timing:** Should be started within 4-6 weeks of surgery
- **Dose:** Highest risk (close/positive margins/ECE)—63-66 Gy in 30-33 fractions (Fig. 30.1)
  High risk (tumor bed)—60 Gy in 30 fractions
  Intermediate risk (operative bed)—57 Gy in 30 fractions
  Low risk—54 Gy in 30 fractions
- **Target: The principal target is the central compartment (hyoid to top of aortic arch and between the carotids).** This typically includes the tumor bed, operative bed, draining lymphatics (levels VI, III-V), paratracheal (consider level II, only if significant nodal disease with ECE), tracheal esophageal groove.
- **Technique:** VMAT, IMRT, and IMPT in experienced centers
- **SIM:** Supine, Aquaplast mask. Wire scar. 3-mm bolus 2 cm around scar
- **IGRT:** Daily kV with weekly CBCT or daily CBCT

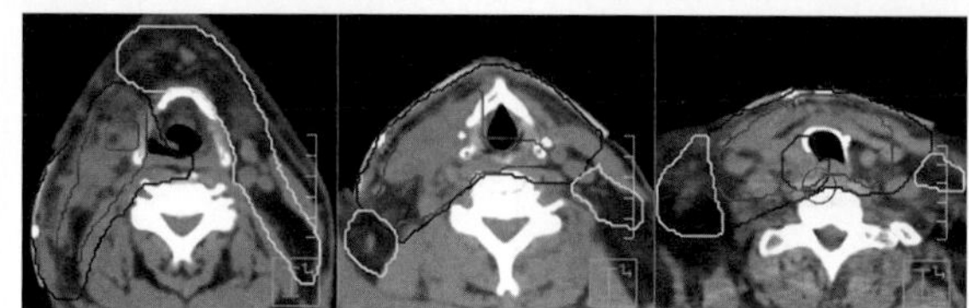

Figure 30.1 A 74-year-old with four previous resections for papillary thyroid cancer. Following surgery, he was found to have a 3-cm right level II node with ECE, 2/10 level right level III nodes up to 2 cm, as well as a right tracheal sidewall mass resected with SM+. Contours shown are GTV-LN (*green*), CTV63 (*purple*), CTV60 (*red*), CTV57 (*blue*), and CTV54 (*yellow*). Treatment was delivered utilizing simultaneous integrated boost in 30 fractions. **See color insert.**

- **Planning directive (for conventional fractionation):**

95% PTV coverage	
Spinal cord	Max < 45 Gy
Brainstem	Max < 45 Gy
Mandible	Max < 60 Gy
Total lung	V20 < 20%
Lens	Max < 5 Gy
Parotids	Mean < 20 Gy, lower for contralateral
Submandibular	Mean < 10 Gy if level II included, then <26 Gy
Larynx	Mean < 35 Gy
Esophagus	Max < 60 Gy (will often be in the CTV)

SURGERY

- Total thyroidectomy or ipsilateral thyroid lobectomy with central neck dissection
- Neck dissection for node positive
  - Radical neck dissection = I-V, CNXI, IJV, SCM
  - Modified radical neck dissection = I-V, preserve one of the above
  - Supraomohyoid = I-III
  - Lateral = II-IV
  - Selective neck dissection = LNs based on site

CHEMOTHERAPY

- **Limited role for traditional chemotherapy**
- **TKIs:** Lenvatinib, vandetanib, cabozantinib, pazopanib, sorafenib
- **Anaplastic thyroid cancer:** RTOG 0912 is looking at paclitaxel/pazopanib with radiation; other targeted agents are heavily investigated. Some ATC can exhibit *BRAF* mutation, which can be targeted similar to melanoma with vemurafenib.

SIDE EFFECT MANAGEMENT

See **Oral Cavity** chapter.

FOLLOW-UP

- History/physical exam and ultrasound or CT of the neck: Every 3-6 months for 3 years → yearly to 5 years. Maintain follow-up with endocrinologist to evaluate thyroid supplementation and target TSH levels.
- Assess compliance with fluoride trays (if applicable) and neck/lymphedema exercises.

UNKNOWN HEAD AND NECK PRIMARY

HOUDA BAHIG • ADAM SETH GARDEN

BACKGROUND

- **Definition:** Metastatic disease in the lymph nodes of the neck for which complete workup failed to determine primary tumor origin—diagnosis of exclusion
- **Incidence/prevalence:** Accounts for 1%-4% of all head and neck cancers. The incidence of cervical node from unknown primary (CUP) has diminished significantly with advances in diagnostic imaging and surgical techniques.
- **Outcomes:** With aggressive radiation approaches, the 5-year overall survival rate is between 80% and 90%; mucosal emergence occurs in <10%, and the most common site of recurrence is distant (20%).
- **Risk factors:** Since CUP is often from undetected oropharyngeal cancer, HPV association is common. Other risk factors include those common for head and neck cancer in general.

TUMOR BIOLOGY AND CHARACTERISTICS

- **Pathology:** Derived from FNA or core biopsy. Open biopsy is discouraged because of risk of tumor spillage.
  - Most common histology is squamous cell carcinoma (75%), of which HPV (HPV-DNA via PCR and/or p16 on IHC) association is identified in up to 75% of patients. EBV association may also be detected.
    - HPV+: Likely oropharynx or nasopharynx primary
    - EBV+: Likely nasopharynx primary
    - HPV−/EBV−: Head and neck primary including all head and neck subsites in addition to skin primary
- Adenocarcinoma histology is most likely associated with subclavicular primary origin (eg, esophageal or lung cancer), after salivary gland or thyroid primary tumors are excluded. Consider thyroglobulin, TTF1, calcitonin, and PAX8 IHC for undifferentiated carcinoma or adenocarcinoma.
- Other histologies include undifferentiated, lymphoma, melanoma, and sarcoma.

ANATOMY

- Most likely occult primary origin is the tonsil or base of the tongue.
- Upper cervical nodes (levels II, III, and V) are likely from HNC primary origin.
- Consider subclavicular primary origin (lung, gastrointestinal, breast) for lower cervical (levels IV and V) and supraclavicular nodes—associated with worse prognosis. Consider skin or salivary gland primary origin for parotid nodes.
- The presence of a level II cystic metastasis is a hallmark of HPV-related SCC.
- Level III metastasis without involvement of level II suggests larynx or hypopharynx primary origin.
- See **Oral Cavity** chapter for discussion of LN levels.

WORKUP

- **History and physical:** The oral cavity, entire pharynx, larynx, and skin, should be carefully examined utilizing palpation and nasopharyngolaryngoscopy.
- **Labs:** CBC, CMP
- **Procedures/biopsy:** FNA or core biopsy of enlarged LN(s). Evaluation of histology with appropriate stains. For the most common histology (squamous), assess HPV status (PCR and/or p16 on IHC) and EBV staining. Exam under anesthesia with panendoscopy, including palatine tonsillectomy, random mucosal biopsies, and biopsy of suspicious sites. Consider bronchoscopy and EGD especially for low LNs (levels IV and V).
- **Imaging:** FDG-PET/CT detects occult primary in 25% of cases and should be done before EUA with panendoscopy. CT and/or MRI of the head and neck, CT of the chest (>T0N2b). CT of the chest, abdomen, and pelvis for lower cervical nodes (levels IV-V)
- **Additional consultations:** Multidisciplinary evaluation with head and neck surgical oncology, radiation oncology, medical oncology, speech, nutrition, dental (fluoride/extractions)

Unknown Primary Staging

(AJCC 8th Edition)

As per AJCC 8th edition, EBV-related cervical adenopathy is staged using nasopharynx cancer staging and HPV-related cervical adenopathy is staged using the HPV-mediated oropharynx cancer staging. HPV-unrelated and EBV-unrelated cervical adenopathy are staged as follows:

Clinical	
N1	Single LN ≤ 3 cm and ECE(−)
N2a	Single LN > 3 cm but ≤6 cm and ENE(−)
N2b	≥2 ipsilateral LN ≤ 6 cm and ENE(−)
N2c	Bilateral or contralateral LN, all ≤6 cm and ENE(−)
N3a	LN > 6 cm and ENE(−)
N3b	Any LN with clinical ENE(+)

Clinical ENE(+): invasion of the skin, infiltration of musculature, dense tethering or fixation of adjacent structures, or invasion (with dysfunction) of cranial nerve, brachial plexus, sympathetic trunk, or phrenic nerve.

Pathologic	
N1	Single LN ≤ 3 cm and ENE(−)
N2a	Single LN ≤ 3 cm and ENE(+) *or* single lymph node >3 cm but ≤6 cm and ENE(−)
N2b	≥2 ipsilateral LN, ≤6 cm and ENE(−)
N2c	Bilateral or contralateral LN, all ≤6 cm and ENE(−)
N3a	LN > 6 cm and ENE(−)
N3b	Single LN > 3 cm and ENE(+) *or* ≥2 ipsilateral or contralateral LN any size and ENE(+) *or* single contralateral LN ≤ 3 cm

Pathologic ENE detected on histopathologic examination is designed as ENE_{mi} (microscopic ENE ≤ 2 mm) or ENE_{ma} (major ENE > 2 mm).

Summative Stage

T	N	M	Stage
T0	N1	M0	III
T0	N2	M0	IVA
T0	N3	M0	IVB
T0	Any N	M1	IVC

Treatment Algorithm

T0N1[a]	1. Selective or comprehensive neck dissection, +/− postoperative RT if ≥2 LN or concurrent chemoRT if ECE on LN dissection pathology 2. Definitive RT[a]
T0N2-3[a]	1. Concurrent chemoRT +/− neck dissection 2. Definitive RT +/− neck dissection 3. Neck dissection + adjuvant radiation +/− systemic therapy 4. Induction chemotherapy followed by RT +/− concurrent systemic therapy (uncommon, mainly if level IV disease)
Stage IVB (M+)	1. Systemic therapy or best supportive care 2. Surgery, RT, or systemic therapy/RT for selected cases with limited metastatic burden

[a]Favored in patients with open biopsy (violated neck)

Radiation Treatment Technique

- **Target:**

Definitive Target Volumes	
CTV_{HD}	GTV nodal (or LN bed after excisional biopsy) + 1 cm
CTV_{ID}	LN levels 2 cm superior and inferior of CTV_{HD}
CTV_{ED}	Remainder LN not included in CTV_{ID} to encompass minimally: Ipsilateral retropharyngeal and levels IB-VI; contralateral levels II-IV; select mucosa (based on HPV/EBV status) • HPV+ histology: oropharynx and nasopharynx mucosa • HPV−/EBV− histology: oropharynx mucosa, nasopharynx mucosa, and consider hypopharynx mucosa and larynx (controversial)
Postoperative Target Volumes	
CTV_{HD}	Tumor bed (determined by imaging and surgical/pathology findings) + 1 cm Consider boosting the resection bed if ECE is detected on pathology.
CTV_{ID}	Operative bed not including CTV_{HD}
CTV_{ED}	Remainder LN not included in CTV_{ID} in involved neck to encompass levels I-V, bilateral RP nodes, and levels II-IV of uninvolved neck • HPV+ histology: Oropharynx and nasopharynx mucosa • HPV−/EBV− histology: Oropharynx mucosa, nasopharynx mucosa, and consider hypopharynx mucosa and larynx (controversial) • Skin primary suspected (pathology reveals squamous cell pathology and HPV−/EBV− especially if history of skin cancers): Consider definitive management of neck with radiation and/or surgery and close observation for the development of a primary. Nasopharynx and oropharynx mucosa.[a]
PTV	CTV + 3-mm margin

- **Dose** (Fig. 31.1):

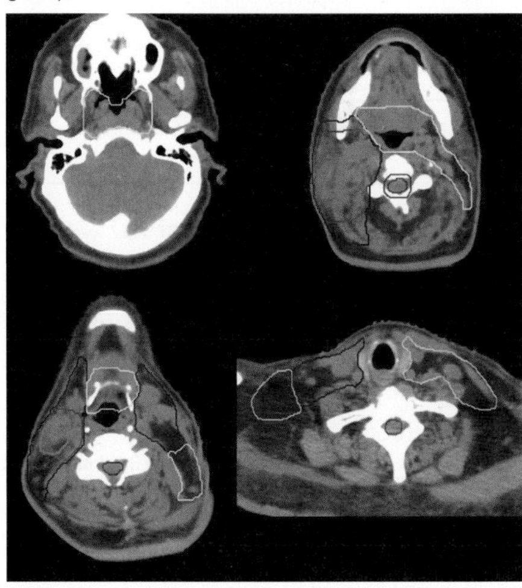

Figure 31.1 Target volumes for CUP with metastasis to left LN levels II-III, showing CTV_{HD} (*red*), CTV_{ID} (*blue*), and CTV_{ED} (*yellow*). **See color insert**.

	Pre-op
CTV_{HD}:	70 Gy in 33 fractions or 66 Gy in 30 fractions
CTV_{ID}:	63 Gy in 33 fractions or 60 Gy in 30 fractions
CTV_{ED}:	56 Gy in 33 fractions or 54 Gy in 30 fractions

Post-op (after neck dissection)	
CTV_{HD}:	60 Gy in 30 fractions
CTV_{ID}:	57 Gy in 30 fractions
CTV_{ED}:	54 Gy in 30 fractions
CTV_{boost}:	63-66 Gy in 30 fractions (consider defining a smaller volume within CTV_{HD} if ECE)

- **Technique:** IMRT, IMPT
- **SIM:** Supine position, arms in shoulder straps to lower shoulders from treatment field, thermoplastic head and neck mask, wire and 3-mm bolus on surgical scar (if LN dissection or excisional biopsy)
- **IGRT:** Daily kV imaging +/– weekly 3D imaging
- **Planning directive:**
  Ensure each PTV coverage by prescription dose with the goal of V100% > 95%, V95% > 99%, V105% < 10%, D_{max} < 120%
  OAR dose should respect the following constraints:

Brainstem:	D_{max} < 45 Gy
Spinal cord:	D_{max} < 45 Gy
Mandible:	D_{max} < CTV_{HD} prescription dose
Parotid:	Mean < 26 Gy
Oral cavity:	Mean < 30 Gy
Larynx:	Mean < 30 Gy *(if larynx/hypopharynx not included in CTV_{ED})*
Cervical esophagus:	Mean < 30 Gy
Submandibular gland:	Mean < 39 Gy *(if level Ib excluded in N0 neck)*
Brachial plexus:	D_{max} < 66 Gy

Chemotherapy

The chemotherapy regimen is extrapolated from data from head and neck cancers with detectable primary.

- **Concurrent:** Single-agent cisplatin, carboplatin, or cetuximab
- **Neoadjuvant:** Docetaxel, cisplatin, and 5-FU

Side Effect Management

See **Oral Cavity** chapter.

Follow-up

- CT of the neck at 8 weeks posttreatment +/– PET/CT at 12 weeks. Failure to achieve complete response mandates neck dissection.
- H&P exam with fiberoptic and skin examination q2-4 mo for years 1-2, q6mo for years 3-5, and q12mo thereafter. Further follow-up imaging as clinically indicated
- TSH q6-12 mo. Annual low-dose chest CT or CXR for patients with smoking history; smoking cessation counseling as indicated

Notable Trials

Surgery alone

- **Mayo Clinic** (*Coster et al. IJROBP* 1992). Retrospective study of 24 patients with unilateral CUP treated by dissection or excisional biopsy; 58% N1 disease; 33% ECE. Primary developed in 4%; neck recurrence in 25%; all but 1 neck recurrence had ECE. Both N1 patients who recurred had ECE. 5-Year OS is 66%. Surgery alone may be sufficient in pN1 and no ECE; consider adjuvant RT if pN2+ or ECE

Radiation

- **Danish** (*Grau et al. Radiother Oncol* 2000). National survey of 277 pts with CUP treated with definitive therapy; 81% treated with bilateral neck + mucosal RT (nasopharynx, hypopharynx, oropharynx, and larynx), 10% treated with ipsilateral RT, 9% with surgery alone. Mucosal primary emergence rate was 19% (50% in lung/esophagus). Emergence of primary was significantly higher with surgery alone vs with RT (54% vs 15%, *P* < .0001). Relative risk of locoregional recurrence was 1.9 for ipsilateral RT vs bilateral + mucosal RT.

- **MD Anderson** (*Kamal et al. Cancer* 2018). Retrospective analysis of 260 pts treated with IMRT to bilateral neck + mucosa. 5-Year OS, regional control, and DMFS were 84%, 91%, and 95%, respectively. 7% had chronic radiation-associated dysphagia. No obvious benefit of adding chemotherapy
- **Beth Israel** (*Hu et al. Oral Oncol* 2017). 60 patients treated with bilateral neck RT + oropharynx mucosa; 82% had neck dissection, 55% received IMRT, and 62% had concurrent chemoradiotherapy. 5-Year regional control, distant metastasis, and overall survival were 90%, 20%, and 79%, respectively. 5-Year primary emergence rate was 10% overall and 3% in nonoropharynx site.

Unilateral vs bilateral radiation

- **Princess Margaret** (*Weir et al. Radiother Oncol* 1995). Retrospective analysis of 144 patients with CUP (85 pts irradiated to involved node region vs 59 pts irradiated to bilateral neck + mucosal sites). 5-Year OS is 41%; trend toward improved survival for treatment of both potential primary sites and nodes ($P = .07$), but no difference in both OS and CSS after adjusting for extent of nodal disease. RT of involved node alone may be adequate in selected patients.
- **Loyola** (*Reddy et al. IJROBP* 1997). Retrospective analysis of 52 patients (36 pts bilateral neck RT + mucosal sites vs 16 pts unilateral neck RT). Control of contralateral neck: 86% for bilateral RT vs 56% with unilateral RT ($P = .03$); mucosal primary emergence 8% for bilateral RT vs 44% for unilateral RT ($P = .0005$). Similar 5-year OS. Bilateral RT + mucosal irradiation is superior for preventing contralateral recurrence and mucosal emergence.

EARLY-STAGE NSCLC

SHERVIN 'SEAN' SHIRVANI • ERIC D. BROOKS • JOE Y. CHANG

BACKGROUND

- **Incidence/prevalence:** The second most common diagnosed cancer and leading cause of cancer death among men and women in the United States.
- **Outcomes:** 5-Year survival estimated at 54% for localized disease, 26% for regional nodal involvement, and 4% for distant disease (SEER). NOTE: 5-Year survival often worse for patients treated with SABR compared with surgery; most patients treated with SABR are medically inoperable and expected to have shorter life expectancy due to greater comorbidities (selection bias). Recent pooled randomized data show SABR yields equivalent or better OS compared with lobectomy and nodal dissection in medically operable patents (STARS/ROSEL trials).
- **Risk factors:** Smoking, radon, ionizing radiation, asbestos, chromium, male sex, family history, acquired lung disease (ie, interstitial pulmonary fibrosis), and other occupational exposures (silica, arsenic, beryllium, coal).
- **Prognostic factors:** Stage, performance status, weight loss, molecular mutations.

TUMOR BIOLOGY AND CHARACTERISTICS

- **Genetic markers:** Higher percentage of clinically relevant mutations that are targetable are found in adenocarcinomas. These include *EGFR* (~20% of adeno cases), *ALK* (~5%), *KRAS*, *ROS-1* (~2%), *BRAF*, *MET*, *RET*, and *PDL-1*.
- **Pathology:** Majority are adenocarcinomas (40% of lung malignancies), then squamous cell carcinomas (30%). Rarer histologies include large cell (15%), neuroendocrine, bronchoalveolar (arising from type II pneumocytes), and carcinoid.

ANATOMY

- Right lung: 3 lobes (upper, middle, lower) and 2 fissures (major, minor)
- Left lung: 2 lobes (upper, lower) and 1 fissure (major)
- Drainage most commonly to ipsi hilar/mediastinal nodes. Hematogenous spread common.
- Lymph node names (numeric classifications) (Fig. 32.1):
  ***Supraclavicular*:** Low cervical, supraclavicular, and sternal notch (LN station 1)
  ***Superior mediastinal*:** Upper paratracheal (2R/L), prevascular (3a), retrotracheal (3p), and lower paratracheal (4R/L)
  ***Aortic*:** Subaortic (5) and para-aortic (6)
  ***Inferior mediastinal*:** Subcarinal (7), paraesophageal (8), and pulmonary ligament (9)
  ***N1*:** Hilar (10), interlobar (11), lobar (12), segmental (13), and subsegmental (14)
- Pancoast tumor (syndrome): Superior sulcus tumor associated with shoulder pain, Horner syndrome (ipsilateral ptosis, miosis, anhidrosis), and atrophy of hand muscles

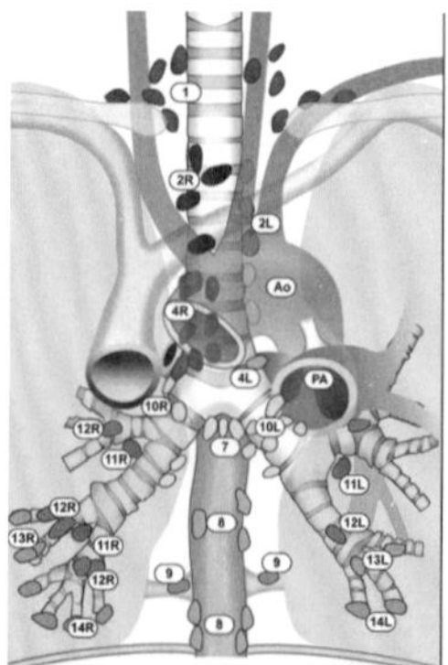

Figure 32.1 Diagram illustrating mediastinal and thoracic lymph node stations. (Adapted from Edge SB, Byrd DR, Compton CC, Fritz AG, Greene FL, Trotti A III. eds. *AJCC cancer staging manual*. 7th ed. New York, NY: Springer; 2010. Copyright © 2010 American Joint Committee on Cancer. Reproduced with permission of Springer in the format Book via Copyright Clearance Center.)

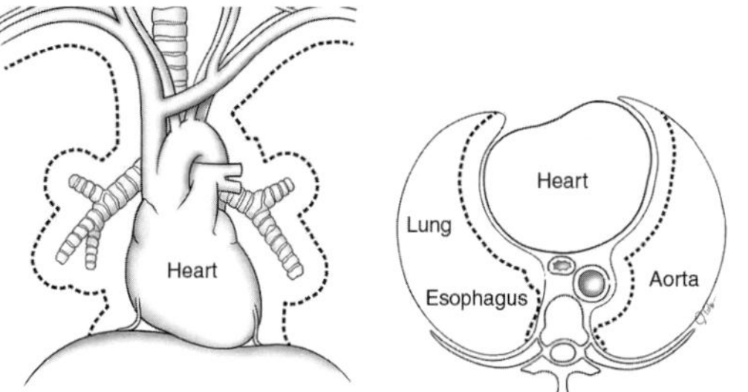

Figure 32.2 Central zone figure. (Reprinted from Chang JY, Bezjak A, Mornex F, et al. Stereotactic ablative radiotherapy for centrally located early stage non-small-cell lung cancer: what we have learned. *J Thorac Oncol.* 2015;10(4):577-585. Copyright © 2015 International Association for the Study of Lung Cancer. With permission.)

- Early-stage (T1-3N0) tumors are divided into central and peripheral lesions. The central zone is defined as the region within 2 cm of the proximal bronchial tree (Fig. 32.2) (which extends from the trachea to the lobar bronchi and other central structures [esophagus, heart, pericardium, great vessels, vertebral body]). Peripheral lesions are beyond this 2-cm zone. Distinction is important for risk of lymph node spread and treatment planning.

WORKUP

- **History and physical:** Typically present with cough, shortness of breath, hemoptysis, weight loss, and/or incidental mass on chest x-ray/CT.
- **Screening:** Annual low-dose CT scan recommended for pts aged 55-74 with ≥30 pack-year smoking history and cessation <15 years ago (*NLST NEJM* 2011).
- **Labs:** CBC, CMP
- **Procedures/biopsy:** Consider CT-guided biopsy if able to obtain tissue of primary. Not necessary if pathology more easily obtained by sampling suspicious nodes during mediastinal staging. Selective sampling of hila/mediastinum (eg, mediastinoscopy, EBUS) is recommended for higher-risk characteristics including central tumors, radiographic suspicion of adenopathy, or ≥T2a tumors but should be considered for all tumors. Pulmonary function testing to evaluate surgical candidacy and to provide baseline.
- **Imaging:** CT of the chest w/ contrast and PET/CT to rule out regional/distant disease for all patients. Brain MRI for all ≥T2a tumors (optional for T1b) or neurologic symptoms. Consider MRI of the shoulder for superior sulcus tumors and octreotide scans if with carcinoid histology.

NSCLC STAGING *(AJCC 8TH EDITION)*

T Stage		**N Stage**	
T1	≤3 cm without main bronchus invasion	N1	Ipsi peribronchial/hilar LN
T1a	≤1 cm	N2	Ipsi mediastinal/subcarinal LN
T1b	>1-2 cm	N3	Scalene/supraclav LN or contra mediastinal/hilar LN
T1c	>2-3 cm	**M Stage**	
T2	>3-5 cm or involves main bronchus but not carina, invades visceral pleura, or associated atelectasis or obstructive PNA	M1a	Nodule in contra lobe, pleura, or pericardium, or malignant pleural or pericardial effusion
T2a	>3-4 cm	M1b	Single extrathoracic metastasis
T2b	>4-5 cm	M1c	Multiple extrathoracic mets
T3	>5-7 cm or separate nodule in the same lobe or invades CW, phrenic nerve, parietal pericardium		
T4	>7 cm or separate nodule in different ipsi lobe or invades the diaphragm, mediastinum, heart, great vessels, trachea, recurrent laryngeal nerve, esophagus, vertebral body, carina		

Stage Grouping

	N0	N1	N2	N3	M1a-b	M1c
T1a-c	IA1-3	IIB	IIIA	IIIB	IVA	IVB
T2a	IB	IIB	IIIA	IIIB	IVA	IVB
T2b	IIA	IIB	IIIA	IIIB	IVA	IVB
T3	IIB	IIIA	IIIB	IIIC	IVA	IVB
T4	IIIA	IIIA	IIIB	IIIC	IVA	IVB

Locally Advanced NSCLC (stage III)

Treatment Algorithm

Stages I-II **(T1-3 satellite nodule, N0M0)**	• Regional/distant disease ruled out during workup. • Surgical candidate (usually postoperative predictive FEV1 >40% and deemed surgical candidate by thoracic surgeon) → lobectomy plus mediastinal lymph node dissection. • Nonsurgical candidate or decline surgery → SABR (aka SBRT). • For special circumstances in which patient tolerance and disease may be limiting, nonpreferred, alternative treatments include sublobar resection, radiofrequency ablation, cryotherapy, chemoradiation, and hypofractionated or conventional radiation.

Radiation Treatment Technique (Stereotactic Ablative Radiotherapy, also Called Stereotactic Body Radiation Therapy)

- **SIM:** Supine with Vac-Lok device and arms above the head. Four-dimensional imaging required. If tumor moves more than 10 mm, consider breath-hold technique or gating if patient is able to hold breath. Scan from base of the skull to top of the kidneys to encompass lung volume across the entire respiratory cycle.
- **Dose:** Goal is BED > 100 (Onishi et al. showed this is required for optimal local control).
  50 Gy to PTV in 4 fractions (peripheral)
  70 Gy to PTV in 10 fractions (central that cannot be safely treated with 50 Gy in 4 fractions, or peripheral lesion abutting the chest wall where 50 Gy in 4 fractions could lead to chest wall injury/pain).
  Note: For large-volume PTV in central regions, consider SIB (70 Gy to iGTV, 50 Gy to PTV in 10 fractions).
- **Target:** iGTV: Tumor across all phases of respiratory cycle (contour on MIP) or, when used, across all breath-hold trials.
  PTV: iGTV + 5 mm.
- **Technique:** 3DCRT, IMRT/VMAT. 6-10 MV photons with heterogeneity correction.
- **IGRT:** Daily cone beam CT with respiratory management.
- **Peripheral tumor planning directive (for 50 Gy in 4 fractions):**
  Chest wall: V30 ≤ 30 cc
  Skin: V30 ≤ 50 cc
  Vessels: V40 ≤ 1 cc, D_{max} ≤ 56 Gy
  Trachea: V35 ≤ 1 cc, D_{max} ≤ 38 Gy
  Bronchial tree: V35 ≤ 1 cc, D_{max} ≤ 38 Gy
  Brachial plexus: V30 ≤ 0.2 cc, D_{max} ≤ 35 Gy
  Esophagus: V30 ≤ 1 cc, D_{max} ≤ 35 Gy
  Heart/pericardium: V40 ≤ 1 cc, V20 ≤ 5 cc, D_{max} ≤ 45 Gy
  Spinal cord: V20 ≤ 1 cc, D_{max} ≤ 25 Gy
  Ipsilateral lung: iMLD ≤ 10 Gy, iV10 ≤ 35%, iV20 ≤ 25%, iV30 ≤ 15%
  Total lung: MLD ≤ 6 Gy, V5 ≤ 5%, V10 ≤ 17%, V20 ≤ 12%, V30 ≤ 7%
- **Central tumor planning directive (for 70 Gy in 10 fractions):**
  Chest wall/skin: V50 ≤ 60 cc, D_{max} ≤ 82 Gy
  Vessels: V50 ≤ 1 cc, D_{max} ≤ 75 Gy

Trachea: V40 ≤ 1 cc, D_{max} ≤ 60 Gy
Bronchial tree: V50 ≤ 1 cc, D_{max} ≤ 60 Gy
Brachial plexus: V50 ≤ 0.2 cc, D_{max} ≤ 55 Gy
Esophagus: V40 ≤ 1 cc, D_{max} ≤ 50 Gy
Heart/pericardium: V45 ≤ 1 cc, D_{max} ≤ 60 Gy
Spinal cord: V35 ≤ 1 cc, D_{max} ≤ 40 Gy
Total lung: MLD ≤ 9 Gy, V40 ≤ 7%

Side Effect Management

- Esophagitis: Magic mouthwash (viscous lidocaine, Benadryl, nystatin), glutamine supplement (eg, Helios), aloe products, and narcotic elixir second line.
- Chest wall pain: OTC analgesics (eg, Tylenol, NSAIDs) or neuropathic agents (select agent based on pain etiology—radicular/neurogenic, myositis/muscular), narcotics second line.
- Pneumonitis: For symptomatic patients (shortness of breath, reduction in O_2 on pulse oxygenation), consider oral steroid taper (typically prednisone starting at 1 mg/kg daily for 2-3 weeks with taper). Bactrim prophylaxis for PCP pneumonia and antacid prophylaxis for gastric ulcers.

Follow-Up

- CT of the chest with contrast q3mo for years 1-2, q6mo for years 3-5, and annually thereafter.
- PET for suspicious CT findings (establish postradiation changes vs recurrence).
- Biopsy for imaging findings consistent with recurrence.

Notable Literature

Stereotactic body radiation therapy—single arm

- RTOG 0236 (*Timmerman et al. JAMA* 2010, update ASTRO abstract 2014): 55 patients with inoperable, stage I NSCLC. *Peripheral only*. 54 Gy in 3 fractions (heterogeneity corrected) over 1.5-2 weeks. 3-Year LC 98%, LRC 87%, DFS 48%, and OS 54%. 17% grade 3 or higher toxicity (4% grade 4 or higher). At 5 years, LC is 98%, LRC 62%, and OS 40%. Importantly, EBUS was not required prior to treatment on this trial.
- RTOG 0813 (*Bezjak et al. ASTRO abstract* 2015 and 2016): Phase I/II trial of 120 patients with inoperable, central (within 2 cm of tracheal/bronchia tree or adjacent to mediastinal/pericardial pleura), stage I NSCLC. 50-60 Gy in 5 fractions. Treatment was given every other day for 1.5 to 2 weeks. Less than 10% dose-limiting treatment toxicity observed but several treatment-related deaths were reported. Final results for oncologic outcomes are pending; however, 7/33 patients treated to 11.5 Gy or 12 Gy/fx had grade 3+ toxicity.
- Phase II SABR Study (*Sun et al. Cancer* 2017): 65 patients, inoperable, stage I, median of 7.2-year follow-up. 7-Year local recurrence was 8.1% and regional recurrence 13.6%. 7-Year PFS was 38.2%, and OS was 47.5%. 4.6% of patients experienced grade 3 or greater events. No grade 4 or 5 events.
- RTOG 0915. Single fraction SBRT randomized phase II (*Videtic et al. IJROBP* 2015). 94 patients, medically inoperable treated to either 34 Gy/1 fx or 48 Gy/4 fx. Adverse event rate between single fraction and multiple fraction regimens similar (10.1% vs 13.3%), along with local control at 1 year (97% vs 92.7%).

Comparison of SBRT vs surgery

- STARS/ROSEL Combined Analysis (*Chang et al. Lancet Oncol* 2015). Unplanned pooled analysis of two randomized controlled trials comparing SBRT and lobectomy. 58 patients randomized. SBRT arm had similar 3-year relapse-free survival (86% vs 80%, P = .54) and improved overall survival (95% vs 79%, HR 0.14, P = .037). Lower grade 3+ event rates with SBRT vs surgery (10% vs 44%). Further studies are warranted to compare these treatment strategies.

STAGE III NSCLC

STEPHEN GRANT • ERIC D. BROOKS • DANIEL GOMEZ

Background

- **Incidence/prevalence:** Stage III NSCLC accounts for ~1/3 of all NSCLC cases.
- **Outcomes:** 5-Year OS for stage III is highly variable and dependent on numerous factors including performance status and comorbidities, estimated to be between 5% and 35% (IIIA, 30%; IIIB, 10%-15%).
- **Demographics and risk factors:** See **Early Stage NSCLC** chapter.

Tumor Biology and Characteristics

See **Early Stage NSCLC** chapter.

Anatomy

See **Early Stage NSCLC** chapter.

Workup

See **Early Stage NSCLC** chapter.

Treatment Algorithm (Stage III)

Resectable	**Neoadjuvant chemo → surgery → PORT** • Allows for tailored RT based on surgical findings, also selects for patients who do not metastasize after chemotherapy, therefore optimizing the benefits of local therapy indications for PORT: N2, (+)margins, residual disease **Neoadjuvant chemoRT → surgery** • May reduce tumor size to decrease extent of surgery • Not a preferred option in patients who would undergo pneumonectomy
Superior sulcus tumor	**Neoadjuvant chemoRT → surgery → completion chemoRT if unresectable** • Preferred approach for borderline resectable T3-4N0-1 tumors (SWOG 9416) **Surgery → chemoRT if unresectable** • Consideration for upfront resectable tumor especially for resectable tumors with significant symptoms (*Gomez et al. Cancer* 2012)
Unresectable[a]	**Definitive chemoRT → adjuvant durvalumab**[b] • Consider RT alone in elderly patients or poor PS.

[a]Includes patients with multiple N2 stations, N3, bulky/invasive LN, lobectomy not feasible, med inoperable
[b]PACIFIC trial: ↑ PFS with durvalumab (anti–PD-L1) compared to placebo following chemoRT

Radiation Treatment Technique

- **Simulation:**
  - Supine, upper body cradle, arms above head, and wedge below knee. A 4DCT preferred. Consider breath-hold if tumor moves >1 cm. Optional fusion with PET
- **Dose:**
  - **Definitive (able to tolerate chemotherapy):** 60 Gy in 30 fractions with concurrent chemotherapy
    Consider simultaneous integrated boost to GTV to 66 Gy.
  - **PORT:** 50.4 Gy in 28 fractions or 50 Gy in 25 fractions
    Increase dose for areas of concern (60-66 Gy for positive margins).
    Add concurrent chemo for gross residual dx.
    Add sequential chemo for N2 disease.
  - **Neoadjuvant:** 45 Gy in 1.8 Gy/fx > surgery if operable or completion to 60-66 Gy radiation if inoperable
  - **RT alone (if unable to tolerate chemotherapy):** 45 Gy in 15 fractions to PTV and SIB to 52.5-60 Gy in 15 fractions to GTV.
  - **Superior sulcus tumors:**
    Neoadjuvant: 45 Gy in 1.8 Gy/fx > surgery if operable or completion to 60-66 Gy radiation if inoperable

Adjuvant: Consider Hyper FX regimen (60 Gy in 1.2 Gy/fx bid) to minimize late radiation effects and reduce risk of brachial plexopathy (*Gomez et al. Cancer* 2012).

- **Target:**
  - **Definitive/neoadjuvant:**

    CTV: GTV contoured on MIP + 8 mm, edited out of the bone and heart, and includes involved nodal stations and, if dose constraints met, ipsilateral hilum (no other elective nodal irradiation except ipsilateral hilum if staging adequate)

    PTV: CTV + 5 mm if daily kV or CTV + 3 mm if daily CBCT
- **Technique:**
  IMRT/VMAT or protons
- **IGRT:**
  Daily kV imaging and weekly CBCT
- **Planning directive (for daily fractionation):**
  Spinal cord: D_{max} < 45 Gy
  Total lung: MLD < 20 Gy, V20 < 35%, V10 < 45%, and V5 < 60%
  Heart: V30Gy < 45%, mean < 26 Gy
  Esophagus: D_{max} < 80 Gy, V70 < 20%, V50 < 40%, and mean < 34 Gy
  Kidney (bilateral): V20Gy < 32%
  Liver: V30Gy < 40%, mean liver <30Gy
  Brachial plexus: D_{max} < 66 Gy

SURGERY

- Surgical resection alone is not sufficient treatment for locally advanced NSCLC.
- Standard surgery is **lobectomy with mediastinal lymph node dissection**.
- Other options depending on the extent of disease include pneumonectomy, segmentectomy, and sleeve resection

SYSTEMIC THERAPY

- Most commonly given alone in the preoperative setting or concurrent with radiation
- **Concurrent chemo:**
  - Cisplatin and etoposide
  - Cisplatin and vinblastine
  - Carboplatin and pemetrexed
  - Cisplatin and pemetrexed
  - Carboplatin and paclitaxel
- **Neoadjuvant and adjuvant chemo:**
  - Multiple platinum-based combinations including cisplatin with etoposide, paclitaxel, pemetrexed, and vincristine
  - If patient can't tolerate cisplatin, consider carboplatin and paclitaxel.
- **Immunotherapy**
  - Adjuvant durvalumab for at least 1 year (if no progression of disease after definitive chemoradiation).

SIDE EFFECT MANAGEMENT

See **Early Stage NSCLC** chapter.

FOLLOW-UP

- History/physical and CT: Every 3 months for 2 years → annually for 3 years
- Postradiation toxicity

  Esophagitis peaks 1-2 weeks after radiation therapy and then resolves weeks-months

  Radiation pneumonitis: Occurs 6 weeks to 1 year following RT with symptoms of dyspnea, cough, and fatigue. Inflammatory changes within RT field on imaging. Treat with high-dose steroid taper.

  Esophageal stricture/fistula (months-years)

  Long-term dyspnea/fibrosis (months-years)

  Brachial plexopathy for apical tumors (years)

NOTABLE LITERATURE AND TRIALS

Evidence supporting trimodality therapy

- **INT 0139** (*Albain et al. Lancet* 2009): Phase III randomized study of 429 operable stage IIIA (N2) patients randomized to surgery (pneumonectomy or lobectomy) vs no surgery following neoadjuvant chemoradiation. All patients received adjuvant cisplatin/etoposide. RT in the surgery arm was 45 Gy/25 fx. Those randomized to no surgery received definitive chemoRT to a total of 61 Gy. Median PFS improved in surgical arm (12.8 vs 10.5 months, $P = .017$), but not 5-year OS (27% surgery vs 20% chemoRT, $P = .10$). Unplanned subgroup analysis showed that pneumonectomy was associated with high mortality risk but that lobectomy was associated with improved OS compared to patients randomized to no surgery.

- **SWOG 9416** (*Rusch et al. JCO* 2007): Phase II single-arm study of 110 superior sulcus tumor patients with T3-4N0-1. Patients received 45 Gy with concurrent cisplatin/etoposide → surgical resection → adjuvant cisplatin/etoposide × 2 cycles. 83 patients underwent complete resection and pathologic complete response seen in 61 patients. 5-Year survival was 44% for all patients and 54% after complete resection.

Postoperative radiation (PORT)

- **PORT Meta-analysis Trialists Group** (*Lancet* 1998). Included 2128 patients who were treated on 9 randomized controlled trial between 1966 and 1994. OS was found to be worse in those who received PORT with an HR of 1.21 ($P = .001$).
- **Adjuvant Navelbine International Trialist Association (ANITA) Trial.** (*Douillard et al. IJROBP* 2008). Retrospective analysis of a prospective adjuvant chemotherapy trial where patients were randomized to surgery +/– chemo. PORT was recommended for pN+ patients but not mandated. 238/840 patients (28%) received PORT to 45-60 Gy. In univariate analysis among all patients, PORT deleterious on OS, but survival benefit was seen in pN2 patients regardless of whether chemotherapy was given.

Evidence supporting definitive chemoradiation approach

- **EORTC 08941** (*van Meerbeeck et al. JNCI* 2007): Phase III prospective randomized trial of 579 operable stage III patients randomizing to induction chemotherapy followed by either surgery or radiation (60-62.5 Gy total). PORT allowed in surgical arm if positive margins (40% of patients received PORT on surgical arm). 5-Year OS (resection, 15.7%; and RT, 14%) and PFS were not significantly different between arms. Radiation was associated with less morbidity.
- **RTOG 9410** (*Curran et al. JNCI* 2011): Three-arm prospective randomized trial of 610 patients with inoperable stage II-IIIB NSCLC. The three arms were the following: arm 1, induction chemotherapy followed by radiation (vinblastine/cisplatin → 63 Gy in 34 fractions in 1.8 Gy × 25 fractions and then 2 Gy × 9 fractions); arm 2, standard daily chemoradiation (cisplatin/vinblastine and 63 Gy in 34 fractions); and arm 3, concurrent bid high-dose chemoradiation (cisplatin/etoposide and 69.6 Gy in 58 fractions bid). Acute toxicity was worse in the bid chemoradiation arm, specifically acute esophagitis grade 3-4: arm 1, 4%; arm 2, 23%; and arm 3, 42% ($P < .001$). However, OS was moderately improved with chemoradiation arms compared to sequential treatment: arm 1, 14.6 months; arm 2, 17 months; and arm 3, 15.6 months.
- **NSCLC Collaborative Group Meta-Analysis** (*Auperin et al. JCO* 2010). Combined data from six eligible RCTs of locally advanced NSCLC, total of 1205 patients. Concurrent chemoRT found to be associated with absolute survival benefit of 4.5% at 5 years ($P = .004$).

Benefit with adjuvant immunotherapy after chemoradiation

- **PACIFIC** (*Antonia et al. NEJM* 2017): Phase III randomized trial of 713 patients with stage III unresectable NSCLC randomized after completion of definitive chemoradiation to adjuvant durvalumab for 1 year (anti–PD-L1 immunotherapy) or observation. PFS was higher with adjuvant durvalumab (16.8 vs 5.6 months, HR = 0.52, $P < .001$). Time to distant metastasis or death was also better with durvalumab (23.2 vs 14.6 months, $P < .001$). Grade 3-4 toxicity was not increased with durvalumab (29.9% vs 26.1% placebo). Patients with and without PD-L1 expression benefited.

Dose escalation for definitive chemoradiation leads to worse outcomes

- **RTOG 0617** (*Bradley et al. Lancet Oncol* 2015): Phase III 2 × 2 randomized trial of stage IIIA-B to dose-escalated chemoradiation (60 vs 74 Gy with carboplatin/paclitaxel). Patients then were randomized for the second time to receive adjuvant cetuximab or nothing. The trial was closed early due to futility. OS was worse in the 74 Gy group (1 year: 80% vs 69.8%, $P = .004$) and adding cetuximab did not improve survival. Reason for the poorer survival in the high-dose group was possibly worse heart dose (no DVH restraints required). Secondary analysis demonstrates correlation of increased heart V40Gy with worse survival (*Chun et al. JCO* 2017).

SMALL CELL LUNG CANCER

ALEXANDER AUGUSTYN • ERIC D. BROOKS • DANIEL GOMEZ

Background

- **Incidence/prevalence:** ~30 000 cases of SCLC per year in the United States (15% of all lung cancer diagnoses). About 1/3 are diagnosed with limited stage disease.
- **Outcomes:** 5-Year survival for stage I, II, III, and IV disease is 31%, 19%, 8%, and 2%, respectively.
- **Demographics:** Average age of diagnosis is 70. Highest incidence in white male smokers
- **Risk factors:** Smoking is the biggest risk factor (>90% of patients are heavy smokers). Increasing age, asbestos, and radon gas exposure are also risk factors.

Tumor Biology and Characteristics

- **Genetics:** TCGA genomic profiling of 110 SCLCs identified loss of *TP53* and *RB1* in nearly all cases. 25% of patients exhibited inactivating NOTCH pathway mutations. Targetable mutations in *EGFR*, *ALK*, *K-RAS*, and *ROS-1* not seen in SCLC
- **Pathology:** Malignant epithelial tumor of small round blue cells of neuroendocrine origin (Fig. 34.1) and scant cytoplasm. Necrosis often extensively seen in pathologic specimens with high mitotic count. SCLC is grouped into two variants: small cell carcinoma and combined small cell carcinoma, which include SCLC cells and any histologic subtype of NSCLC. On pathology, positive staining seen for synaptophysin, chromogranin A, IGF-1, and CD56 and typically negative for TTF1 and keratin (which are positive in NSCLC)
- **Imaging:** Enhance significantly on contrasted CT and highly PET-avid as well (Fig.34.1). Typically presents centrally as opposed to peripherally

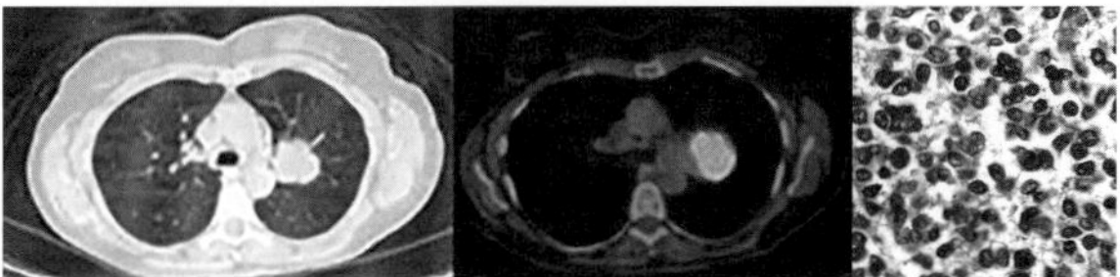

Figure 34.1 Representative CT (*left*) and PET (*middle*) images obtained from a patient presenting with cough/weight loss. The LUL mass and L hilar LNs were biopsied with pathology returning as SCLC. Note the small, round blue cells with scant cytoplasm and large nuclei which is classic for SCLC (*right image*).

Workup

- **History and physical:** High frequency of bulky mediastinal lymphadenopathy leads to shortness of breath, hoarse voice, dysphagia, and/or superior vena cava syndrome. Evaluate for neurologic symptoms, paraneoplastic syndromes, and bone pain.
- **Labs:** CBC, CMP, LFTs, and LDH. SCLC is the most common solid malignancy associated with paraneoplastic syndromes: Syndrome of inappropriate antidiuretic hormone SIADH seen in 11%-15% of patients. Ectopic Cushing syndrome (5%) and Lambert-Eaton syndrome (1%-3%) are also observed.
- **Procedures/biopsy:** Bronchoscopy +/– FNA with biopsy if central, CT-guided, or thoracentesis for peripheral lesions. If cT1-T2N0 disease with no evidence of distant metastases, consider mediastinal staging.
- **Imaging:** CT of the chest with contrast and PET/CT done for staging (identifying distant metastases, distinguishing between limited stage and extensive stage). MRI of the brain w/ contrast performed on all patients as the brain is a sanctuary site with respect to chemotherapy and frequently the first site of failure in patients with SCLC

Anatomy

- See Early NSCLC section.

SMALL CELL LUNG CANCER STAGING (AJCC 8TH EDITION)

(Same as NSCLC; however, use of historical "limited" and "extensive" stage definitions is frequently made)

T Stage		N Stage	
T1	≤3 cm without main bronchus invasion	N1	Ipsi peribronchial/hilar LN
T1a	≤1 cm	N2	Ipsi mediastinal/subcarinal LN
T1b	>1-2 cm	N3	Scalene/supraclav LN or contra mediastinal/hilar LN
T1c	>2-3 cm	**M Stage**	
T2	>3-5 cm or involves the main bronchus but not carina, invades visceral pleura, or associated atelectasis or obstructive pneumonia	M1a	Nodule in contra lobe, pleura, or pericardium or malignant pleural or pericardial effusion
T2a	>3-4 cm	M1b	Single extrathoracic metastasis
T2b	>4-5 cm	M1c	Multiple extrathoracic mets
T3	>5-7 cm or separate nodule in the same lobe or invades CW, phrenic nerve, parietal pericardium		
T4	>7 cm or separate nodule in different ipsi lobe or invades the diaphragm, mediastinum, heart, great vessels, trachea, recurrent laryngeal nerve, esophagus, vertebral body, carina		

Stage Grouping

<table>
<tr><th></th><th>N0</th><th>N1</th><th>N2</th><th>N3</th><th>M1a-b</th><th>M1c</th></tr>
<tr><td>T1a-c</td><td>IA1-3</td><td rowspan="3">IIB</td><td rowspan="3">IIIA</td><td rowspan="3">IIIB</td><td rowspan="5">IVA</td><td rowspan="5">IVB</td></tr>
<tr><td>T2a</td><td>IB</td></tr>
<tr><td>T2b</td><td>IIA</td></tr>
<tr><td>T3</td><td>IIB</td><td rowspan="2">IIIA</td><td rowspan="2">IIIB</td><td rowspan="2">IIIC</td></tr>
<tr><td>T4</td><td></td></tr>
</table>

Locally Advanced SCLC (stage III)

VA LUNG CANCER STUDY GROUP STAGING

- Historical definitions:
  - **Limited stage:** Intrathoracic disease that can be encompassed within a reasonable radiation field, excluding those with pleural or pericardial effusions. However, applicability of these definitions to modern techniques is questionable. Overall, "limited" = localized; "extensive" = metastatic
  - **Extensive stage:** All others

TREATMENT ALGORITHM

Limited stage	• For solitary pulmonary nodule and medically operable based on PFTs → mediastinoscopy → proceed to surgery (lobectomy preferred) if negative lymph node involvement. Adjuvant platinum and etoposide 4-6 cycles followed by PCI. For positive nodes after resection, proceed to concurrent chemoRT followed by PCI. • For locally advanced disease → chemoRT followed by PCI. If poor performance status, can consider chemotherapy alone or supportive care
Extensive stage	• Platinum and etoposide ×4-6 cycles → for partial or complete response, consolidative chest RT. Weigh risks/benefits and consider PCI. • Patients with symptomatic brain mets or cord compression, provide palliative RT +/– steroids and 4-6 cycles of platinum/etoposide → for partial or complete response, consolidative chest RT

Chemotherapy Treatment Guidelines

- **LS-SCLC:** Acceptable regimens for limited stage disease (maximum 4-6 cycles)
  Cisplatin or carboplatin with etoposide
  During concurrent chemoradiation, cisplatin/etoposide is recommended.
- **ES-SCLC:** Acceptable regimens for extensive stage disease (maximum 4-6 cycles)
  Cisplatin or carboplatin with etoposide

Radiation Treatment Technique

- **SIM:** 4DCT, supine, both arms abducted holding T-bar, upper Vac-Lok, wingboard, and knee wedge. Consider breath-hold technique if motion is >1 cm on 4D CT scan (Fig. 34.2).
- **Dose: Limited stage:** 45 Gy in 30 fractions twice a day (at least 6 hours apart) at 1.5 Gy/fx (preferred MDACC approach).
  If bid fractionation is not feasible, acceptable alternative is 1.8-2.0 Gy/d to a dose of 60-70 Gy. Radiation should be delivered concurrently with chemotherapy, ideally beginning during cycle 1.
  Extensive stage: 30 Gy in 10 fractions or 45 Gy in 15 fractions daily.
- **Target:** Paradigm similar to NSCLC. GTV defined by most recent PET/CT. If chemo is given first, can limit GTV to postchemo tumor volume. Use prechemo PET/CT involved LN stations. Historically, elective nodal radiation was used, but it is omitted in current trials as rate of nodal failure is low when using PET/CT for staging.
  Margins: 5- to 10-mm CTV, 5-mm PTV expansion for daily CBCT.
- **Technique:** IMRT (Fig. 34.3)
- **IGRT:** For free breathing treatment setup, daily kV imaging, and weekly CBCT
  For breath-hold treatment setup, CBCT before each fraction
- **Planning directive (either daily or BID fractionation)**
  Ensure coverage of PTV by >95% of prescription dose
  Spinal cord D_{max} < 36 Gy (bid), <45 Gy (daily).
  Mean lung dose <20 Gy, V20 < 35%, V10 < 45%, and V5 < 60%
  Heart V30 < 45 Gy, mean heart dose <26 Gy
  Esophagus D_{max} < 80 Gy, V70 < 20%, V50 < 40%, mean dose <34 Gy
  Kidney (bilateral) V20 < 32%
  Liver V30 < 40%, mean liver dose <30 Gy
  Brachial plexus D_{max} < 50.6 Gy (bid), <3 cc, >44.5 Gy (bid), D_{max} < 66 Gy (daily)
  Chest wall V40 < 150 cc (bid) (Figs. 34.2 and 34.3)

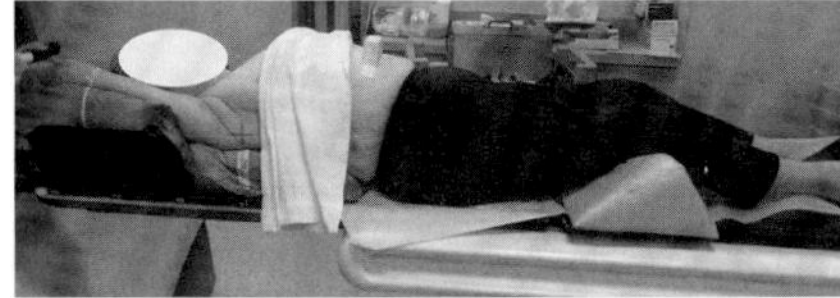

Figure 34.2 Typical SCLC/NSCLC simulation setup showing a patient positioned supine with a wingboard, upper Vac-Lok device, both hands gripping a T-bar. Opaque markers mounted on a box are taped to the patient's abdomen to assess breathing.

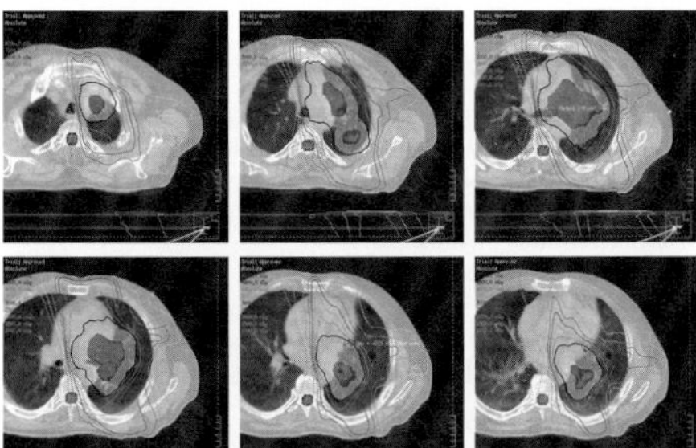

Figure 34.3 Limited stage SCLC IMRT plan. 45 Gy isodose line showed in *blue* surrounding PTV (*sky blue color wash*), CTV (*tan*), and GTV (*red*). Note sparing of contralateral lung. **See color insert.**

Prophylactic Cranial Irradiation (PCI)

- **Indication**
  - For limited stage, PCI should be discussed for patients with a partial or complete response following chemoRT, as it decreases the risk of developing brain metastasis by about 50% and improves OS based on clinical studies. Restage after completion of chemoRT and if no progression (local or distant) then consider starting PCI 6-12 weeks after chemoRT completion.
  - For extensive stage, a thorough discussion should take place in context of conflicting data (*Takahashi et al. Lancet Oncol* 2017; *Slotman et al. NEJM* 2017). Patients should be informed that it will reduce the risk of developing subsequent brain metastases with questionable OS benefit.
- **SIM:** Supine, holding A-bar, aquaplast mask with isocenter placed at midbrain.
- **Dose:** 25 Gy in 10 fractions
- **Target:** Whole brain, ensure coverage of cribriform plate and inferior edge should extend to C1/C2 vertebral bodies.
- **Technique:** 3DCRT. Beam arrangement typically opposed laterals or right and left anterior obliques (gantry angled to 85 and 275 degrees) to spare lens exposure due to beam divergence.
- **IGRT:** Usually no image guidance, setup to marks only. Consider daily MV or kV imaging.

Surgery

- High local recurrence rates (35%-50%) suggest that surgery may offer benefit in local control.
- Surgical resection generally only recommended for patients with a solitary pulmonary nodule, no evidence of local/regional lymphadenopathy, no distant metastatic disease, and no contraindications to surgery. Lobectomy preferred
- The survival of patients undergoing surgery for pathologic stage I, II, and III disease was 48%, 39%, and 15% at 5 years.
- No randomized trials exist for adjuvant therapy; however, most patients receive adjuvant chemotherapy and adjuvant radiation for those found to have pathologic N1 or N2 disease.

Side Effect Management

- Nausea: Zofran, Compazine, Reglan, low-dose dexamethasone, Haldol, IV fluids
- Pneumonitis: For symptomatic patients (eg, shortness of breath, drop in pO_2), consider oral steroid taper (typically prednisone starting at 1 mg/kg daily for 2-3 weeks, remember Bactrim prophylaxis for PCP pneumonia and antacid prophylaxis for ulcers)
- Esophagitis: Magic mouthwash (viscous lidocaine, Benadryl, nystatin), glutamine supplement (eg, Helios), aloe products, narcotic elixir second line
- Dermatitis: Aquaphor or other moisturizing cream, gel sheets
- Chest wall pain: Analgesics, physical therapy
- Neurocognitive side effects of PCI: Memantine 20 mg bid (start 20 mg daily ×1-2 weeks and then increase) to reduce risk of late neurocognitive side effects in patients with >6 months expected survival

Follow-Up

- History/physical and CT: Every 3 months for 2 years → annually for 3 years.
- Postradiation toxicity
  - Esophagitis peaks 1-2 weeks after radiation therapy and then resolves weeks-months
  - Radiation pneumonitis: Occurs 6 weeks to 1 year following RT with symptoms of dyspnea, cough, and fatigue. Inflammatory changes within RT field on imaging. Treat with high-dose steroid taper.
  - Esophageal stricture/fistula (months-years)
  - Long-term dyspnea/fibrosis (months-years)
  - Brachial plexopathy for apical tumors (years)

Notable Trials

Chemoradiation vs chemotherapy alone

- RT Meta-analysis (*Pignon et al. NEJM* 1992): Meta-analysis evaluated 13 trials with 2140 patients comparing chemo vs chemoRT and identified a 5% increase in 3-year overall survival with chemoRT (8.9 → 14.3%; *P* = .001). Local control improved from 16% to 34%. A trend was seen toward a larger reduction in mortality among younger patients (<55 years). Chemotherapy was predominately cyclophosphamide or doxorubicin based, not cisplatin + etoposide, which is standard of care.

Daily vs twice daily thoracic radiation in limited stage disease

- INT 0096 (*Turrisi et al. NEJM* 1998): Evaluated biologic advantage of bid treatment based on empiric data that the dose-response curve for SCLC lacks a shoulder. Prospective randomized phase III trial comparing daily vs twice daily concurrent chemoRT. Patients with limited stage disease were randomized to daily thoracic RT to 45 Gy in 1.8-Gy fractions over 5 weeks vs thoracic RT to 45 Gy in 1.5-Gy fractions BID. All patients receiving concurrent cis/etoposide. PCI was offered to those with a complete response after 12 weeks. OS at 5 years was improved by 10% with bid fractionation (16% vs 26%, $P = .04$), along with decreased rate of local failure in bid arm (36% vs 52%, $P = .06$). However, there was increased incidence of grade 3 esophagitis in bid fractionation arm (27% vs 11%, $P < .001$).
- CONVERT Trial (*Faivre-Finn et al. Lancet Oncol* 2017). Randomized 547 limited stage SCLC patients to either BID chemoRT (45 Gy/30 fx) or daily chemoRT (66 Gy/33 fx). Primary endpoint was 2-year OS and was found to be nonsignificant (56% BID vs 51% daily, $P = .14$). Toxicities were similar aside from increased grade 4 neutropenia in BID group (49% vs 38%, $P = .05$). Grade 3 esophagitis nonsignificant between both arms (19% in both)

Role of consolidative chemoRT in extensive stage disease

- Yugoslavia trial (*Jeremic et al. JCO* 1999): Phase III trial enrolled 210 patients treated w/ 3 cycles of cisplatin/etoposide. Pts w/ distant CR + local CR/PR randomized to RT (54 Gy in 36 fractions over 18 days) with concurrent carboplatin/etoposide followed by 2 more cycles of PE vs no radiation and 4 additional cycles of cisplatin/etoposide. PCI done for all patients with distant CR. Median survival improved in chemoRT consolidation arm (17 vs 11 months, $P = .041$).
- Netherlands trial (*Slotman et al. Lancet* 2015): Phase III study randomizing 498 ES-SCLC patients who had any response to cisplatin/etoposide to thoracic RT and PCI vs PCI alone. All patients received 4-6 cycles of cisplatin/etoposide. Thoracic RT was started within 7 weeks of chemotherapy to a dose of 30 Gy in 10 fraction targeting the postchemo GTV with a 15-mm margin. For those who received prechemoradiation, the involved hilar and mediastinal nodes were included. OS was improved at 2 years in thoracic RT arm (13% vs 3%, $P = .004$). Consolidative thoracic RT improved 6-month PFS (24% vs 7%, $P = .001$) and resulted in 50% reduction in intrathoracic recurrences.

Evidence for prophylactic cranial irradiation in SCLC

- PCI Meta-Analysis (*Auperin et al. NEJM* 1999). A total of 987 patients included from seven RCTs who received PCI vs no PCI in SCLC patients who achieved complete response to therapy (12%-17% had ES-SCLC). 3-Year OS was 21% vs 15% in favor of PCI ($P = .01$). 3-Year local control in the brain was 33% for PCI arm vs 59% in no PCI arm ($P < .001$). Larger RT doses (8, 24-25, 30, 36-40 Gy) led to greater decrease in risk of mets, but no impact on survival.
- EORTC 08993-22993 (*Slotman et al. NEJM* 2007). Phase III RCT of PCI vs no PCI in ES-SCLC with any response to platinum-based therapy. PCI doses ranged from 20 to 30 Gy in 10 fractions. 1-Year OS found to be improved with PCI (27.1% vs 13.3%, $P = .003$) with reduced incidence of brain mets (14.6% vs 40.4%, $P < .001$).
- Japanese Trial (*Takahashi et al. Lancet* 2017). Phase III RCT of PCI vs no PCI in ES-SCLC patients with any response to platinum-based doublet chemotherapy. PCI dose 25 Gy/10 fx. At 1 year, PCI reduces incidence of brain mets (32.9% PCI vs 59% no PCI, $P < .0001$), without improvement in median survival (11.6 months PCI vs 13.7 months no PCI, $P = .094$). Importantly, unlike the EORTC 08993-22993 study, patients received MRI for upfront staging. Close MRI surveillance was performed (q3mo) on all pts.

THYMOMA AND THYMIC CARCINOMA

SAMANTHA M. BUSZEK • ERIC D. BROOKS • QUYNH-NHU NGUYEN

BACKGROUND

- **Incidence/prevalence:** Rare, ~0.15/100 000, the most common neoplasm of the anterior mediastinum
- **Outcomes:** 5-Year OS by Masaoka stage: stage I, 95%; stage II, 90%; stage III, 60%; and stage IV, 11%-50%. Thymic carcinoma, 20%-30%
- **Demographics:** Median age 40-60 years; equal in males and females
- **Risk factors:** May be related to autoimmune disorders including myasthenia gravis. No other known etiologic risk factors

TUMOR BIOLOGY AND CHARACTERISTICS

- **Pathology:** Histologic subtypes include benign, medullary, and spindle cell, mixed; moderately malignant, lymphocyte-rich, lymphocytic, predominantly cortical, organoid, cortical, epithelial, atypical, squamoid, and well-differentiated thymic carcinoma; and highly malignant, thymic carcinoma (<1% of thymic tumors).

ANATOMY

Thymus originates from thymic *epithelial* cells (third pharyngeal pouch); involved in processing and maturation of T lymphocytes to recognize foreign Ag from self-Ag

- Thymomas: 1%-2% lymph node metastasis rate and 1% distant metastasis (mostly to the lung)
- Thymic carcinomas: 30% lymph node metastasis rate and 12% distant metastasis (lung, bone, liver)
- Lymph node drainage to the lower cervical, internal mammary, and hilar nodes
- **Differential of mediastinal mass**
  Anterior: Thymoma, thymic carcinoma, carcinoid, germ cell tumor, lymphoma, and goiter
  Middle: Cysts > lymphomas, teratomas > sarcomas, and granuloma
  Posterior: Neurogenic tumors (PNET, schwannomas, neurofibroma, neuroblastoma, ganglioneuroma) and pheochromocytoma

WORKUP AND STAGING

- **History and physical:** 1/3 asymptomatic (incidental), 1/3 myasthenia gravis, and 1/3 thoracic symptoms (cough, SOB, CP, SVC). Ask for B symptoms (rule out lymphoma). Thymoma diagnosed clinically if mediastinal mass + symptoms of myasthenia, red cell aplasia, or hypogammaglobulinemia
- **Labs:** LDH, ESR, and AFP/HCG (rule out germ cell tumor). Paraneoplastic syndromes include myasthenia gravis (35%-50%), due to autoAb to postsynaptic AChR; **symptoms**, easy fatigability, double vision, and ptosis; **diagnosis**, Tensilon test (edrophonium); **treatment**, AChE inhibitors (pyridostigmine) or thymectomy. May also present with red cell aplasia (5%), immune deficiency syndromes (ie, hypogammaglobulinemia, 5%), autoimmune disorders (collagen vascular, dermatologic, endocrine), and other malignancies (lymphomas, GI/breast carcinoma, Kaposi sarcoma)
- **Imaging/procedures:** CT of the chest with contrast preferred. MRI optional. PET/CT if lymphoma or thymic carcinoma suspected, PFTs. If thymoma is suspected, straight to surgery (avoid biopsy if resectable to avoid seeding)

NEW THYMOMA AND THYMIC CARCINOMA STAGING

(AJCC 8TH EDITION)

T Stage		N Stage	
T1a	Encapsulated or unencapsulated, w/ or w/o extension into mediastinal fat	N0	None
T1b	Extension into mediastinal pleura	N1	Anterior (perithymic) nodes

T Stage	
T2	Pericardium
T3	Lung, brachiocephalic vein, SVC, chest wall, phrenic nerve, hilar (extrapericardial) pulmonary vessels
T4	Aorta, arch vessels, main pulmonary artery, myocardium, trachea, or esophagus

N Stage	
N2	Intrathoracic or cervical nodes
M Stage	
M0	None
M1a	Separate pleural or pericardial nodule(s)
M1b	Pulmonary intraparenchymal nodule or distant organ mets

Summative Stage

<table>
<tr><th></th><th>N0</th><th>N1</th><th>N2</th><th>M1a</th><th>M1b</th></tr>
<tr><td>T1a</td><td rowspan="2">I</td><td rowspan="5">IVA</td><td rowspan="5">IVB</td><td rowspan="5">IVA</td><td rowspan="5">IVB</td></tr>
<tr><td>T1b</td></tr>
<tr><td>T2</td><td>II</td></tr>
<tr><td>T3</td><td>IIIA</td></tr>
<tr><td>T4</td><td>IIIB</td></tr>
</table>

Masaoka Stage	
	Completely encapsulated (micro and macro)
IIA	Microscopic transcapsular invasion
IIB	Macroscopic invasion into fatty tissue or adherent to pleura/pericardium
III	Macroscopic invasion into other organs (ie, pericardium, vessels, lung)
IVA	Mets to pleura/pericardium

TREATMENT ALGORITHM[a]

- Prognosis: associated with completeness of resection
- If myasthenia gravis, signs and symptoms should be controlled medically before surgery

WHO Designations	
Type A-AB	Benign thymoma
Type B1-B3	Malignant thymoma
Type C	Thymic carcinoma

Masaoka Stage	Recommended Treatment
Stage I	Surgical resection
Stage II	Surgical resection Consider PORT particularly for high risk factors (close/positive margins, high grade, pleural adhesion)
Stage III	Surgical resection → Consider PORT
Stage IV	Induction chemo → surgery → consider PORT
Thymic carcinoma	**Operable:** Max surgery → consider chemoRT for cases of limited disease **Inoperable:** Consider induction chemo, RT, or chemoRT

[a]With new AJCC staging, these recommendations may change.

RADIATION TREATMENT TECHNIQUE

- **SIM:** 4DCT, supine, upper Vac-Lok device. Consider breath-hold if tumor moves >1 cm.
- **Dose:** Unresectable: 60-70 Gy (45-50 Gy to PTV and 60-70 Gy SIB to GTV)
  PORT: R0 resection = 45-50 Gy; R1 resection = 54 Gy; R2 resection = 60-70 Gy
- **Target:** GTV: grossly visible tumor/tumor bed (clips can be useful if placed)
  CTV: Entire pretreatment superior-inferior extent of disease, posttreatment lateral extent (respect anatomic boundaries and follow pleural spaces)
  PTV: 0.5-1 cm based on IGRT

- **Technique:** IMRT or VMAT
- **Planning directive (for conventional fractionation):**

RT Alone	chemoRT	Neoadjuvant chemoRT
Lung: V20 ≤ 40% Heart: V30 ≤ 45% mean < 26 Gy Spinal cord: D_{max} < 45 Gy Esophagus: V50 < 50%	Lung: V20 ≤ 35%, V10 ≤ 45% V5 ≤ 65% Heart: V30 ≤ 45% mean < 26 Gy Spinal cord: D_{max} < 45 Gy Esophagus: V50 < 40%	Lung: V20 ≤ 30%, V10 ≤ 40% V5 ≤ 55% Heart: V30 ≤ 45% mean < 26 Gy Spinal cord: D_{max} < 45 Gy Esophagus: V50 < 40%

CHEMOTHERAPY

- **Induction:** Can downstage if unresectable
  First line: Cytoxan/adriamycin/cisplatin (CAP) +/– prednisone
- **Adjuvant:** Thymoma with gross residual disease or thymic carcinoma with R1-R2 resection
  Possible chemotherapy regimens include
  VP-16/ifosfamide/cisplatin (VIP)
  Cisplatin/VP-16 (EP)
  Carboplatin/paclitaxel
  Cisplatin/adriamycin/vincristine/Cytoxan (ADOC)

SIDE EFFECTS

See **Early Stage NSCLC** chapter.

FOLLOW-UP

- History/physical q3-12mo + annual CT of the chest for life (late recurrences can occur for >10 years)

NOTABLE LITERATURE

Adjuvant radiation therapy after surgical resection

- Peking 1999 (*Zhang Chin Med J (Engl)* 1999): 29 patients randomized trial (stage I, age <65). Surgery vs surgery → adjuvant RT. RT AP and/or two anterior oblique wedge fields. Lymphocytic predominant, 50 Gy/25 fx; epithelial/mixed, 60 Gy/30 fx. Outcome: no recurrence or mets in either group; 10-year OS surgery 92% vs surgery + RT 88% (NS). Conclusion: Adj RT not necessary for stage I thymoma
- ITMIG 2016 (*Rimner et al. JCO* 2016): 1263 patients with stage II-III thymoma and R0 resection were analyzed from a retrospective database consisting of patients from 39 centers (international). Those who received PORT after R0 resection were compared to those who did not receive PORT. Patients who received PORT had significantly longer 10-year OS (86% vs 79%, P = .002). However, patients receiving PORT were younger, more likely to have myasthenia gravis, had more stage III disease, were male, had larger tumors, had malignant thymomas, and were less likely to receive chemotherapy. Recurrence-free survival was not affected by giving PORT. As such, selection bias must be taken into account for possibilities in survival benefit; however, PORT remained a significant factor on multivariate analysis and for both Stage II and III thymoma. As such, this provides evidence and support for PORT in stage II-III completely resected thymoma.

MESOTHELIOMA

NIKHIL G. THAKER • ERIC D. BROOKS

BACKGROUND

- **Incidence/prevalence:** Approximately 3000 cases diagnosed annually in the United States. Overall incidence in decline in the United States due to less asbestos exposure.
- **Outcomes:** Median survival is ~12 months (range 4-20 months). MS 8 months sarcomatoid, 19 months epithelioid, and 13 months mixed subtype. Stage I MS = 20 months, Stage II MS = 19 months, Stage III MS = 16 months, Stage IV MS = 11 months *(Rusch et al. J Thorac Oncol* 2012)
- **Demographics:** Peak incidence in fifth to seventh decades.
- **Risk factors:** 70%-80% related to asbestos exposure (commonly found in insulation, ship building, construction work, and brake pads and therefore 90% male predominance). Rod/needle (amphibole) greater risk factor than serpentine (chrysotile). Latency is 20-40 years due to chronic pleural irritation leading to malignant transformation. Smoking + asbestos increases risk.

TUMOR BIOLOGY AND CHARACTERISTICS

- **Genetics:** Four distinct molecular subtypes: sarcomatoid, epithelioid, biphasic-epithelioid (biphasic-E), and biphasic-sarcomatoid (biphasic-S) based on RNA-seq. Mutations in BAP1, NF2, TP53, SETD2, DDX3X, ULK2, RYR2, CFAP45, SETDB1, and DDX51. Loss of tumor suppressor genes p14, p16, and NF-2. Alterations in Hippo, mTOR, histone methylation, RNA helicase, and p53 signaling pathways
- **Pathology:** Sarcomatoid (15%-25%), epithelioid (40%-60%, best prognosis), and mixed subtypes (25%-35%). May be confused with adenocarcinoma (IHC or electron micro required to differentiate).
- **Imaging:** Appears as a pleural thickening, possibly with pleural plaques, calcifications, involvement of interlobar fissures on x-ray and CT imaging

ANATOMY

- Mesothelium is a membrane composed of simple squamous epithelium, which forms the lining of pleura (thoracic cavity), mediastinum, pericardium, peritoneum, tunica vaginalis testis, and tunica serosa uteri.
- The inner lining of the pleura is the visceral pleura and outer lining is the parietal pleura. Parietal pleura includes the mediastinal and diaphragmatic pleura.
- Pleura extends from SCV fossa (thoracic inlet) superiorly to the insertion of the diaphragm inferiorly.
- Mesothelioma spreads by direct extension and seeding into the pleural space, through the chest wall, into the mediastinum, to the peritoneum, and to the lymph nodes. It has a tendency to grow along tracks of biopsies or chest tubes. Lymph node drainage:
  - Peribronchial, internal mammary nodes (IMN), hilar, and ipsi and contralateral mediastinum
  - Spreads to level 8 (lower paraesophageal), level 9 (pulmonary ligament), and diaphragmatic nodes more frequently than NSCLC
  - Axillary and/or supraclav (SCV) nodes at risk if with chest wall involvement

WORKUP

- **History and physical:** Ask about asbestos exposure. Evaluate performance status. Typically present with weight loss and respiratory symptoms
- **Labs:** CBC, CMP, and PFTs
- **Procedures/biopsy:** Historically, biopsy is done via thoracentesis, but if VATS is being done, obtain biopsy at that time. Perform pulmonary function tests to evaluate operability. VATS to r/o c/l or peritoneal dz. Mediastinoscopy to r/o N2/N3 disease. Renal scan prior to RT
- **Imaging:** CT of the chest/abdomen with contrast for pleural effusions or calcified pleural plaques. Chest MRI with contrast and PET/CT scan optional and typically done to determine chest wall/diaphragm invasion.

MALIGNANT PLEURAL MESOTHELIOMA STAGING

(AJCC 8TH EDITION)

T Stage		N Stage	
T1	Limited to the ipsi parietal pleura w/wo involvement of visceral pleura, mediastinal pleura, diaphragmatic pleura	N1	Mets in the ipsi bronchopulmonary, hilar or mediastinal (including the internal mammary, peridiaphragmatic, pericardial fat pad, or intercostal) LNs
T2	Involving any of the ipsi pleural surfaces with at least one involvement of diaphragmatic muscle, extension into underlying lung parenchyma	N2	Mets to contralateral mediastinum, ipsi or contralateral SCV LNs
T3	*Locally advanced but potentially resectable tumor.* Involving any of the ipsi pleural surfaces with at least one: involvement of the endothoracic fascia, extension into the mediastinal fat, solitary completely resectable focus of tumor extending into the soft tissues of the chest wall, nontransmural involvement of the pericardium	**M Stage**	
T4	*Locally advanced technically unresectable tumor.* Involving all of the ipsi pleural surfaces with at least one: diffuse extension or multifocal masses of tumor in the chest wall (with or without rib destruction), invasion through the diaphragm to the peritoneum, extension to contralateral pleura, extension to mediastinal organs, extension into the spine, extension through to the internal surface of the pericardium (with or without a pericardial effusion or involving the myocardium).	M1	Metastasis to distant organ

Summative Stage

<table>
<tr><th></th><th>N0</th><th>N1</th><th>N2</th><th>M1</th></tr>
<tr><th>T1</th><td>IA</td><td rowspan="2">II</td><td rowspan="3">IIIB</td><td rowspan="4">IV</td></tr>
<tr><th>T2</th><td rowspan="2">IB</td></tr>
<tr><th>T3</th><td>IIIA</td></tr>
<tr><th>T4</th><td colspan="3">IIIB</td></tr>
</table>

TREATMENT ALGORITHM

Stage I-III and epithelioid (medically operable)	Surgical resection (EPP) → chemotherapy → RT Surgical resection (P/D) → chemotherapy → RT (on protocol) Chemotherapy → surgical resection (EPP) → RT Chemotherapy → surgical resection (P/D) → observation vs RT (on protocol)
Sarcomatoid, mixed histology, medically inoperable, Stage IV	Chemotherapy (PS 0-2) vs best supportive care (PS 3-4)

Surgery

- Surgical resection possible in only a minority of patients with T1-3N0-1
- Extrapleural pneumonectomy (EPP) provides the greatest cytoreduction and includes the en bloc resection of the parietal and visceral pleura, lung, pericardium, and ipsilateral diaphragm. Mediastinal lymph node sampling of at least three stations is recommended. Graft is placed in the region of the diaphragm.
- Pleurectomy and decortication (P/D) is the complete removal of the pleura, and all gross tumor +/– en bloc resection of the pericardium and/or diaphragm with reconstruction, P/D can be considered for patients with more extensive disease (greater nodal burden, more invasive disease) or medically high risk. Allows expansion of the ipsi lung and reduces recurrent pleural effusions
- Pleurodesis with talc can be palliative.

Radiation Treatment Technique

- **SIM:** Supine, arms up, with a wingboard, upper body Vac-Lok device, and T-bar. 4DCT scan. Wire scar/drain sites. Consider 5-mm bolus (3 cm) around the scar/drain sites. Scan from thoracic inlet (beg. of ribs around T1) through below the ribs (at least L2 or as inferiorly as possible). If PD or biopsy only, get quantitative perfusion scan to assess lung function (FEV1 [% contribution contralateral lung] should be >30% predicted).
- **Dose:** 45-50.4 Gy in 28 fractions at 1.8 Gy/fx, consider SIB to gross disease, positive margin, and PET-avid regions to 60 Gy (2.4 Gy/fx) to increase the likelihood of local control.
  Palliation: Several possible regimens, including 45 Gy in 15 fractions, 30 Gy in 10 fractions, or 20 Gy in 5 fractions. ≥4 Gy for skin nodules/pain from chest wall invasion
  Prophylactic: 7 Gy × 3 to drain sites (*Boutin et al. Chest* 1995 and NCCN), although may not reduce rate of seeding (*Clive et al. Lancet Oncol* 2016), not done routinely at MDACC
- **Target:** Ipsilateral hemithoracic pleural surfaces, including the parietal/visceral pleura, diaphragm, and involved nodal stations (Fig. 36.1). Modify contours to include scars and drains with ~2.5 cm margin. Approach center of the sternum anteromedially and approach/abut the spinal canal posteromedially. Include the diaphragm crus/insertion (~L2) inferiorly. Utilize surgical clips, scars, and drain sites. High-risk areas for contouring misses: costophrenic, costodiaphragmatic, anteromedial pleural reflection, and cardiophrenic angles. If treatment after P/D or biopsy alone, consider

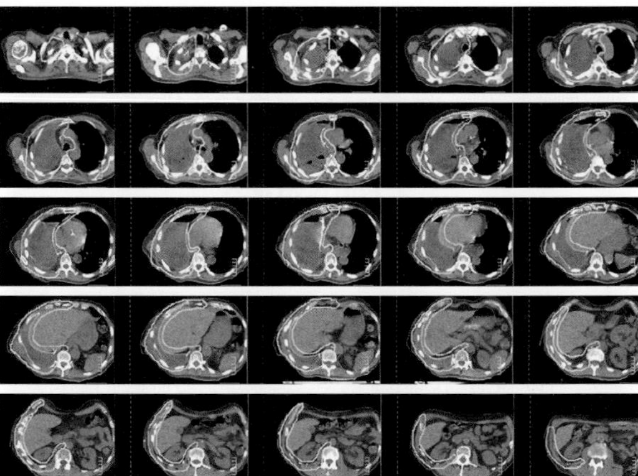

Figure 36.1 IMRT/VMAT contours for right-sided mesothelioma.

1 cm outside chest wall, 0.6 cm into lung parenchyma (+/– inclusion of fissures) with "donut" technique.

- **Technique:** IMRT/VMAT (Fig. 36.2)

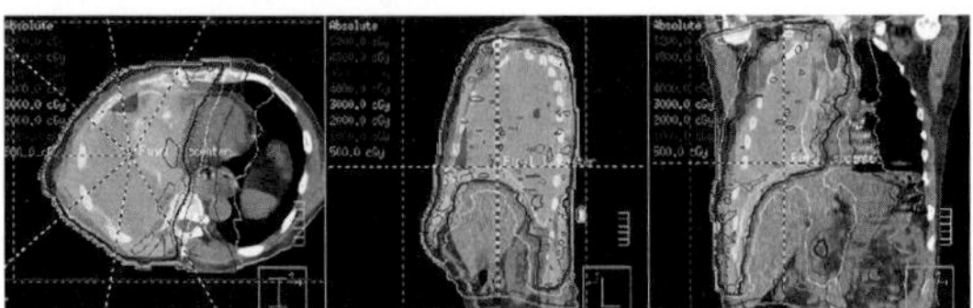

Figure 36.2 IMRT/VMAT plan for right-sided mesothelioma.

- **IGRT:** Daily kV imaging with once or twice weekly CBCT up to daily CBCT (depending on setup stability)
- **Planning directive (for 45 Gy in 25 fractions sp EPP and with optional boost to 54-60 Gy for R1/R2 resection AND hemithoracic RT on protocol sp P/D):**
  Target: V95% or D95% of the PTV is 45 Gy; D99%-100% of CTV gets 45 Gy.
  Contralateral lung: MLD < 8 Gy, V20 < 7%
  Liver: V30 < 50%, Mean < 30 Gy
  Contralateral kidney: V15 < 20%
  Ipsilateral kidney: V20 < 33% (compromise coverage if necessary based on renal scan results)
  Stomach: Mean < 30 Gy
  Esophagus: V55Gy < 70%, V60Gy < 30%, Mean < 34Gy
  Heart: V40Gy < 70%, V45Gy < 30, V30Gy < 45%, Mean < 26Gy%
  Spinal cord: D_{max} < 50 Gy, V45Gy < 10%
  Major vessels: 5 cc < 70 Gy, 10 cc < 60 Gy
  Brachial plexus: D_{max} < 60 Gy, 1 cc < 50 Gy, 10 cc < 40 Gy

  For palliative cases, utilize standard lung constraints (see NSCLC sections).

CHEMOTHERAPY

- **Agents:** Cisplatin and pemetrexed +/– bevacizumab

SIDE EFFECT MANAGEMENT

- Nausea: Zofran, Compazine, Reglan, low-dose dexamethasone, Haldol, IV fluids
- Pneumonitis: For symptomatic patients (eg, shortness of breath, drop in pO_2), consider oral steroid taper (typically prednisone starting at 1 mg/kg daily).
- Esophagitis: Magic mouthwash (viscous lidocaine, Benadryl, nystatin), glutamine supplement (eg, Helios), aloe products, narcotic elixir second line
- Dermatitis: Aquaphor or other moisturizing cream, gel sheets
- Chest wall pain: Analgesics, physical therapy

FOLLOW-UP

- CT of the chest/abdomen/pelvis: at 6 weeks, then q3mo for 2 years and then q6-12mo thereafter. PET/CT scan can also be used at 3 months and then PRN for suspicious findings on CT imaging.

NOTABLE LITERATURE

EPP +/– hemithoracic RT

- SAKK Trial (*Lancet Oncol* 2015). Questioned whether hemithoracic RT improves outcomes following EPP and chemo in mesothelioma in a randomized trial (phase II). Fifty-four patients received neoadjuvant cisplatin and pemetrexed followed by EPP and were eligible for randomization to hemithoracic RT vs observation. RT provided no LRR benefit, OS benefit, and added toxicity and detracted from baseline QOL compared to observation. However, this included unfavorable histologies (eg, sarcomatoid)—although this was only 4% of the population—and the trial was likely not powered enough to detect meaningful differences. However, the study results suggest that the role of radiation needs to be discussed thoroughly with patients and evaluated with further protocols moving forward. The rationale for continued use of RT in the EPP setting comes from retrospective studies showing reasonable outcomes with multidisciplinary management.

Intensity-modulated radiation therapy s/p EPP

- Harvard (*Allen et al. IJROBP* 2006). 13 patients treated with IMRT to 54 Gy. Most also received heated intraoperative cisplatin. 46% fatal pneumonitis. Beams passing through contralateral lung. Pulmonary death: MLD 15.2 Gy, V20 17.6%. No pulmonary death: MLD 12.9 Gy, V20 10.9%
- MD Anderson (*Rice et al. IJROBP* 2007). 63 patients s/p EPP, Stages III-IV. IMRT to 45-50 Gy. MS: 14.2 months. LRR 13%, DM 54% (only 7 received chemo). Pulmonary death: 9.5%. Pulmonary death: MLD 10.2 Gy, V20 9.8%. No pulmonary death: MLD 7.6 Gy, V20 3.6%. Recommended constraints: MLD < 8.5 Gy, V20 < 7%
- MD Anderson (*Gomez et al. J Thorac Oncol* 2013). 86 patients s/p EPP and adjuvant IMRT (45-50 Gy). Median OS 14.7 months. Grade 5 pulmonary toxicity, $n = 5$. Grade 3+ toxicity: skin 17%, lung 12%, heart 2.3%, and GI 16%. LRR 16%, DM 59%

Intensity-modulated radiation therapy s/p P/D

- MD Anderson (*Chance et al. IJROBP* 2015). Hemithoracic IMRT post P/D vs post EPP. Retrospective. 48 patients (24 each group). Nearly all had neoadjuvant chemotherapy. Epithelioid and sarcomatoid/mixed histologies (~75% epithelioid). P/D IMRT associated with improved OS 28.4 vs 14.2 months, improved PFS 16.4 vs 8.2 months
- MSKCC (*Gupta et al. IJROBP* 2005). 125 patients s/p P/D followed by RT. Median dose 42.5 Gy. MS 13.5 months, 2-year OS 23%. LC 42%. RT dose <40 Gy, nonepithelioid, left-sided disease, and use of implant worse. 12 pts with pneumonitis, 8 pts with pericarditis, and 2 pts died from grade 5 toxicity.

Chemotherapy

- University of Chicago (*Vogelzang et al. JCO* 2003). Randomized phase III trial. 456 pts, unresectable disease. Pemetrexed/cisplatin vs cisplatin alone. Response rate: 41% vs 17%. TTP 6 vs 4 months. OS 12 vs 9 months

ESOPHAGEAL CANCER

LISA SINGER • ERIC D. BROOKS • DANIEL GOMEZ

Background

- **Incidence/prevalence:** The seventh leading cause of cancer death in men in the United States; 16 940 cases diagnosed each year (15 690 estimated deaths); lifetime risk 0.5%
- **Outcomes:** 5-Year survival for local, regional, and distant disease 42.9%, 23.4%, and 4.6%, respectively (SEER)
- **Demographics:** More common in men; squamous cell carcinoma prevalent in developing nations (>90%). Adenocarcinoma more common in developed countries including the United States (~70% cases). Typically diagnosed between ages 50 and 70. Men account for 80% of the diagnoses.
- **Risk factors:** Squamous cell carcinoma risks include tobacco, smoking, alcohol, asbestos, and possibly HPV. Adenocarcinoma risks include obesity, hiatal hernia, elevated BMI, and Barrett esophagus/GERD.

Tumor Biology and Characteristics

- **Genetics:** HER-2 (25% of adenocarcinomas+), COX-2, EGFR overexpression; *TP53* mutations common
- **Pathology:** Squamous cell carcinoma or adenocarcinoma; Barrett esophagus is replacement of squamous with columnar epithelium and is associated with progression to adenocarcinoma.

Anatomy

- The esophagus extends from the pharynx to the stomach, the trachea anteriorly.
- Total length of the esophagus estimated to be 25 cm.
- Cardia marks the junction of the stomach and esophagus.
- Locations of esophageal tumors and lymph node drainage summarized below.

Name		Location (Landmarks)	Elective Nodal Coverage
Cervical		15-18 cm from upper incisors (C6 is distal hypopharynx)	Periesophageal, mediastinal, supraclavicular
Upper thoracic		18-24 cm from incisors (carina at ~24 cm)	
Mid thoracic		24-32 cm from incisors	Periesophageal, mediastinal
Lower thoracic/GEJ		32-40 cm from incisors	Periesophageal, mediastinal, perigastric, celiac
GEJ Tumor Classifications	Siewert type 1	1-5 cm superior to cardia	Recommend covering LN stations described in *Matzinger et al. Radiother Oncol* 2009
	Siewert type 2	At cardia or up to 1 cm superior, 2 cm inferior	
	Siewert type 3	2-5 cm inferior to cardia	

Workup

- **History and physical:** Typically present with progressive dysphagia, weight loss, and/or worsening heartburn
- **Screening:** Indicated for patients with documented Barrett esophagus (usually via biannual EGDs) (Fig. 37.1). Risk of development to esophageal cancer is 0.1%-0.4% per year.

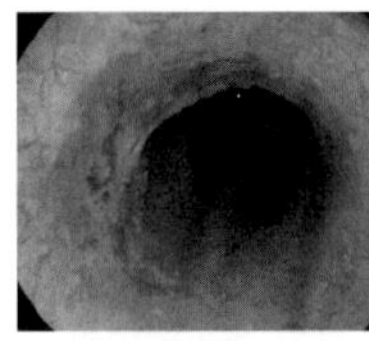

Figure 37.1 Image taken from surveillance upper endoscopy of a 63-year-old male with long-standing history of Barrett esophagus. Note the ulcerated mucosal lesion, which was biopsied and consistent with superficially invasive esophageal adenocarcinoma.

- **Labs:** CBC and CMP. Consider HER-2 tested for adenocarcinoma if metastatic.
- **Procedures/biopsy:** EGD and EUS +/– FNA (most sensitive for nodal staging). Consider bronchoscopy to rule out tracheal invasion of tumors located above the carina.
- **Imaging:** CT of the chest/abdomen/pelvis with contrast and PET/CT to rule out regional/distant disease for all patients

Esophageal TNM Cancer Staging *(AJCC 8th edition)*

T Stage		N Stage	
T0	No primary tumor	N0	No regional LNs involved
Tis	High-grade dysplasia	N1	Metastasis to 1-2 regional LNs
T1a	Invades lamina propria or muscularis mucosae	N2	3-6 regional LNs
T1b	Invades submucosa	N3	7+ regional LNs
T2	Invades muscularis propria	**M Stage**	
T3	Invades adventitia	M0	No distant metastasis
		M1	Distant metastasis
		G Category	
T4a	Invades pleura, pericardium, azygos vein, diaphragm, peritoneum	GX	Cannot assess differentiation
		G1	Well-differentiated
T4b	Invades other adjacent structures such as aorta, vertebral body, trachea	G2	Moderately differentiated
		G3	Poorly differentiated
Squamous Cell Carcinoma L Category (Location of Tumor Epicenter)			
LX	Location unknown		
Upper	Cervical esophagus to lower border azygos vein		
Middle	Lower border azygos vein to lower border inferior pulmonary vein		
Lower	Lower border inferior pulmonary vein to stomach, including GEJ		

Summative Stage (AJCC 8th Edition)

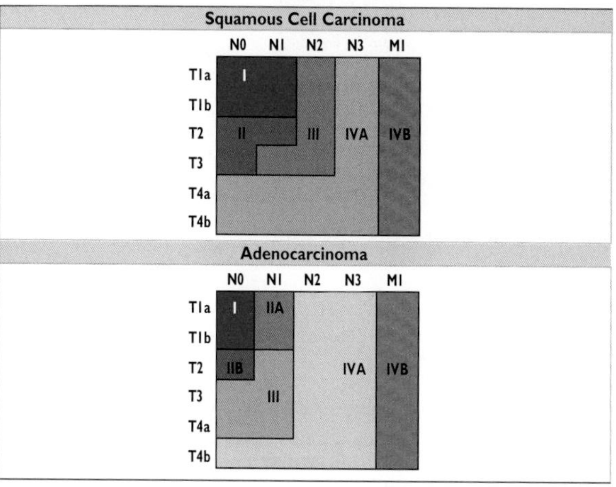

Treatment Algorithm

cTis-T1b, N0	Esophagectomy, endoscopic resection or ablation if patient can tolerate and extent of disease permits
cT1bN1 and higher, operable	Preoperative chemoradiation and then surgery (or definitive chemoradiation) Surgery upfront with post-op chemoRT if LN+[a], ≥pN1+, +margins
cT1bN1 and higher, cervical location squamous histology	Definitive chemoradiation preferred. Surgery can be very morbid in this location. Consider boost of the primary tumor to 66-70 Gy.
cT1bN1 and higher, inoperable	Definitive chemoradiation
M1	Palliative RT, chemotherapy, or best supportive care

[a]**Note:** Postoperative chemoradiation only recommended for ≥pN1+ if adenocarcinoma histology, observation recommended for ≥pN1+ squamous cell histology.

Radiation Treatment Technique

- **SIM:** NPO ×3 hours. Supine, arms up if tumor below carina (arms down if tumor above carina), immobilization device, iso at carina; scan from the mandible through stomach and celiac axis. Consider oral contrast to delineate tumor and head and neck mask for cervical primaries. 4DCT for GEJ tumors to account for movement.
- **Dose:** 50.4 Gy in 1.8 Gy/fx with concurrent chemotherapy
  Consider 66-70 Gy boost to GTV only for definitively treated squamous tumors.
- **Target:** GTV = PET/CT + primary and nodal disease at EGD/EUS
  CTV = 3-4 cm mucosal margin superiorly/inferiorly and 1 cm radial margin, trimmed from surrounding structures (Fig. 37.2)
  PTV = 5 mm margin with daily kV imaging
- **Technique:** IMRT and proton therapy (under investigation)
- **IGRT:** Daily kV imaging, consider weekly CBCT
- **Planning directive (for conventional fractionation):**
  PTV: 50.4 Gy in 28 fractions
  GTV (squamous undergoing definitive treatment): 66.6 Gy in 37 fractions (sequential boost)
  Esophagus minus GTV: D_{max} < 70 Gy, V50 < 50%

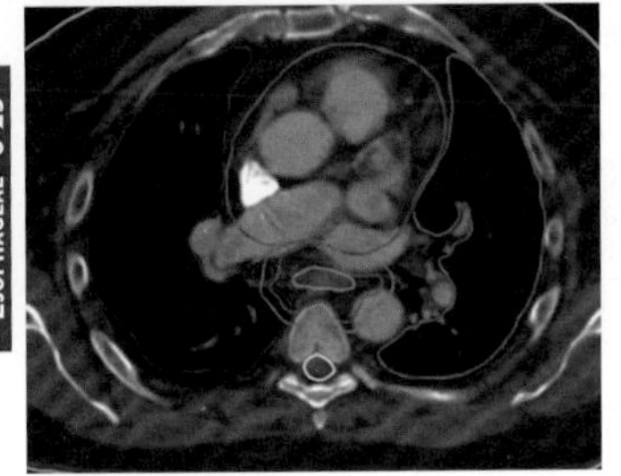

Figure 37.2 Representative cross-sectional image illustrating typical contours for an esophageal adenocarcinoma patient. GTV, CTV, and PTV contours showed in *orange*, *red*, and *pink*, respectively. **See color insert**.

Heart V30 < 45%, mean < 26 Gy
Total lung mean dose <20 Gy; V5 < 65%, V10 < 45%, V20 < 25%
Liver minus GTV: Mean dose <32 Gy, V20 < 50%, V30 < 30%
Kidney V20 < 33% each kidney
Spinal cord D_{max} < 45 Gy
Stomach D_{max} < 54 Gy

SURGERY

- **Approaches to esophagectomy:**
  - Transhiatal esophagectomy: Upper midline laparotomy and L neck incision; often uses gastric pull-through approach for cervical anastomosis; usually avoids thoracotomy
  - Transthoracic esophagectomy, Ivor-Lewis approach: R thoracotomy of the abdomen and upper abdominal laparotomy incisions allow for direct visualization of thoracic esophagus but limit length of proximal esophagus that can be removed.
  - Transthoracic esophagectomy, modified Ivor-Lewis approach: L thoracoabdominal incision only with anastomosis in L chest
- **Conduits:** Following esophagectomy. Connection between the remaining esophagus and stomach, colon, or jejunum
- **Lymph node dissection**: Should include at least 15 LNs if no preop chemoRT

CHEMOTHERAPY

- **Concurrent with RT, preoperative or definitive:** Paclitaxel/carboplatin or 5-FU/cisplatin, or 5-FU/oxaliplatin
- **Adjuvant:** Capecitabine or oxaliplatin
- **Perioperative (thoracic adenocarcinoma or GEJ):** 5-FU/cisplatin, ECF (epirubicin, cisplatin, 5-FU)

RT SIDE EFFECT MANAGEMENT

- Nausea: Zofran, Compazine, Reglan, low-dose dexamethasone, Haldol, and IV fluids
- Esophagitis: Magic mouthwash (viscous lidocaine, Benadryl, nystatin), glutamine supplement (eg, Helios), aloe products, and narcotic elixir second line.
- Thrush: Nystatin swish/swallow, fluconazole
- Weight loss: Nutrition consult/diet modifications, opiates if needed; may require feeding tube
- Leukopenias due to chemotherapy: Weekly labs with transfusion/Neupogen PRN
- Pneumonitis: ~6 weeks to 1 year after RT and may present with cough, dyspnea, and fever. Prescribe steroid taper (60 mg for 2-3 weeks with taper) and/or NSAIDs. Patient may even require O_2.
- Late effects: Tracheoesophageal fistula (5%-10%) if esophageal tumor invades trachea; presents as choking with PO intake, coughing, or recurrent pneumonias; treatment may involve stent or surgery (Ke et al. *J Thorac Dis* 2015). RT induced pericarditis and coronary artery disease in long-term survivors.

Follow-Up (Per NCCN)

- History/physical: Every 3-6 months for 1-2 years → every 6-12 months for 3-5 years
- CT of the chest/abdomen with contrast: Every 4-6 months for the first year and every 6-9 months for the next 2 years
- EGD: Every 3-6 months × 2 years and then 6-12 months in definitive chemoRT or early-stage surgical patients

Notable Literature

Outcomes with definitive chemoradiation

- RTOG 85-01 (*Herskovic et al. NEJM* 1992; *Cooper et al. JAMA* 1999): Phase III trial randomizing 129 patients with cT1-3, N0-N1, M0 squamous cell carcinoma, or adenocarcinoma of the esophagus to RT alone (50 Gy + 14 Gy boost) vs chemoRT (30 Gy + 20 Gy boost with 5FU and cisplatin); 5-year OS 0% vs 27% in RT alone vs chemoRT. No significant differences in late effects but acute toxicity worse in chemoRT arm
- INT-0123/RTOG 94-05 (*Minsky et al. JCO* 2002): Phase III trial randomizing patients to 50 Gy or high-dose (65 Gy) chemoRT with concurrent 5FU and cisplatin; trial stopped due to interim analysis demonstrating equivalent 2-year OS and LR with decreased treatment-related death in standard vs high-dose arms (2% vs 10%).

Neoadjuvant chemoradiation improves overall survival

- CROSS Trial (*van Hagen et al. NEJM* 2012; *Shapiro et al. Lancet Oncol* 2015): Phase III trial randomizing patients with resectable squamous cell or adenocarcinomas of the esophagus or GEJ to surgery alone or pre-op chemoRT (41.4 Gy/23 fx with carboplatin/paclitaxel) followed by surgery. 366 patients randomized. Median OS improved with preop chemoRT (49.4 vs 24 months, $P = .003$). Furthermore, R0 resection rates improved with chemoRT (92% vs 69%, $P < .001$). pCR rate 29% overall (49% for SCC and 23% for adenocarcinoma)

COLORECTAL CANCER

AHSAN FAROOQI • CHAD TANG • PRAJNAN DAS

BACKGROUND

- **Incidence/prevalence:** The third most common diagnosed cancer and third leading cause of death among men and women in the United States. Approximately 39 220 cases are diagnosed annually in the United States.
- **Outcomes:** 5-Year survival across all stages estimated at 67% (SEER data)
- **Demographics:** Lifetime risk 1 in 20 (5%). Highest incidence in Western countries
- **Risk factors:** Increasing age, familial syndromes (FAP, HNPCC, Peutz-Jeghers syndrome, juvenile polyposis), personal or family history of polyps, obesity, sedentary lifestyle, EtOH consumption, tobacco use, inflammatory bowel disease, low-fiber diet, and Western diet

TUMOR BIOLOGY AND CHARACTERISTICS

- **Genetics:** TCGA genomic profiling identified ~16% of colorectal cancers hypermutated. Frequent mutations in *APC*, *TP53*, *SMAD4*, *PIK3CA*, and *KRAS* (*Cancer Genome Atlas Network Nature* 2012). Four consensus molecular subtypes proposed include CMS1 (hypermutated microsatellite unstable, 14%), CMS2 (epithelial with marked WNT and MYC signaling, 37%), CMS3 (epithelial and metabolically dysregulated, 13%), and CMS4 (mesenchymal, 23%) (*Guinney et al. Nature Med* 2015).
- **Pathology:** Majority adenocarcinomas (>90%). Minority neuroendocrine, mesenchymal tumors or lymphomas. IHC testing for mismatch repair proteins (MLH1, PMS2, MSH2, and MSH6) commonly conducted and predictive of response to immunotherapy (*Le et al. Science* 2017). Consider testing for *BRAF* and *KRAS* mutations.
- **Imaging:** MRI accurate tool for local staging and for assessment of pelvic lymphadenopathy. Tumors typically visualized on high-resolution T2-weighted sequences, with increased signal on DWI sequence. Endorectal US can help distinguish between T1 and T2 tumors.

ANATOMY

- Rectum: Begins at the rectosigmoid junction at the level of S3. Total length of the rectum estimated to be between 12 and 15 cm. Squamous mucosa ends at the dentate line (~2 cm from anal verge). Internal anal sphincter ends 2 cm superior to dentate line (~4 cm from anal verge).
- Colon: Cecum is the junction between the small and large intestines (intraperitoneal) → ascending colon (retroperitoneal) → transverse colon (intraperitoneal) → descending colon (retroperitoneal) → sigmoid colon (intraperitoneal).
- Lymph node drainage:
  - Upper half rectum: Superior hemorrhoidal → IMA → para-aortic
  - Lower half rectum: Inferior + middle hemorrhoidal → internal iliac, obturator presacral nodes
  - Involvement of anal canal: Superficial inguinal nodes
  - Invading anterior structures (prostate, bladder, vagina) → external iliac

WORKUP

- **History and physical:** DRE for all patients and pelvic exam in women
- **Labs:** CBC, CMP, CEA
- **Procedures/biopsy:** Colonoscopy with biopsy of primary(ies)
- **Imaging:** Contrast-enhanced CTs of the chest/abdomen/pelvis (important to image the liver) for all patients. MRI of the pelvis w/ contrast typically done as well (if available). Contrast-enhanced PET/CT is not routinely indicated.

COLON AND RECTAL CANCER STAGING *(AJCC 8TH EDITION)*

T Stage		N Stage	
Tis	Carcinoma in situ (intramucosal)	N1a	1 regional LN involved
T1	Invades the submucosa	N1b	2-3 regional LNs involved
T2	Invades the muscularis propria	N1c	Tumor deposit

T3	Invades through the muscularis propria into the pericolorectal tissue	N2a	4-6 regional LNs involved
		N2b	≥7 regional LNs involved
		M Stage	
T4a	Invades through visceral peritoneum	M1a	Metastasis to 1 distal organ
		M1b	Metastasis to ≥1 distal organ
T4b	Tumor directly invades or adheres to adjacent organs or structures	M1c	Metastasis to peritoneal surface ±distal organ involvement

Summative Stage

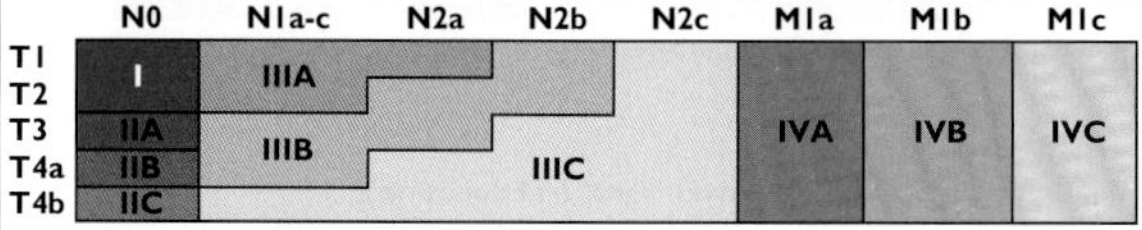

	N0	N1a-c	N2a	N2b	N2c	M1a	M1b	M1c
T1	I	IIIA				IVA	IVB	IVC
T2	I	IIIA				IVA	IVB	IVC
T3	IIA	IIIB				IVA	IVB	IVC
T4a	IIB	IIIB		IIIC		IVA	IVB	IVC
T4b	IIC					IVA	IVB	IVC

Note: TisN0M0 is Stage 0

Treatment Algorithm for Rectal Cancer

Stage I	Surgical resection → chemoRT or observation (observation considered if pT1-2N0M0 with R0 resection)
Stage II-III	ChemoRT → surgical resection → chemotherapy
Stage IVa (oligometastatic)	Chemotherapy → +/– chemoRT or short-course radiation → surgical resection of primary and definitive local treatment of metastatic disease (in either order) → chemotherapy
Stage IVb	Chemotherapy or best supportive care

Treatment for colon cancer is surgical + adjuvant chemo without routine use of adjuvant RT. Local control benefit of adjuvant RT was seen in T4 tumors invading adjoining structures, associated with perforation or fistula, or in the setting of residual disease (*Willett et al. Cancer J Sci Am* 1999). However, this was not confirmed when tested in the phase III Int 0130 trial comparing adjuvant chemo to chemo+RT (*Martenson et al. JCO* 2004) in T4 or T3N+ patients. Consider RT to metastatic sites if oligometastatic with good PS.

Radiation Treatment Technique for Rectal Cancer

- **SIM:** Prone on a bellyboard, Vac-Lok device, comfortably full bladder, and marker on anal verge (wire perineal scars if post-op). Scan from mid lumbar spine to middle femur, isocenter midline at top of femoral heads.
- **Dose:** 45 Gy in 25 fractions at 1.8 Gy/fx → cone-down boost to 50.4 Gy in 1.8 Gy/fx
  Recurrent after prior RT: 39 Gy in 1.5 Gy/fx bid
  Short course: 25 Gy at 5 Gy/fx
- **Target:** Pre-op: GTV, mesorectum, internal iliac, obturator, presacral nodes
  Post-op: Tumor bed, anastomosis, mesorectum, internal iliac, obturator, presacral nodes

Considerations: If T4 disease (invasion into anterior structures including the bladder, vagina, prostate), cover external iliac nodes. If locally advanced or recurrent, consider intraoperative radiation therapy (10-15 Gy, electrons, or HDR brachytherapy)

- **Technique:** 3DCRT: 3-field PA and opposed laterals, use IMRT for short-course radiation (Fig. 38.1).

Initial Fields: 45 Gy in 25 Fractions	
Superior	L5/S1 border
Inferior	Bottom of obturator foramen *or* 3 cm below tumor
Anterior	3 cm anterior to sacral promontory
Posterior	1 cm behind sacrum
Lateral	2 cm beyond pelvic inlet
Cone-Down Boost: 5.4 Gy in 25 Fractions	
2-cm expansion on GTV expanding posteriorly to include the sacrum using opposed laterals	

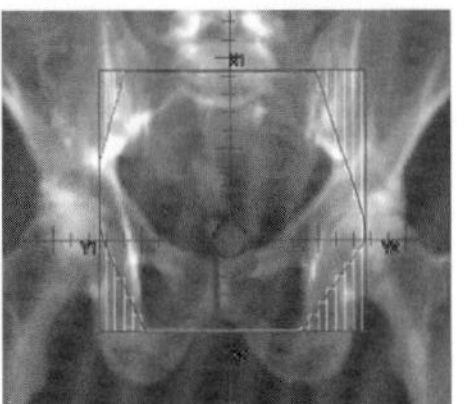
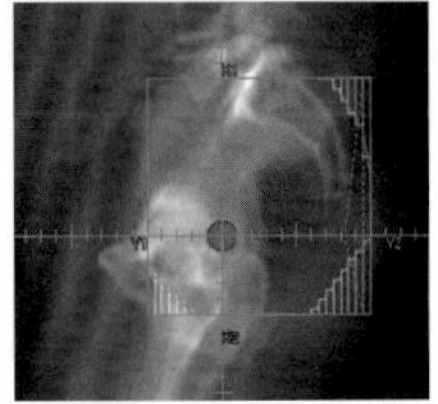

Figure 38.1 Standard PA and lateral fields.

- **IGRT:** Weekly kV imaging
- **Planning directive (for conventional fractionation):**
  Ensure coverage of GTV by 50.4 Gy isodose line
  Spinal cord D_{max} < 45 Gy
  Femoral heads V45 < 20%
  Bowel "bag" V45 < 195 cc
  Bladder V50 < 30%

Surgery

- Transanal excision (TAE): Sphincter-preserving, full-thickness local excision with adequate margin. Consider for low-lying (<10 cm) T1N0 lesions <30% circumferential involvement, <3 cm in size, clear margins, low-intermediate grade, and no LVI. Consider post-op chemoRT or radical surgery if path shows high-risk features, staging is upgraded, or there are inadequate margins.
- Low anterior resection (LAR): Sphincter-preserving total mesorectal excision (TME). Dissection and anastomosis below peritoneal reflection with ligation of superior and middle hemorrhoidal arteries. Adequate LN dissection removes ≥12 LNs.
- Abdominoperineal resection (APR): Total mesorectal excision (TME) with complete removal of the rectum and anal canal and permanent colostomy. Adequate LN dissection removes ≥12 LNs.

Chemotherapy

- **Concurrent:** Capecitabine (825 mg/m^2 bid, 5 days a week) or continuous infusion 5-FU (225 mg/m^2/d)
- **Adjuvant/neoadjuvant:** FOLFOX (folinic acid, oxaliplatin, 5-FU), or capecitabine, or CAPOX (capecitabine + oxaliplatin)

Side Effect Management

- Nausea: First-line Zofran (8 mg q8h PRN) → second-line Compazine (10 mg q6h prn) → ABH (lorazepam 0.34 mg, diphenhydramine 25 mg, and haloperidol 1.5 mg) 1 capsule q6h
- Diarrhea: First-line Imodium titrating to a max of 8 pills/day → second-line alternating Lomotil 2 pills and Imodium 2 pills every 3 hours
- Cystitis: *Urgency/frequency and dysuria.* UA to r/o UTI. Treat if positive.
- Skin care: First-line sitz baths, Aquaphor, and Domeboro powder → second-line Silvadene cream and hydrogel dressings (Cool Magic)
- Proctitis: *Diarrhea/abdominal pain.* first-line alternating Lomotil and Imodium (as above) → second-line steroid enemas.
- Hand and foot syndrome: Redness, swelling, and pain in the hand and foot. Consult with medical oncology about reducing concurrent capecitabine dose.

Follow-up

- History/physical and CEA: Every 3-4 months for 3 years → every 6 months for 2 years
- CT of the chest/abdomen/pelvis: Every year
- Colonoscopy: At years 1 and 3 and every 5 years thereafter
- Vaginal dilators for women

Notable Trials

Neoadjuvant chemoradiation

- German rectal trial (*Sauer et al. NEJM* 2004; *Sauer et al. JCO* 2012): Two-arm prospective randomized phase III trial comparing patients undergoing neoadjuvant chemoRT followed by surgery vs surgery followed by adjuvant chemoradiation. Both groups received adjuvant chemotherapy with bolus 5-FU. No OS survival difference but 10-year local recurrence is 7.1% vs 10.1% (*P* = .048, HR 0.60) favoring neoadjuvant approach. Grade 3-4 acute toxicities reduced (27% vs 40%, *P* = .001) along with grade 3-4 long-term toxicities (14% vs 24%, *P* = .01) in neoadjuvant-treated patients. Increased sphincter preservation among unfavorable patients in neoadjuvant group
- NSABP R-04 trial (*O'Connell et al. JCO* 2014; *Allegra et al. JNCI* 2015): Four-arm prospective randomized phase III trial comparing concurrent infusional 5-FU vs capecitabine, vs 5-FU + oxaliplatin, vs capecitabine + oxaliplatin. No significant difference in pathologic complete response, locoregional control, and overall survival. Increased diarrhea with oxaliplatin

Short-course (SC) radiation

- Dutch Trial (*Kapiteijn et al. NEJM* 2001; *van Gijn et al. Lancet Oncol* 2011): Two-arm prospective randomized phase III trial comparing SC + surgery (TME required) vs surgery alone. SC consisted of 25 Gy in 5 fractions given over 1 week. Surgery could include APR, LAR, or Hartmann procedure. 10-Year local recurrence improved with neoadjuvant SC (5% vs 11%, *P* < .0001).
- Polish Trial (*Bujko et al. Ann Oncol* 2016): cT3-T4 patients randomized prospective phase III trial comparing neoadjuvant SC RT followed by 3 cycles of FOLFOX4 to neoadjuvant long-course chemoRT to 50.4 Gy/28 fx combined with concurrent bolus 5-FU and leucovorin. Primary endpoint was R0 resection rate (77% SC vs 71% long course, *P* = .07). 3-Year OS favoring SC (73% vs 65%, *P* = .0046)
- TROG 01.04 (*Ngan et al. JCO* 2012): Two-arm randomized phase III trial comparing SC followed by surgery and adjuvant chemotherapy to long course chemoRT followed by surgery and adjuvant chemotherapy. Trial was powered to detect a 3-year local recurrence rate of 15% for SC and 5% for long course. At 3 years, local recurrence was not significantly different between the arms (7.5% SC vs 4.4% long course, *P* = .24).

ANAL CANCER

EMMA B. HOLLIDAY

Background

- **Incidence/prevalence:** Very rare; it makes up only 1% of all GI malignancies, but the incidence is increasing. 8200 new cases diagnosed in 2017 leading to 1100 deaths
- **Outcomes:** 5-Year survival for T2-T4; M0 was 71%-78% (RTOG 9811).

By stage (*Gunderson et al. IJROBP* 2013):

T2N0 5-y OS 87%, LRF 17%	T2N+ 5-y OS 70%, LRF 26%
T3N0 5-y OS 74%, LRF 18%	T3N+ 5-y OS 57%, LRF 44%
T4N0 5-y OS 57%, LRF 40%	T4N+ 5-y OS 42%, LRF 60%

- **Risk factors:** Female gender, older age (most 50-60+), and increased number of sexual partners, receptive anal intercourse, smoking, immunosuppression (including HIV)

Tumor Biology and Characteristics

- **HPV association:** 80%-90% of anal cancers are HPV+; HPV16 is present in 70% of tumors. HPV+ anal cancers have a better prognosis. HPV vaccination has been shown to decrease the incidence of premalignant anal lesions in men who have sex with men (*Lawton et al. Sex Transm Infect* 2013), but there has been no evidence of benefit for widespread cancer/premalignancy screening programs (*Leeds et al. World J Gastrointest Surg* 2016).

- **Pathology:** ~90% squamous cell carcinoma and ~10% adenocarcinoma (have much worse prognosis and typically treated with rectal cancer paradigm of neoadj chemoRT → APR)
- **Imaging:** Primary anal tumors are not typically well visualized on cross-sectional imaging. So anoscopy is very important.

Anatomy

- The anal region includes the anal canal (3-5 cm from the anal verge) and the anal margin (5-6-cm radius of perianal skin around the anal verge). Dentate line represents separation between columnar and squamous epithelium and occurs ~2 cm into the anus
- Lymph node drainage:
  - Anal margin: Superficial inguinal nodes
  - Anal canal below the dentate line: Superficial inguinal nodes
  - Anal canal above the dentate line: Anorectal, perirectal, paravertebral nodes → internal iliac nodes
  - Invasion into anterior structures (prostate, bladder, vagina): External iliac nodes

Workup

- **History and physical:** DRE and inguinal nodal exams for all patients
- **Labs:** CBC, CMP, LFTs, HIV testing, Pap smear/cervical screening for all females if they are not up to date. PSA and prostate cancer screening for all males
- **Procedures/biopsy:** Anoscopy with biopsy of primary
- **Imaging:** Contrast-enhanced CTs of the chest and abdomen for systemic staging and a CT or an MRI recommended for pelvis. We favor a contrast-enhanced PET/CT for both locoregional and systemic staging, and pelvic MRI reserved for patients with bulky T3 or T4 disease for whom better visualization of the tissue planes is desired.

Anal Cancer Staging *(AJCC 8th edition)*

T Stage		**N Stage**	
Tis	Carcinoma in situ (intramucosal)	N1a	Inguinal, mesorectal, internal iliac LNs
T1	≤2 cm	N1b	External iliac LNs
T2	>2-5 cm	N1c	Both N1a and N1b
T3	>5 cm	**M Stage**	
T4a	Invades adjacent organs: vagina, uterus, urethra, bladder, or prostate	M1	Metastasis to distal sites (including para-aortic LNs)

Summative Stage

<table>
<tr><th></th><th>N0</th><th>N1</th><th>M1</th></tr>
<tr><td>T1</td><td>I</td><td rowspan="2">IIIA</td><td rowspan="4">IV</td></tr>
<tr><td>T2</td><td>IIA</td></tr>
<tr><td>T3</td><td>IIB</td><td rowspan="2">IIIC</td></tr>
<tr><td>T4</td><td>IIIB</td></tr>
</table>

Treatment Algorithm

M0 anal canal cancer	Definitive chemoradiation
M1 anal canal or anal margin cancer	Systemic chemotherapy (5-FU/cisplatin) +/– local RT vs clinical trials
T1N0, well-differentiated anal margin cancer	Local excision → observation if adequate margins If inadequate margins, re-excision preferred or can consider local RT +/– concurrent chemotherapy
T1N0, poorly differentiated or T2-T4, N0 or any T, N+ anal margin cancer	Definitive chemoradiation

Radiation Treatment Technique

- **SIM:** Supine, frog-legged position, and custom immobilization device for the lower body. Place radiopaque BB at the anal verge to help delineate tumor during treatment planning, place wire around any perianal extension, and consider bolus. Consider full bladder to displace small bowel. Use vaginal dilator for women to displace the anterior vaginal wall. Use scrotal shelf for men to minimize skin toxicity. Position and immobilize penis midline.
- **RTOG0529 dose:**

	Dose/Fractions (dose per fraction)	
	Primary Tumor Involved nodes	**Elective Nodal Volume**
Primary Tumor Stage		
T2	50.4 Gy/28 fx (1.8 Gy/fx)	42 Gy/28 fx (1.5 Gy/fx)
T3/T4	54 Gy/30 fx (1.8 Gy/fx)	45 Gy/30 fx (1.5 Gy/fx)
Nodal Size		
≤3 cm	50.4 Gy/30 fx (1.68 Gy/fx)	
>3 cm	54 Gy/30 fx (1.8 Gy/fx)	

- **MDACC dose:**

	Dose/Fractions (dose per fraction)	
	Primary Tumor Involved Nodes	**Elective Nodal Volume**
Primary Tumor Stage		
T1	50 Gy/25 fx (2 Gy/fx)	43 Gy/25 fx (1.72 Gy/fx)
T2	54 Gy/27 fx (2 Gy/fx)	45 Gy/27 fx (1.67 Gy/fx)
T3/T4	58 Gy/29 fx (2 Gy/fx)	47 Gy/29 fx (1.62 Gy/fx)
Nodal Size		
<2 cm	50 Gy/25 fx[a] (2 Gy/fx)	
2-5 cm	54 Gy/27 fx[a] (2 Gy/fx)	
>5 cm	58 Gy/29 fx[a] (2 Gy/fx)	

[a]*The tumor, involved LNs, and elective nodal volume are treated using one IMRT plan with a simultaneous integrated boost technique. The number of fractions should be determined by the largest of either the primary tumor or the involved LN. For example, a T2 tumor with a 1.5-cm inguinal node would be treated in 27 fractions. The primary tumor would receive 54 Gy, the inguinal node would receive 50 Gy, and the elective nodal volume would receive 45 Gy.*

- **Target:** CTVp (primary) = anal GTV + 1 cm
  CTVn (involved nodes) = nodal GTV + 5 mm
  CTVe (elective nodal volume) = Should extend at least 2 cm inferior to anal GTV and include the entire mesorectum to the pelvic floor. Nodal areas include inguinal, perirectal, presacral, internal, and external iliacs to the level of the bifurcation of the common iliacs (~L5/S1)
  PTV margin with daily kV IGRT is 5 mm from CTV.
- **Technique:** IMRT
- **Target delineation:**
  Primary and nodes:
  Utilize information from physical exam, CT, PET/CT or MRI, and endoscopy reports to delineate the GTVp and GTVn.

CTVp = GTVp + 1 cm	CTVn = GTVn + 5 mm
PTVp = CTVp + 5 mm	PTVn = CTVn + 5 mm

Elective nodal volume:

In the **low pelvis**, the CTVe should extend inferiorly at least 2 cm below GTVp (may include perianal skin).

Should include the entire mesorectum to the pelvic floor.

+/– extension into ischiorectal fossa (RTOG atlas states only extend a few mm beyond levators if no ischiorectal fossa involvement; Australasian atlas includes the entire ischiorectal fossa.)

The inguinal nodal area should be covered from the inguinal ligament superiorly to the lesser trochanter inferiorly. The lateral border is the iliopsoas (I), the medial border is the adductor longus (AL) and pectineus (P), the posterior border is the

I and P, and the anterior border is the sartorius (S).

In the **mid pelvis**, the CTVe should extend to the lateral pelvic sidewall (muscle or bone). There should be an extension of ~1 cm into the bladder and cover the posterior internal obturator vessels.

In the **high pelvis**, the perirectal coverage should extend to the rectosigmoid junction. The superior border of CTVe should extend to where the common iliacs bifurcate into internal and external iliacs (~L5/S1). The internal, external, and presacral nodal basins should be covered. A margin of ~7 mm in soft tissue around the external iliac vessels should be added excluding muscle and bone.

Resources:

RTOG Atlas (used for RTOG 0529): https://www.rtog.org/CoreLab/ContouringAtlases/Anorectal.aspx

Australasian GI Trials Group Atlas: *Ng et al. Int J Radiat Oncol Biol Phys* 2012.

Inguinal Nodal Atlas: *Kim et al. Pract Radiat Oncol* 2012.

- **IGRT:** daily kV imaging and/or daily CBCT to ensure consistent bladder filling and soft tissue alignment
- **Planning directive:**
  Ensure coverage of GTV by prescription Gy isodose line.
  Femoral heads V45 < 20%
  Small bowel V50 < 10 cc, D_{max} < 54 Gy
  Bowel bag V45 < 195 cc (*Kavanaugh et al. Int J Radiat Oncol Biol Phys* 2010)
  Bladder V50 < 30%
  Genitalia V30 < 20%, V20 < 67%

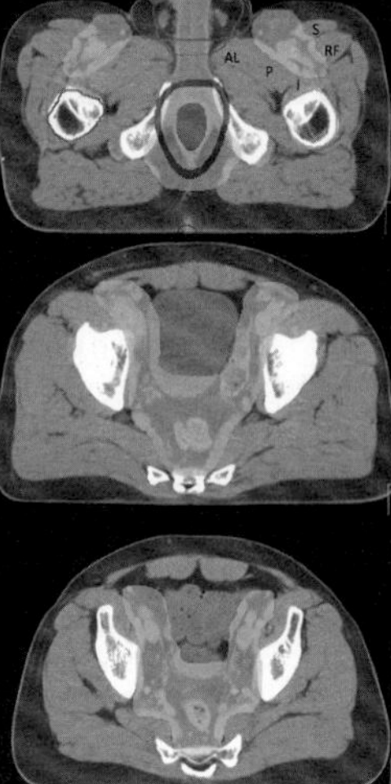

Figure 39.1 RTOG Atlas (used for RTOG 0529) https://www.rtog.org/CoreLab/ContouringAtlases/Anorectal.aspx. **See color insert.** (Australasian GI Trials Group Atlas: Ng et al., *Int J Radiat Oncol Biol Phys*, 2012.; Inguinal Nodal Atlas: Kim et al., *Pract Rad Onc*, 2012.)

Chemotherapy

- **Concurrent:**
  - **Most widely accepted regimen:** Continuous-infusion 5-FU 1000 mg/m^2/d IV days 1-4 and 29-32. Mitomycin C 10 mg/m^2 IV bolus days 1 and 29 or Mitomycin C 12 mg/m^2 (capped at 20 mg) on day 1
  - **MDACC preferred regimen:** Weekly bolus cisplatin 20 mg/m^2 and continuous-infusion 5-FU 300 mg/m^2 administered Monday-Friday on the days of radiation (NCCN cat 2B recommendation)
  - **Other NCCN-listed regimens:** Capecitabine 825 mg/m^2 PO bid, Monday-Friday on the days of radiation. Mitomycin C 10 mg/m^2 days 1 and 29 or mitomycin C 12 mg/m^2 IV bolus on day 1.

Side Effect Management

- Nausea: First-line Zofran (8 mg q8h prn) → second-line Compazine (10 mg q6h prn) → ABH (lorazepam 0.34 mg, diphenhydramine 25 mg, and haloperidol 1.5 mg) 1 capsule q6h
- Diarrhea: First-line Imodium titrating to a max of 8 pills/day → second-line alternating Lomotil 2 pills and Imodium 2 pills every 3 hours
- Cystitis: *Urgency/frequency and dysuria*. UA to r/o UTI. Treat if positive. If negative, consider Pyridium OTC or prescription for dysuria.
- Dermatitis—Grades 1-2: sitz baths, Aquaphor, and Domeboro powder → Grades 2-3: Silvadene cream and hydrogel dressings (Cool Magic) → Grade 4: treatment break and surgical consult
- Proctitis/anal pain: treat diarrhea and dermatitis as above. Consider topical lidocaine, steroid suppositories, or steroid enemas. Many patients require opiate pain medications.

Follow-up

- Skin and toxicity check at 6 weeks posttreatment with a DRE
- First restaging at 12 weeks posttreatment includes DRE, anoscopy, and CT of the chest/abdomen/pelvis. If disease is persistent, reevaluate in 4 weeks and continue monitoring until complete clinical response (CR). If no complete CR by 6 months, consider biopsy.
  **It is important not to biopsy prematurely as only 52% of patients on ACT II achieved a complete CR by 11 weeks from the start of treatment, but 72% of the patients who didn't achieve a complete CR by 11 weeks had achieved a complete CR by 26 weeks.*
- Once complete CR achieved, DRE q3mo, anoscopy q6mo, and CT of the chest/abdomen/pelvis annually if initially T3, T4, or N+ disease
- If biopsy-proven locally recurrent disease, perform systemic restaging and proceed to salvage abdominoperineal resection +/– inguinal nodal dissection. If metastatic disease is found, treat with cisplatin/5-FU systemic therapy or enroll on a clinical trial.

Notable Trials

chemoRT vs RT alone

- UKCCCR ACT I (*Northover et al. Br J Cancer* 2010): 577 patients with T2-T4M0 anal squamous cell carcinoma randomized to either RT or chemoRT with 5-FU/MMC. RT included 45 Gy in 20-25 fractions followed by reassessment at 6 weeks. If >50% response, boost with 15 Gy or 25 Gy Ir-192. If <50%, proceed to APR. Trend toward improved overall survival (OS) (33% vs 28% at 12 years, $P = .12$), but significantly improved local control (LC) (66% vs 41% at 12 years, $P < .0001$), colostomy-free survival (CFS) (30% vs 20% at 12 years, $P = .004$), and disease-free survival (DFS) (30% vs 18% at 12 years, $P = .004$)
- EORTC (*Bartelink et al. JCO* 1997): 103 patients with T3-T4 and N1-N3 anal squamous cell carcinoma randomized to either RT or chemoRT with 5-FU/MMC. RT included 45 Gy in 25 fractions followed by reassessment at 6 weeks. If CR, boost 15 Gy; if PR, boost 20 Gy; if no response, proceed to APR. No difference in 5-year OS or DFS, but 5-year LC and CFS were improved with chemoRT (68% vs 50%, $P = .02$ and 68% vs 40%, $P = .002$, respectively).

Optimal concurrent chemoRT regimen

- RTOG 9811 (*Gunderson et al. JCO* 2012): 649 patients with T2-T4 and M0 anal squamous cell carcinoma randomized to either chemoRT with 5-FU/MMC or induction cis/5-FU ×2 → chemoRT with cis/5-FU. RT included 45 Gy in 25 fractions followed by a 10-14 Gy boost for T3/T4 or N+ disease or residual T2 disease after the first 45 Gy. No difference in LC or CFS, but DFS and OS were better in the 5-FU/MMC arm (68% vs 58%, $P = .006$, and 78% vs 71%, $P = .026$, respectively).
- UKCCCR ACT II (*James et al. Lancet Oncol* 2013): 940 patients with M0 anal squamous cell carcinoma randomized in a 2 × 2 design to chemoRT with either 5FU/MMC or cis/5-FU and +/– maintenance cis/5-FU. RT included 50.4 Gy in 28 fractions. LC at 26 weeks was no different. 3-Year CFS, DFS, and OS were all no different. Only 44% of patients randomized to maintenance chemo completed it. G3 hematologic toxicity was 16% with cis/5FU compared with 26% with 5-FU/MMC.

Induction chemotherapy and additional RT boost

- ACCORD 03 (*Peiffert et al. JCO* 2012): 307 patients with M0 squamous cell carcinoma >4 cm or N+ randomized in a 2 × 2 design to +/– neoadj cis/5FU followed by chemoRT with cis/5-FU followed by either a 15 Gy boost or a 20-25 Gy boost. RT included 45 Gy in 25 fractions followed by reassessment at 3 weeks. If any clinical response was seen, the boost was given according to the fractionation arm. If no response, the patient was taken off trial and given an APR. There was no difference in 5-year LC, OS, CFS (primary endpoint), or DFS among all arms.

PANCREATIC CANCER

SHALINI MONINGI • LAUREN ELIZABETH COLBERT • PRAJNAN DAS

BACKGROUND

- **Incidence/prevalence:** The 12th most commonly diagnosed cancer and the 4th most common cause of cancer death. Estimated ~50 000 new cases diagnosed per year in the United States
- **Outcomes:** The 5-year survival is 8%.
- **Demographics:** Lifetime risk is 1 in 65. Slightly higher incidence in males vs females (1.25:1). More common in developed nations. Typically diagnosed between ages 50 and 70 years
- **Risk factors:** Increasing age, familial-associated genetic changes (p16 and BRCA2), obesity, ETOH consumption, chronic pancreatitis, diabetes, red meat, tobacco use, exposure to 2-naphthylamine and benzidine

TUMOR BIOLOGY AND CHARACTERISTICS

- **Genetics:** The most common mutated oncogenes in PCA include *KRAS*, *CDKN2A*, *TP53*, and *SMAD4*.
- **Pathology:** Majority are ductal adenocarcinomas (80%). Other less common subtypes include mucinous cystadenocarcinoma, acinar cell carcinoma, and adenosquamous carcinoma.
- **Imaging:** Predominately hypointense compared with a normal pancreas on CT scans with contrast. Hypointense on T1-weighted MRI. Associated imaging findings include pancreatic duct dilatation, abrupt changes in duct caliber, and parenchymal atrophy distal to the lesion.

ANATOMY

- The pancreas is divided into the head, neck, body, and tail.
- Retroperitoneal structure, with pancreatic duct merging with the common bile duct to drain into the second portion of the duodenum at the ampulla of Vater.
- The pancreas is next to numerous critical GI structures including the duodenum, jejunum, stomach, spleen, liver/gallbladder, and both the celiac and SMA axes, which makes treatment difficult.
- Lymphatic drainage is to peripancreatic, celiac, SMA, porta hepatis, and para-aortic lymph nodes.
- Bony landmarks:
  Celiac artery at the level of T12
  SMA at the level of L1
  Pancreas is seen at the level of L1-L2.

WORKUP

- **History and physical:** Examination focusing on abdominal symptoms including bloating, abdominal pain, and history of pancreatitis. Evaluation of systemic symptoms including jaundice, weight loss, and back pain.
- **Labs:** CBC, CMP, LFTs, and CA19-9
- **Procedures/biopsy:** Endoscopic ultrasound with biopsy if able. Consider endoscopic evaluation with endoscopic retrograde cholangiopancreatography (ERCP) or percutaneous transhepatic cholangiography (PTC) for evaluation and biopsy. If jaundice, consider stent placement. If resectable, consider staging laparoscopy in high-risk patients.
- **Imaging:** CT of the chest and abdomen with contrast, pancreas protocol (early arterial, pancreatic, and portal venous phase)

Pancreatic Cancer Staging (AJCC 8th Edition)

T Stage		N Stage	
Tis	Carcinoma in situ (includes high-grade pancreatic intraepithelial neoplasia [PanIN-3])	Nx	One regional LN involved
T1	Tumor ≤2 cm in greatest dimension	N0	No regional lymph nodes involved
T1a	Tumor ≤0.5 cm in greatest dimension	N1	Metastasis in 1-3 regional lymph nodes
T1b	Tumor ≥0.5 cm and <1 cm in greatest dimension	N2	Metastasis in 4 or more regional lymph nodes
T1c	Tumor 1-2 cm in greatest dimension		
T2	Tumor >2 cm and ≤4 cm		
T3	Tumor >4 cm in greatest dimension		
		M Stage	
T4	Tumor involves the celiac axis, superior mesenteric artery, and/or common hepatic artery	M1	Distant metastasis

	N0	N1	N2	M1
T1	IA			
T2	IB	IIB		
T3	IIA			IV
T4			III	

Definitions of Resectability (Katz J Am Coll Surg 2008)

	Potentially Resectable	Borderline Resectable	Locally Advanced
Portal vein/SMV	TVI < 180 degrees	TVI ≥ 180 degrees and/or reconstructable occlusion	Unable to reconstruct
Hepatic artery	No TVI	Reconstructable short-segment TVI of any degree	Unable to reconstruct
Superior mesenteric artery	No TVI	TVI < 180 degrees	TVI ≥ 180 degrees
Celiac trunk	No TVI	TVI < 180 degrees	TVI ≥ 180 degrees

TVI, tumor-vessel interface.

Treatment Schema

PCA Stage	Treatment
Resectable PCA	*Pre-op approach:* Chemo → chemoRT or SBRT → surgery *Adjuvant approach:* Surgery → chemo → restage → consider post-op chemoRT in selected cases
Borderline PCA	Chemo → chemoRT or SBRT → assess for resectability → surgery
Locally advanced PCA	Chemo → restage → consider chemoRT or SBRT[a]

[a]Stereotactic body radiation therapy (SBRT) is contraindicated when significant bowel (duodenum) invasion.

Radiation Treatment Technique

Conventional RT

- **SIM:** Supine, wingboard, T-bar, Vac-Lok, and Iso at T-12 right of midline. Scan from carina to iliac crest. IV contrast
- **Dose:** Pre-op: Capecitabine + 50-50.4 Gy, 1.8-2 Gy/fx
  Post-op: Capecitabine + 50-50.4 Gy, 1.8-2 Gy/fx
- **Target:** Pre-op: Tumor, involved nodes, celiac, SMA, +/− porta hepatis (for pancreatic head only)
  Post-op: Tumor bed, celiac, SMA, porta hepatis (for pancreatic head only), para-aortics (*Goodman et al. IJROBP* 2012)
  Locally advanced: Tumor, involved nodes, celiac, SMA
- **Technique:** 3D or IMRT

SBRT

- **SIM:** Arms extended overhead, upper Vac-Lok, T-bar, and wingboard. IV contrast, breath-hold scans. Patient is NPO 3 hours prior to SIM and treatment. Fiducials
- **Dose:** 33-36 Gy in 5 fractions (Fig. 40.1)
- **Target:** GTV and tumor-vessel interface (TVI)
- **Technique:** 6× photons delivered by VMAT

Contouring and Target Delineation for Pancreatic SBRT[a]	
GTV	Primary tumor
TVI	The circumferential extent of major vessels in direct contact with GTV
PRV	Stomach/duodenum/small bowel + 3 mm
PTV1	GTV + TVI + 3 mm
PTV2	PTV1 − PRV
PTV3	(TVI + 3 mm) − PRV
Treatment Planning	
36 Gy delivered to the interface of the tumor and vessel, PTV3	
33 Gy delivered to the main target, PTV2	
25 Gy delivered to the areas of overlap of 3 mm of critical structures, PTV1	

[a]Adapted from Alliance trial A021501 contouring guidelines.

- **IGRT:** Daily cone beam CT and kV.
  Respiratory motion management, for example, breath hold
  We strongly recommend implanting fiducials for SBRT cases.

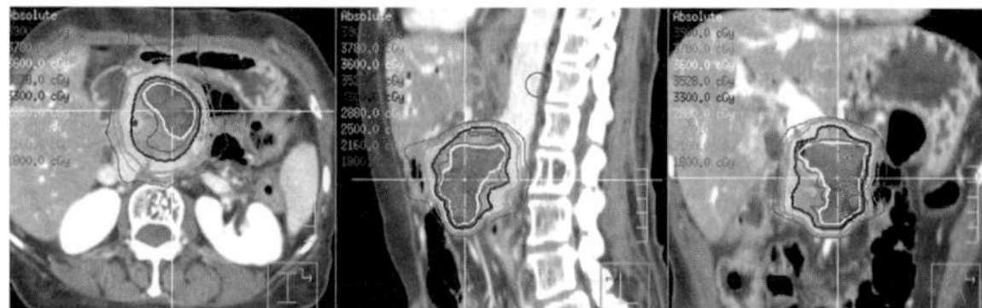

Figure 40.1 Representative cross-sectional axial, sagittal, and coronal images (L→R) from a SBRT treatment plan for locally advanced pancreatic cancer. The *white* isodose line represents 36 Gy encompassing the *red color* wash, which delineates PTV3 (tumor-vessel interface minus PRV). The *sky-blue* isodose line represents 25 Gy, which is encompassing the *yellow contour* that represents PTV1 (gross tumor + TVI + 3 mm). This patient had fiducials placed, which was used daily for image guidance along with CBCT. **See color insert.**

- **Planning Directive (for SBRT) and Conventional RT:**

SBRT	Conventional RT
Spinal cord V20 < 1 cc	spinal cord: ≤45 Gy
Duodenum V20 < 20 cc; V35 < 1 cc	Duodenum: Max dose 54 Gy (consider V54 ≤ 1 cc if needed)
Liver V12 < 50%	Liver: Mean < 28 Gy; V20 < 50%; V30 < 33%
Stomach V20 < 20 cc	Stomach: Max dose < 54 Gy
Kidneys V12 < 25%	Kidney: V20 < 33% for each kidney, mean < 18 Gy

Surgery

- Pancreaticoduodenectomy (Whipple procedure):
  En bloc removal of the distal stomach, 1st and 2nd position of the duodenum, head of the pancreas, common bile duct, and the gallbladder
  Anastomoses:
  - Pancreas to jejunum
  - Gallbladder to jejunum
  - Stomach to jejunum

Chemotherapy

- **Concurrent with standard dose RT:** Capecitabine
- **Neoadjuvant:** FOLFIRINOX (5-fluorouracil, leucovorin, irinotecan, and oxaliplatin) or gemcitabine and nab-paclitaxel
- **Metastatic:** FOLFIRINOX or gemcitabine and nab-paclitaxel

Side Effect Management

- Nausea: First-line Zofran (8 mg q8h prn) → second-line Compazine (10 mg q6h prn) → ABH (lorazepam 0.34 mg, diphenhydramine 25 mg, and haloperidol 1.5 mg) 1 capsule q6h
- Diarrhea: First-line Imodium titrating to a max of 8 pills/day → second-line alternating Lomotil 2 pills and Imodium 2 pills every 3 hours. Patients will be evaluated and receive CREON (pancrelipase) prior to initiation of therapy.
- Fatigue: Supportive care
- Chronic side effects: Ulcer formation, bowel perforation, and bowel stenosis. Refer to GI specialists.

Follow-up

- History/physical and CT of the abdomen and chest: Every 3 months

Notable Trials

Resected pancreatic cancer

- ESPAC 1 Trial (*Lancet* 2001): Prospective trial that randomized 541 patients with resected pancreatic cancer to observation, chemotherapy alone (5-FU), chemoradiation alone (40 Gy split course given in two 20 Gy increments), or chemoradiation followed by additional chemotherapy. There was no benefit to chemoRT (HR 1.18, $P = .24$), but median survival improved with adjuvant chemotherapy (19.7 months vs 14 months, $P = .0005$). There are many criticisms of the trial design including lack of central QA and selection bias.
- CONKO-001 Trial (*JAMA* 2007, 2013): Prospective randomized trial of 354 patients with either N0 or N1 disease s/p R0-R1 resection. Patients were randomized to observation or adjuvant therapy with 6 cycles of gemcitabine. Results showed a 5-year OS benefit with adjuvant gemcitabine (21% vs 9%, $P = .01$), which was maintained at 10-year follow-up update (12.2% vs 7.7%, $P = .01$).
- ESPAC 4 Trial (*Lancet* 2017): Prospective randomized trial of 451 patients with gross total resection of T1-4N0-N1M0 pancreatic tumors. Randomized to receive either adjuvant gemcitabine or adjuvant gemcitabine and capecitabine. Improved overall survival with gemcitabine + capecitabine (median survival 28 months vs 25.5 months, $P = .032$).

Locally advanced pancreatic cancer

- LAP 07 Trial (*JAMA* 2016): Prospective randomized trial of 442 patients with locally advanced unresectable pancreatic adenocarcinoma. 2 × 2 randomization, first between gemcitabine and gemcitabine with erlotinib. For those without progression, they were again randomized to receiving additional chemotherapy with or without RT (54 Gy and capecitabine at 1600 mg/m^2/d). Of 269 patients with no progression after 4 months, median survival is equivalent between the chemo and chemo+RT arms. However, there was a local control benefit with additional of chemoRT (32% vs 46%, $P = .03$).
- Phase II SBRT (*Herman Cancer* 2015): Evaluated 49 patients with locally advanced PCA. All patients received 6.6 Gy ×5 SBRT following gemcitabine. Median OS was 13.9 months with 1 year freedom from local progression of 78%.

GASTRIC CANCER

LAUREN ELIZABETH COLBERT • PRAJNAN DAS

BACKGROUND

- **Incidence/prevalence:** 22 000 new cases in the United States annually. More common in East Asia (Japan, China, Korea) relative to the United States
- **Outcomes:** 5-Year survival across all stages estimated at 67% (SEER data)
- **Demographics:** 35% gastric fundus, 25% gastric body, 40% distal/antrum
- **Risk factors:** HNPCC, Li-Fraumeni, E-cadherin alteration (CDH1), Bloom syndrome (BLM/RECQL3), BRCA1/BRCA2, xeroderma pigmentosum, Cowden (PTEN), GERD/gastritis/Barrett esophagus, pernicious anemia, diet high in salted meats and nitrates and low in fruits and vegetables, smoking

TUMOR BIOLOGY AND CHARACTERISTICS

- **Genetics:** 60% have p53 loss and should have HER2 overexpression seen in 22% of patients on ToGA trial (*Bang et al. Lancet* 2010); other subtypes include EBV+, microsatellite instability (MSI)+, genomically stable (GS), and chromosomal instability (CIN) (*TCGA* 2014). Many are associated with *H. pylori* and EBV; others have CDH1 mutation or mismatch repair w/ MLH1 silencing (CIMP phenotype).
- **Pathology (Lauren histologic classification):**
  - **Intestinal subtype:** Male predominant; arises from precursor lesions; better prognosis, more localized; EBV, MSI, or CIN subtype; arises in GEJ/cardia
  - **Diffuse subtype:** Female predominant; no precursor lesions; worse prognosis, more invasive; GS subtype; locations diffuse

ANATOMY

- From cranial to caudal: Esophagus → GE junction → cardia → fundus → body → antrum/pyloric antrum → pylorus → duodenum (Fig. 41.1)
- Siewert classification: Type I—5-1 cm proximal (above) to GEJ, Type II—Epicenter of tumor located between 1 cm proximal and 2 cm distal of GEJ, Type III—2-5 cm distal to GEJ
- Lymph node drainage:
  - Fundus/cardia → perigastric, celiac, left gastric, splenic, hepatic
  - Body → Perigastric, celiac, left gastric, splenic, hepatic, sub-/suprapyloric, pancreaticoduodenal
  - Antrum/pylorus → perigastric, celiac, left gastric, hepatic, sub-/suprapyloric, pancreaticoduodenal
- Vascular supply (from celiac artery)
  - Left gastric: Lesser curvature
  - Right gastric: Lesser curvature/inferior stomach
  - Right gastroepiploic: Greater curvature
  - Left gastroepiploic: Upper greater curvature
  - Short gastric arteries: Fundus/proximal stomach

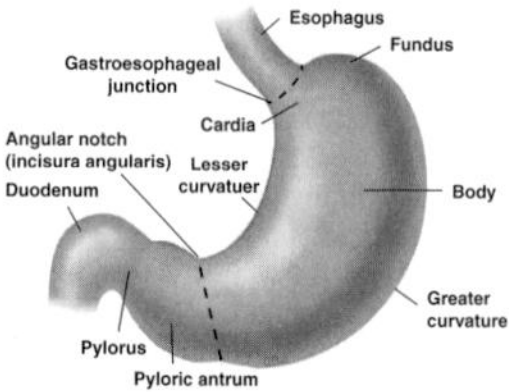

Figure 41.1 Anatomy of the stomach. (Reproduced with permission from Mansfield PF. Clinical features, diagnosis, and staging of gastric cancer. In: UpToDate, Post TW (Ed), UpToDate, Waltham, MA. (Accessed on [Date].) Copyright © 2019 UpToDate, Inc. For more information visit www.uptodate.com.)

WORKUP

- **History and physical:** Standard H&P with evaluation of left-sided supraclavicular lymph nodal station (Virchow node)
- **Labs:** CBC, CMP
- **Procedures/biopsy:** Esophagogastroduodenoscopy (EGD) with biopsies (>6 preferred) along with endoscopic ultrasound (EUS) (depth of tumor + LN involvement; ~85%-90% accurate; nodal Sn/Sp are ~83%/67%). Nutritional assessment/counseling. Consider Her2-neu testing if metastatic disease documented/suspected. **Need laparoscopy evaluation** particularly if T4 or undergoing neoadjuvant therapy (20%-30% of pts with >T1 tumors and negative imaging + peritoneal implants)
- **Imaging:** Recommend CT of the chest, abdomen, and pelvis with IV and oral contrast. NCCN recommends PET/CT if there is no evidence of M1 disease (false negative ~40% of the time, particularly in diffuse subtype).

Gastric Cancer Staging (AJCC 8th edition)

T Stage	
T0	No evidence of primary tumor
Tis	Carcinoma in situ; intraepithelial tumor without invasion of lamina propria
T1a	Tumor invades lamina propria, muscularis mucosae, or submucosae
T1b	Tumor invades submucosa
T2	Tumor invades muscularis propria
T3	Tumor penetrates subserosal connective tissue without invasion of visceral peritoneum or adjacent structures
T4a	Tumor invades serosa (visceral peritoneum)
T4b	Tumor invades adjacent structures

N Stage	
N0	No regional lymph node metastasis
N1	Metastasis in 1-2 regional lymph nodes
N2	Metastasis in 3-6 regional lymph nodes
N3a	Metastasis in 7-15 regional lymph nodes
N3b	Metastasis in 16 or more regional lymph nodes

M Stage	
M0	No distant metastasis
M1	Distant metastasis

Summative Stage

<table>
<tr><th></th><th>N0</th><th>N1</th><th>N2</th><th>N3a</th><th>N3b</th><th>Any N, M1</th></tr>
<tr><td>T1</td><td>IA</td><td>IB</td><td>IIA</td><td>IIB</td><td rowspan="2">IIIB</td><td rowspan="6">IV</td></tr>
<tr><td>T2</td><td>IB</td><td>IIA</td><td>IIB</td><td>IIIA</td></tr>
<tr><td>T3</td><td>IIA</td><td>IIB</td><td>IIIA</td><td rowspan="2">IIIB</td><td rowspan="3">IIIC</td></tr>
<tr><td>T4a</td><td>IIB</td><td>IIIA</td><td>IIIA</td></tr>
<tr><td>T4b</td><td>IIIA</td><td>IIIB</td><td>IIIB</td><td></td></tr>
<tr><td>Any T, M1</td><td colspan="5"></td></tr>
</table>

Treatment Algorithm

T1N0	Surgery (gastrectomy vs endoscopic mucosal resection)
T2+ N+ (combined modality)	Surgery → chemo → ChemoRT → chemo—**INT 0116, ARTIST** Surgery → chemo (cape/ox ×6)—**CLASSIC** Induction chemo → pre-op chemoRT → surgery—**MDACC** Periop chemo (ECF ×3 → surgery → ECF ×3)—**MAGIC**
Stage IV	Chemotherapy Palliative chemoRT

Radiation Treatment Technique

Preoperative

- **SIM: Supine, arms up, upper Vac-Lok, 3 hours NPO**, +/–4DCT, scan carina to pelvic brim, Iso@T12
- **Dose:** 45 Gy in 25 fractions at 1.8 Gy/fx
- **Target: GTV:** based on EGD/CT/PET + 3 cm mucosal expansion = mucosal target volume (MTV) (Fig. 41.2)
  CTV = MTV + involved nodes + elective nodes + 1 cm
  PTV = CTV + 0.5 cm

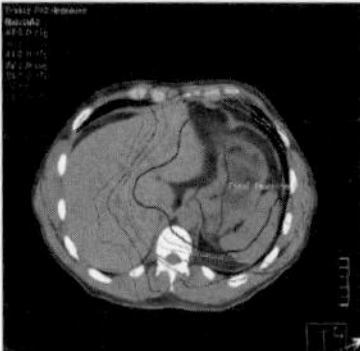
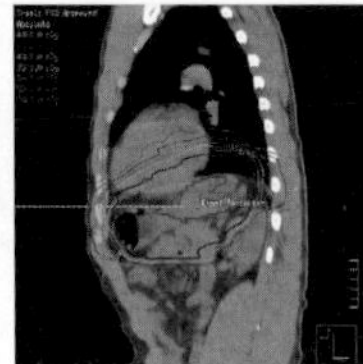
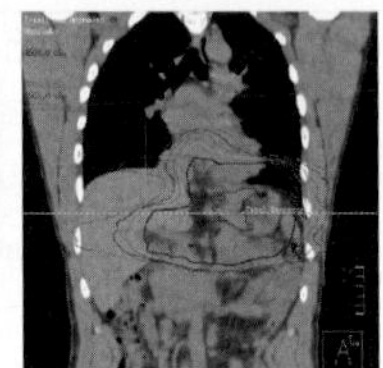

Figure 41.2 Representative axial, sagittal, and coronal cross-sectional images (L → R) illustrating a typical IMRT treatment plan for preoperative radiation for gastric adenocarcinoma. The 45-Gy isodose line is shown in *blue*, which encompasses the MTV (*red line*), involved and elective nodes, with a 1-cm expansion. This patient's primary tumor was located at the GEJ extending 4 cm into the cardia. **See color insert**.

Elective Nodes

GEJ/fundus/cardia	Perigastric, celiac, left gastric artery, splenic artery, splenic hilar, hepatic artery, porta hepatis
Body	Perigastric, celiac, left gastric artery, splenic artery, splenic hilar, hepatic artery, porta hepatis, sub-/suprapyloric, pancreaticoduodenal
Antrum/pylorus	Perigastric, celiac, left gastric artery, hepatic artery, porta hepatis, sub-/suprapyloric, pancreaticoduodenal

- **Technique:** IMRT

Adjuvant/post-op

- **Dose:** 45 Gy in 25 fractions at 1.8 Gy/fx, consider boost if R1/R2 resection
- **Target:** Draw tumor bed using pre-op imaging, op report, and pathology. Same nodal regions as pre-op, cover anastomosis (may be high in the thorax), cover gastric remnant.
- **Technique:** IMRT
- **IGRT:** Daily kV imaging
- **Planning directive (for conventional fractionation):**
  Cord Max < 45 Gy
  Lung: V20 < 25%, V10 < 45%, V5 < 65%, MLD < 20 Gy
  Heart: V30 < 25%, ALARA
  Kidney: Each kidney V20 < 33%, mean < 18 Gy
  Liver: V30 < 30%, V20 < 50%, mean < 25 Gy

Surgery

- For distal tumors (body/antrum) → subtotal gastrectomy; proximal → total gastrectomy
- D1 Dissection—removes involved proximal or distal or entire stomach + perigastric LNs
- D2 Dissection—D1 + celiac, L gastric, hepatic, splenic, splenic hilum (celiac + branches)
- D3 Dissection—D2 + PA +/– porta hepatis
- Billroth I anastomosis (end-to-end gastrojejunal w/ gastric resection margin) or Billroth II (end-to-side anastomosis, gastric resection margin NOT used)

Chemotherapy

- **Concurrent pre-op:** Infusional 5-FU based (+/– oxaliplatin) OR paclitaxel/carboplatin
- **Concurrent post-op:** 5-FU alone (infusional or capecitabine)
- **Perioperative/postoperative:** 5-FU + cisplatin OR fluoropyrimidine + oxaliplatin OR epirubicin, cisplatin + 5-FU

Side Effect Management

- Nausea: Use PPI, first-line Zofran (8 mg q8h prn) → second-line Compazine (10 mg q6h prn) → ABH (lorazepam 0.34 mg, diphenhydramine 25 mg, and haloperidol 1.5 mg) 1 capsule q6h

- Anorexia: Maintain hydration, IVF if necessary, dietary counseling including protein heavy intake
- Skin care: Aquaphor
- Hand and foot syndrome: *Redness, swelling, and pain in hand and foot.* Consult with medical oncology about reducing concurrent capecitabine dose.

Follow-up

- History/physical: Every 3-6 months for 2 years → every 6-12 months for 5 years
- EGD: As clinically indicated
- CT C/A/P w/ contrast (or PET/CT): Every 6-12 months for 2 years and then annually

Notable Trials

Post-op chemoRT

- **Intergroup 0116** (*Macdonald NEJM* 2001; *Smalley JCO* 2012): Two-arm randomized b/w surgery vs surgery + post-op chemoRT (5-FU/LV ×1 before, 2 during, 2 after). Included Stage IB-IV, R0 resection, PS $\leq$ 2, and maintaining 1500 kcal/day diet. Mostly D0 and D1 dissections (10% D2). Improved median OS with post-op chemoRT: 39 months vs 27 months ($P = .0046$) and 3-year RFS 48% vs 31% ($P < .001$). Subgroup analysis showed lack of benefit in women with diffuse subtype.
- **CRITICS** (*Dikken BMC Cancer* 2011; *Verheij ASCO* abstract 2016): Prospective randomized trial of 788 patients from Netherlands, Denmark, and Sweden. Patients had Stage IB-IV gastric cancer and received neoadjuvant chemo ECC/EOC ×3 + gastrectomy/D1 dissection → post-op chemo (3× ECC/EOC) vs post-op chemoRT (45 Gy/25 fx + cape/cis) → 5-year OS similar (41.3% chemoRT vs 40.9% CHT, $P = .99$), heme toxicity higher in CHT arm vs chemoRT (44% vs 34%, $P = .01$).
- **ARTIST** (*Lee JCO* 2012; *Park JCO* 2015): Prospective randomized trial of 458 patients with Stage IB-IV gastric cancer following D2 dissection. Patients randomized to receive post-op chemo (cape/cis ×6) vs post-op chemo + chemoRT (cape/cis ×2 → RT 45Gy/cape → cape/cis ×2). Median OS similar between arms; however local recurrence lower with RT (13% vs 7%, $P = .003$). Subgroup analysis showed improved DFS in node+ patients with chemoRT (76% vs 72%, $P = .04$) or those with intestinal subtype (94% vs 83%, $P = .01$).

Pre-op chemoRT

- **CROSS trial** (*van Hagen NEJM* 2012; *Shapiro Lancet Oncol* 2015): Two-arm randomized esophageal + GE junction (75% adeno, 23% SCC) T1-T3, N0-N1 to surgery alone vs pre-op chemoRT + surgery (41.4 Gy w/ carbo/tax). Median OS 49 months (chemoRT) vs 24 months (sx), higher for SCC but both groups benefit. R0 resection rate 92% (chemoRT) vs 69% (sx alone).
- RTOG 9904 (*Ajani JCO* 2006): Phase II trial of 49 total patients with localized gastric adenocarcinoma. A negative laparoscopic evaluation was required. Patients received 2 cycles of induction 5-FU, leucovorin, and cisplatin followed by concurrent chemoRT (with infusional 5-FU and weekly paclitaxel). Resection was attempted following completion of neoadjuvant therapy. pCR and R0 resection rates were 26% and 77%, respectively. Patients with pCR had improved survival at 1 year (82% vs 69%). D2 performed in 50% of patients.

Periop chemo

- **MAGIC** (*Cunningham NEJM* 2006): Prospective randomized trial of 503 patients with gastric/GEJ cancer $\geq$ Stage II randomized to surgery alone vs periop chemo + surgery (pre-op ECF ×3 and post-op ECF ×3). 5-Year OS 36% (chemo + sx) vs 23% (sx alone), $P = .009$, with 0% pCR rate.
- **FFCD** (*Ychou JCO* 2011): Prospective randomized trial of 224 patients with GEJ + gastric/GEJ cancer, $\geq$Stage II → sx alone vs periop chemo + sx (5-FU/cis ×2-3 pre-op and ×3-4 post-op). 5-Year OS improved with chemotherapy 38% vs 24% ($P = .02$) along with DFS 34% vs 19% ($P = .003$). Overall 38% grade 3-4 toxicity in chemotherapy + sx arm, with 3% pCR rate

Post-op chemo

- **CLASSIC** (*Bang Lancet* 2012; *Noh Lancet Oncol* 2014): Prospective randomized trial of 1035 patients with Stage II-IIIB gastric, required D2 dissection. Randomized between surgery alone vs surgery + post-op chemo (cape/oxali ×6 months). Improved 5-year DFS with chemo 68% vs 53% ($P < .0001$) and 5-year OS 78% vs 69% ($P = .0015$)

HEPATOBILIARY CANCER

LAUREN ELIZABETH COLBERT • PRAJNAN DAS

Hepatocellular Carcinoma (HCC)

- **Incidence/prevalence:** Fifth most common cancer worldwide, third leading cause of cancer mortality. Screening programs are effective—those w/ risk factors should be screened with US and AFP q6-12mo.
- **Risk factors:** Cirrhosis from any cause, including hepatitis (B > C; accounts for 75% of cases), alcoholic, autoimmune, and NASH-related
- **Evaluation/workup:** Need to know Child-Pugh score (albumin, total bili, INR, ascites, encephalopathy); imaging w/ triphasic CT or MRI; hepatitis serologies; labs including AFP and LFTs

Treatment Algorithm for HCC

Resectable, operable candidate	Child-Pugh A (occ. B) → Surgical resection; 5-y OS 40%-80%
Liver transplant candidate	Child-Pugh B-C okay; Based on **Milan criteria** (solitary lesion ≤5 cm, or 3 lesions each ≤3 cm, no vascular invasion, no LN) → transplant list. Can use SBRT, EBRT, or other local therapies as bridge to transplant
Unresectable/not transplant candidate	Transcatheter arterial chemoembolization (TACE), radiofrequency ablation (RFA), Sir-Spheres Y-90, SBRT/EBRT, sorafenib (median OS 10.7 mo vs 7.9 mo in phase III trials; (*Llovet NEJM* 2008), nivolumab (*El-Khoueiry Lancet* 2017)

Choosing Local Therapy

RFA	Tumor ≤4 cm, CP A/B, >1 cm from the liver capsule, vessels, diaphragm, dome of the liver
TACE	NO portal vein thrombosis (need vascular access)
Radiation	Portal vein thrombosis okay, large tumors okay (as long as adequate preserved functional liver)

Cholangiocarcinoma

- **Incidence/prevalence:** 10% intrahepatic, 60% perihilar, 30% distal. Extrahepatic includes perihilar and distal. The second most common primary hepatobiliary malignancy after HCC. Estimated 6000 cases per year in the United States
- **Risk factors:** Anything causing chronic inflammation of the gallbladder or gallbladder tracts: Primary sclerosing cholangitis, liver flukes, chronic calculi
- **Evaluation/workup:** Triphasic CT or MRI with contrast. MRCP or ERCP (particularly if obstruction, need stenting), CA19-9, AFP, CEA, and LFTs. Evaluate for resectability (hepatic duct involvement, encasement of portal vein, stage III-IV disease, late-stage cirrhosis, medically unfit for surgery are all reasons to pursue alternate treatment options).

Treatment Algorithm for Cholangiocarcinoma

Distal	More likely to be resectable → requires pancreaticoduodenectomy→ adjuvant chemo or chemoRT if R1 or N+ (*Horgan JCO* 2012)
Intrahepatic	Surgery when feasible. If unresectable → RT Unresectable dz: survival improved with ablative RT (BED > 80.5; *Tao JCO* 2016)
Perihilar	If resectable requires hepatic lobectomy + involved bile ducts + nodal dissection → adjuvant chemo or chemoRT if R1 or N+. Often unresectable. Definitive RT if unresectable

Anatomy

- The liver has eight independent segments.
- The middle hepatic vein divides the liver into right and left lobes.
- The portal vein divides the liver into upper and lower segments.
- Dual blood supply by portal vein and hepatic artery

Radiation Treatment Technique for HCC/Cholangiocarcinoma

- **SIM:** NPO for 3 hours, with IV contrast, 5-6 repeat deep inspiration breath-hold scans for reproducibility; start scans 30 seconds after IV contrast administration to get variable contrast phases
- **Dose:** Depends on tumor location, size, and anatomy; goal BED > 80 if possible. SBRT (50 Gy in 4-5 fractions), dose-escalated hypofractionated IMRT (60-67.5 Gy in 15 fractions) or standard fractionation (54-50.4 Gy in 28 fractions). Consider lower doses for post-op cases with R0 resection. Need >5 mm from GI mucosa. Preserve >700-800 cc functional liver
- **Target:** Tumor defined on liver protocol CT/MRI and breath-hold scans from simulation to accommodate respiratory movement; contour GI mucosal avoidance structure based on anatomic movement + 5 mm
  If extrahepatic cholangiocarcinoma, consider elective treatment of portal and celiac vein LN basins to 45 Gy in 25 fractions.
- **Technique:** IMRT, SBRT, or protons; use daily CT on rails or fiducials with CBCT for cases with escalated dose/SBRT
- **Constraints:**

Structure	4 or 5 Fractions (50 Gy)	15 Fractions (60-67.5 Gy)	25 or 28 Fractions
Spinal cord	D_{max} < 18 Gy; 10 cc < 15 Gy	D_{max} < 30 Gy	D_{max} < 45 Gy
Liver (minus GTV)	700 cc < 15 Gy; mean < 16 Gy	Child-Pugh A 700 cc < 24 Gy; mean < 24 Gy Child-Pugh B 700 cc < 18 Gy; mean < 18 Gy	Child-Pugh A 700 cc < 28 Gy; mean < 28 Gy Child-Pugh B 700 cc < 24 Gy; mean < 24 Gy
Kidneys	V15 < 67% for contralateral, V15 < 35% for both	V20 < 33% for each	V20 < 33% for each
Stomach	D_{max} < 28 Gy	D_{max} < 45 Gy	D_{max} < 55 Gy
Duodenum	D_{max} < 28 Gy	D_{max} < 45 Gy	D_{max} < 55 Gy,
Small bowel	D_{max} < 28 Gy	D_{max} < 45 Gy	D_{max} < 55 Gy
Large bowel	D_{max} < 30 Gy	D_{max} < 50 Gy	D_{max} < 60 Gy
Heart	V40 < 10%	V40 < 10%	V40 < 10%
Common bile duct	D_{max} < 55 Gy	D_{max} < 70 Gy	D_{max} < 80 Gy

Notable Trials

SWOG 0809 (*Ben-Josef JCO* 2015): Phase II trial of 79 patients with extrahepatic cholangiocarcinoma or gallbladder cancer s/p radical resection. Patients received four cycles of IV gemcitabine and capecitabine, followed by chemoRT with capecitabine (54-59.4 Gy to tumor bed, 45 Gy to regional lymphatics). 2-Year OS 65%, including 67% and 60% in R0 and R1 patients, respectively. Grade 3 side effects were observed in 52% and grade 4 in 11%. Overall survival was higher than expected with this regimen (predicted to be ~45% for this population using historical data).

GENERAL BREAST CANCER

AMY C. MORENO • WENDY WOODWARD

Background

- **Incidence/prevalence:** See other breast cancer chapters.
- **Outcomes:** See other breast cancer chapters.
- **Risk factors:** Increasing age, personal or family history of breast cancer, genetic mutations (BRCA1/2, p53 [Li-Fraumeni], PTEN [Cowden], STK11 [Peutz-Jeghers], ATM [ataxia-telangiectasia]), prior chest radiotherapy, estrogen exposure (obesity, hormone therapy/contraceptive use, early menarche, late menopause, nulliparity), alcohol consumption

Breast Cancer Screening Guidelines

- **American Cancer Society:** Annual mammogram (MMG) ages 45-54, biennial MMG beginning at age 55
- **U.S. Preventive Task Force:** Biennial screening MMG from ages 50 to 74. Recommends against breast self-examination
- **High-risk patients:** BRCA carriers/untested 1° relatives: age 25-30 or 10 years earlier than affected 1° relative; women with 1° relative with premenopausal BCA or women with lifetime risk of BCA ≥ 20%
- **Breast MR imaging:** Not required for screening, useful for women with dense breasts

Tumor Biology and Characteristics

- **Genetics:** BRCA1: 60%-80% lifetime risk of breast cancer and 40% risk for ovarian cancer
  BRCA2: 40%-50% lifetime risk of BCA and 10%-20% risk for ovarian cancer. Genetic counseling recommended if high-risk features present for hereditary breast cancer
- **Pathology:** See other breast cancers.
- **Imaging:** See other breast cancers.

BI-RADS Categories for MMGs			
1	Negative	4	New suspicious abnormality (biopsy)
2	Stable benign findings	5	New finding highly suggestive of malignancy (biopsy and treat)
3	New finding, likely benign (recommend biopsy or repeat MMG in 6 mo)	6	Known biopsy, proven malignancy

Anatomy

Field borders are not to rigidly supercede volume-based target definitions edited for patient- and tumor-specific factors.

- **Breast anatomic breast borders:** Inferior border of clavicular head or 2nd anterior rib (superior) and loss of apparent breast parenchyma or 6th anterior rib (inferior), midaxillary line (lateral), and sternum-rib junction (medial). Breast contouring should include all of the glandular breast tissue and the clinically apparent breast mound.
- **Regional nodal borders** (normal volumes are described in the RTOG atlas and should be considered a starting place and edited for clinical risk):
  - Axillary: level 1 (inferior and lateral to pectoralis minor), level 2 (subpectoral and constrained by pectoralis minor, includes Rotter nodes), and level 3 (medial and superior to pectoralis minor, should always be contoured if targeted and should be entirely within the SCV field when treating with 3D)
  - Internal mammary: superior aspect of medial 1st rib (superior) to superior aspect of 4th rib (inferior). IM nodes should be contoured if targeted.
  - Supraclavicular: cricoid (superior), inferior border of clavicular head (inferior). Medial border should cover the volume even if it includes the trachea.

Breast Cancer Staging *(AJCC 8th edition)*

T Stage		N Stage	Clinical	Pathologic
Tis	Ductal carcinoma in situ	N0	No regional LN(s) involved	pN0: None pN0(i+): ITCs only pN0(mol+): Positive by RT-PCR only
T1mi	Tumor size (TS) ≤ 1 mm	N1mi	Micromets (~200 cells, >0.2 mm but ≤2 mm)	
T1a	TS > 1 mm but ≤5 mm	N1	Mobile ipsilateral level I-II axillary LN(s)	pN1a: 1-3 axilla LN(s) pN1b: Ipsi IM LN(s) pN1c: pN1a + pN1b
T1b	TS > 5 mm but ≤10 mm	N2a	Matted/fixed ipsi level I-II axillary LN(s)	4-9 axillary LN(s)
T1c	TS > 10 mm but ≤20 mm	N2b	Only ipsi IM LN(s) involved	
T2	TS > 20 mm but ≤50 mm	N3a	Ipsi infraclavicular LN(s)	≥10 axillary LN(s) or infraclavicular LN(s)
T3	TS > 50 mm	N3b	Ipsi IM and axillary LN(s)	
T4a	Extension to chest wall (invasion of pectoralis in the absence of chest wall invasion does not qualify)	N3c	Ipsi supraclavicular LN(s)	
T4b	Ulceration and/or ipsilateral satellite nodules and/or edema without meeting criteria for T4b	**M Stage**		
		M0	No distant metastases cM0(i+): tumor cell deposits ≤2 cm detected only by microscopic or molecular techniques	
T4c	Both T4a and T4b present			
T4d	Inflammatory carcinoma (see **IBC** chapter)	M1	Distant metastases present	

Summative Stage: Prognostic Stage Groups should now be used in countries that routinely test for receptors and grade, See AJCC 8th edition

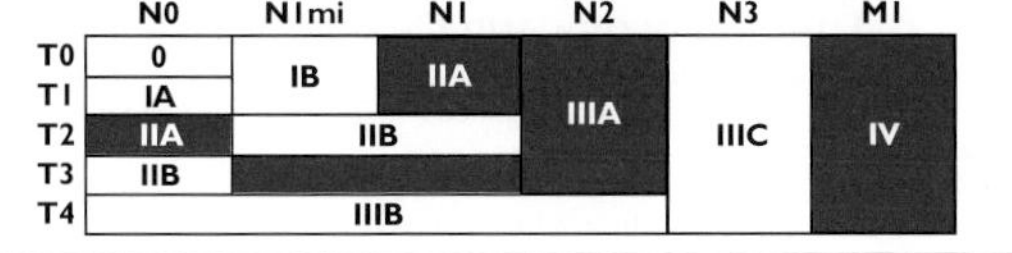

Abbreviations: Ipsi, ipsilateral; IM, internal mammary; ITCs, isolated tumor cells.

Systemic Therapy

Preference at our institution is for neoadjuvant chemotherapy (NAC) if the decision to give chemotherapy is known. NAC is the first option in a patient who wants BCS but cannot proceed due to tumor size.

	ER/PR+ HER2–	ER/PR +/– HER2+	ER/PR– HER2–
DCIS	+ Hormone therapy	+/– Hormone therapy (for ER+ only)	Observation
Primary <5 mm or microinvasive N0	+/– Hormone therapy[a]	+/– Herceptin-based chemotherapy[a] +/– Hormone therapy (ER+ only)[a]	+/– Chemotherapy[a]

Primary 0.5-5 cm N0	+/– Chemotherapy (Oncotype DX[b] or other genomic study) + Hormone therapy	+ Herceptin-based chemotherapy +/– Hormone therapy (ER+ only)	+ Chemotherapy
Primary >5 cm and/or ≥N1mi	+ Chemotherapy + Hormone therapy	+ Herceptin-based chemotherapy +/– Hormone therapy (ER+ only)	+ Chemotherapy

[a]Choice of hormone therapy, chemotherapy, or Herceptin-based chemotherapy is unclear and depends on discussion of factors including patient preference, age, and pathology factors (size, grade, margin, etc.).
[b]if Oncotype DX score <18, then no chemotherapy; score 18-30, then unclear; score >30, then chemotherapy.

- Chemotherapy (for Her2–): AC (Adriamycin, cyclophosphamide) ×4, ddAC (dose-dense AC, administered twice for every 4-week cycle) ×4, or FAC (fluorouracil, Adriamycin, and cyclophosphamide) ×4 → paclitaxel q1wk ×12
- Herceptin-based chemotherapy (for Her2+): THP (paclitaxel, Herceptin, pertuzumab) ×6, then consider ddAC q2wk ×4 pre-/postop → maintenance Herceptin q3wk (total 1 year)
- Alternate Her2+ regimen: TCHP (paclitaxel, carboplatin, Herceptin, pertuzumab) ×6 → maintenance trastuzumab q3wk (total 1 year)
- Hormone therapy: tamoxifen or aromatase inhibitor for 5-10 years

DUCTAL CARCINOMA IN SITU (DCIS)

AMY C. MORENO • WENDY WOODWARD

Background

- **Incidence/prevalence:** Approximately 70 000 cases diagnosed annually in the United States. DCIS accounts for 15%-30% of all detected breast cancer.
- **Outcomes:** Mortality from DCIS is very low. 20-Year breast cancer–specific mortality is 3.3% (*Narod et al. JAMA Oncol* 2015).
- **Risk factors:** See **General Breast Cancer** chapter.

Tumor Biology and Characteristics

- **Genetics:** See **General Breast Cancer** chapter.
- **Pathology:** Subtypes of DCIS include comedonecrosis and noncomedo (cribriform, papillary, medullary, and solid type).
- **Imaging:** On mammogram, characteristically appears as linear or granular calcifications. May underestimate size by 1-2 cm. On *ultrasound*, typically presents as hypoechoic mass with ductal extension. On *MRI*, regional branching or linear enhancement is seen on T1.

Workup

- **History and physical:** Including bilateral breast examination and axilla palpation. Consider genetics evaluation.
- **Labs:** β-HCG (if premenopausal)
- **Procedures/biopsy:** Core needle biopsy of suspicious breast lesions, pathology staining of biopsy for ER/PR status. Two commercially available genomic tests may further refine risk estimates: DCISionRT and Oncotype DX.
- **Imaging:** Bilateral diagnostic mammogram (MMG), breast ± regional LN basin ultrasound, consider MRI for dense breasts.

Treatment Algorithms

Screen detected, low-intermediate grade, <2.5 cm, ≥3-mm margins	BCS → observation or hormone therapy[a]
Age ≥ 50, <2.5 cm, low-intermediate grade, ≥3-mm surgical margins, ER positive	BCS → APBI → hormone therapy
No eligibility restrictions	BCS → WBI → observation or hormone therapy[a]
No eligibility restrictions	Total mastectomy +/– SLNB → observation or hormone therapy[a]

[a]If ER/PR+

Radiation Treatment Technique for WBI

- **SIM:** Supine, upper Vac-Lok device, ipsilateral arm abducted/externally rotated over the head. Use slant board (5-15 degrees) to make breasts fall downward but balance with degree of inframammary fold (can worsen skin reactions). Consider wiring surgical scar and treatment borders, inspiration breath-hold for left-sided tumors to reduce heart/lung doses, and prone simulation for larger BMI and/or pendulous breasts.
- **Dose:** 40.05 Gy in 15 fx → boost to 10-16 Gy* in 2 Gy/fx or 42.5 Gy in 16 fx if a boost was intended but not feasible (eg, complicated surgical bed)
- **Target:** Clinical breast mound including all glandular breast tissue (Fig. 44.1)
- **Considerations:** Boost doses: *10 Gy for negative SM, 14 Gy for close SM, and 16 Gy for positive SM (reexcision preferred but if not possible [ie, positive SM at fascia] give higher boost dose)
- **Technique:** Opposed lateral tangents and appositional electron field for boost

Initial WBI Field Treatment Borders Finalize using RTOG consensus guidelines and CT/volume-based contouring	
Superior	Typically 2 cm below humeral head if not using high tangents
Inferior	2 cm below inframammary fold
Anterior	Flash ipsilateral breast
Posterior	≤2 cm of ipsilateral lung
Medial	Sternum (avoid treating contralateral breast)
Lateral	Midaxilla (cover entire ipsilateral breast)
Cone-Down Tumor Bed Boost	
2-cm expansion around tumor bed, 2-cm margin to block edge. Typically use appositional electron field. Resimulate during treatment with breast compression device if needed to flatten tumor bed and improve setup reproducibility	

- **IGRT:** Weekly MV imaging once setup is stable
- **Planning directive for WBI:**
  - Breast: V98 ≥ 100%, V100 > 90%
  - Entire breast/CW covered by 98% isodose line (IDL)
  - Entire tumor bed covered by 100% IDL
  - Boost target covered by 90% IDL
  - Heart: V5 ≤ 40% (≤50% for left-sided tumors)
    Expected mean heart dose for left intact breast with no IMC < 1 Gy
  - Total lung: V20 < 35%
    V40 < 20%
  - Evaluate each beam separately for adequate coverage
  - Avoid 106% hot spots, consider using wedges or field-in-fields

Systemic Therapy

- Chemotherapy not part of management for DCIS
- Consider endocrine therapy for 5 years for estrogen receptor (ER)-positive DCIS.
  - **Tamoxifen** 20 mg PO daily for premenopausal women
  - **Aromatase inhibitors (anastrozole, letrozole)** for pre- or postmenopausal women

Surgical Definitions and Pathology Information

- **Breast-conserving surgery (BCS) or lumpectomy:** Removal of tumor and surrounding area of breast tissue to ensure negative margins

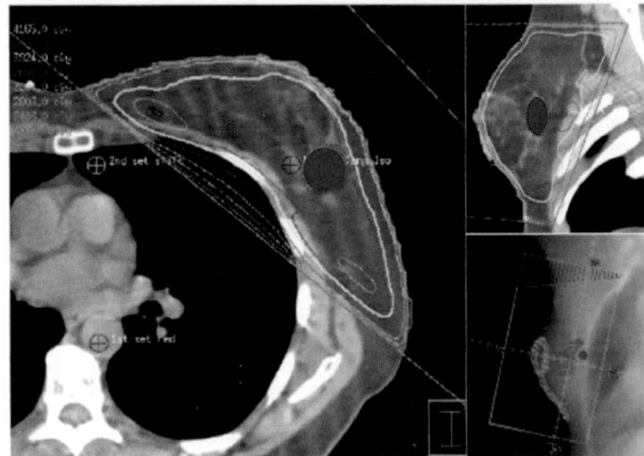

Figure 44.1 CT-based XRT planning images and DRR of the left lateral tangent beam. Contours: *Maroon*, tumor bed. Isodose lines on CT images: *White*, 98% IDL.

- **Total or skin-sparing mastectomy:** Complete removal of the breast ± overlying skin
- **Sentinel lymph node biopsy (SLNB):** Not indicated in DCIS. May be offered if high risk for occult invasive disease and if mastectomy is planned. Blue dye and/or radioactive tracer is injected into the ipsilateral breast to help locate typically 1-3 sentinel nodes for removal
- **Pathology report:** Review ER/PR status, tumor grade, tumor size, extent (multifocal?), surgical margin status (either positive, close [0-1.9 mm], or negative [≥2 mm])

Side Effect Management

- **Skin care:** Aquaphor → Cool Magic → Mepilex dressings

Follow-up

- History and physical: Every 6-12 months ×5 years, then annually
- Bilateral diagnostic mammogram: Every year

Notable Trials

WBI after lumpectomy results in ~50% reduction in ipsilateral breast recurrence

- **NSABP B17/B24** (*Wapnir et al. JNCI* 2011): BCS vs BCS + WBI, margins negative (50 Gy in 25 fractions, 9% received boost). 15-Year ipsilateral breast tumor recurrence reduced with BCS + WBI (IBTR; DCIS or invasive): 19% vs 9% (HR 0.48, $P < .001$). No difference in OS or CSS
- **EORTC 10853** (*Donker et al. JCO* 2013): BCS vs BCS + WBI (50 Gy in 25 fractions, 5% received boost). 15-Year IBTR reduced with BCS + WBI: 30% vs 17% (HR 0.52, $P < .001$). No difference in OS or CSS
- **SweDCIS** (*Warnberg et al. JCO* 2014): BCS vs BCS + WBI (48-50 Gy total dose, boost not recommended). 20-Year IBTR risk reduced with BCS + WBI: 32% vs 20%. No difference in OS or CSS
- **EBCTCG DCIS meta-analysis** (*Correa et al. JNCI* 2010): RT after BCS decreases any IBTR by ~50% (28.1% w/o RT vs 12.9% w/ RT). Proportional reduction in ipsilateral breast events greater in older vs younger women (≥50 vs <50). RT reduced absolute 10-year risk of IBTR by 15% regardless of patient age, extent of BCS, use of TAM, margin status, tumor grade, or size

Tamoxifen after lumpectomy further reduces ipsilateral breast recurrence

- **UK/ANZ** (*Cuzick et al. Lancet Oncol* 2011): 2 × 2 comparing BCS ± WBI ± tamoxifen (TAM) given 20 mg PO daily for 5 years. 10-Year IBTR reduced with WBI: 19% vs 7% (HR 0.32, $P < .001$). 10-Year IBTR reduced with TAM: 20% vs 16% (HR 0.68, $P = .04$)

- **NSABP B17/B24** (*Wapnir et al. JNCI* 2011): BCS + WBI vs BCS + WBI + tamoxifen. 15-Year contralateral breast tumor occurrence reduced with BCS + WBI + tamoxifen (IBTR): 11% vs 7% (HR 0.68, *P* = .023). No difference in OS or CSS

Omission of RT after BCS for good-risk DCIS

- **ECOG 5194** (*Solin et al. JCO* 2015): BCS vs BCS + WBI (31% received TAM) in "low-risk" patients: grade 1-2 DCIS measuring ≤2.5 cm **or** high-grade DCIS measuring ≤1 cm, all required normal post-op MMG and margins ≥3 mm. High-grade patients had unacceptable 25% 12-year IBTR (13% invasive) compared with lower/intermediate-grade patients who had an acceptable 14% IBTR (8% invasive). **Additional conclusion:** High-grade DCIS is a poor prognostic factor for radiation omission.
- **RTOG 9804** (*McCormick et al. JCO* 2015): BCS vs BCS + WBI in "low-risk" patients. Grade 1-2 DCIS ≤ 2.5 cm with margins ≥3 mm. TAM 20 mg PO daily given in both arms (69% overall compliance). 7-Year local failure rate reduced with BCS + WBI: 6.7% vs 0.9%, but 6.7% was deemed an acceptable risk. Grade 1-2 toxicities were lower in observation arm: 76% vs 30%.

Hypofractionated whole breast radiation is safe for DCIS

- **MDACC randomized clinical trial** (*Shaitelman et al. JAMA Oncol* 2015): 287 women age ≥40 with stage 0-II BCA (22% DCIS) randomized to HF-WBI (42.56 Gy/16 fx + boost) vs CF-WBI (50 Gy/25 fx + boost) after BCS. Decreased acute grade 2 toxicity with HF-WBI (47% vs 78%; *P* < .001) and improved QOL and less fatigue with HF-WBI vs CF-WBI

EARLY-STAGE BREAST CANCER (ESBC)

JAY PAUL REDDY • WENDY WOODWARD

Background

- **Definition:** Stage I/II patients (T1/2 N0/1mic/1)—T3N0 (stage IIB) is included in **LABC** chapter.
- **Incidence/prevalence:** Most commonly diagnosed cancer among women and second leading cause of death in the United States. Approximately 250 000 new cases of invasive breast cancer (BCA) annually and 40 000 deaths annually. Lifetime risk is 1 in 8 (12%).
- **Outcomes:** 5-Year survival ~90%
- **Risk factors:** See **General Breast Cancer** chapter.
- **Screening guidelines:** See **General Breast Cancer** chapter.

Tumor Biology and Characteristics

- **Pathology:** Majority invasive ductal carcinoma (~90%). Remaining 10% is invasive lobular carcinoma, which is bilateral in up to 30% of cases. Pathologic evaluation for tumor grade, size, extent (multifocal?), surgical margin (SM) status (either positive, close [0-1.9 mm], or negative [≥2 mm]). IHC testing for ER (≥1% threshold), PR, Her2 (IHC: 3+ on ≥10% breast tissue threshold, if Her2+ utilize FISH testing and test if ratio > 2.0), and Ki-67
- **Molecular subtypes (incidence and receptor-based surrogates):**
  - Luminal A–like (70%): grades 1-2, high ER+/PR+, Her2–, low Ki-67
  - Luminal B–like (10%): grade 3, low ER+/PR+, +/–Her2+, high Ki-67
  - Her2-like (10%): grade 3, ER/PR–/+, Her2+, high Ki-67
  - Basal-like (10%): grade 3, triple negative (TNBC), BRCA1 associated. Basal-like further subclassed.

Note: gene expression and receptor subtypes not perfectly correlated.

- **Multigene panels and signature scores:** Routinely utilize recurrence scores including Oncotype DX DCIS recurrence score. Retrospective analyses of the NSABP data suggest that recurrence score is prognostic for LRR in node-negative and node-positive ER+ patients (*Paik et al. NEJM* 2004).
- **Imaging:** *MMG*, linear or granular microcalcifications, masses, skin thickening, nipple retraction, or distortions. *Ultrasound*, hypoechoic mass with irregular margins and ductal extension ± infiltration of surrounding tissue. *MRI*, regional branching, mass, or linear enhancement on T1
- **Anatomy:** See **General Breast Cancer** chapter.

Workup

- **History and physical:** Including bilateral breast examination and axilla palpation. Consider genetics evaluation.
- **Labs:** β-HCG (if premenopausal), for stage IIB add CBC and LFTs
- **Procedures/biopsy:** Core needle biopsy of suspicious breast lesions, pathologic staining of biopsy for ER/PR status and Her2 expression. Consider obtaining Oncotype DX score if indicated.
- **Imaging:** Bilateral diagnostic MMG, breast and regional LN basin ultrasound. Consider MRI for dense breasts, suspected multicentric/multifocal disease, occult primary, or chest wall invasion. If abnormal LFTs, or symptoms, bone scan and/or CT of the chest, abdomen, and pelvis.

Treatment Algorithms

- **Overall treatment:** Both adjuvant and neoadjuvant chemotherapy are equally valid, consider neoadjuvant if patient desires BCS but cannot due to size of primary disease. Institutional preference is for neoadjuvant approach.
- **Adjuvant systemic therapy approach:** Mastectomy/BCS + SLNB ± ALND → systemic therapy (if any) → radiation → completion hormone/Herceptin therapy (if any)
- **Neoadjuvant systemic therapy approach:** Systemic therapy (if any) → mastectomy/BCS + SLNB ± ALND → radiation → completion hormone/Herceptin therapy (if any)

Radiation options

- **Whole breast irradiation (WBI):** See **DCIS** chapter. *In a patient with involvement of 1-2 LNs identified on SLNB and who did not have an ALND, consider contouring level I-II LNs and modifying WBI tangents to encompass.*
- **WBI + regional nodal irradiation (RNI):** See **LABC** chapter.
- **Postmastectomy radiation therapy (PMRT):** Chest wall radiation and RNI, see **LABC** chapter.
- **Accelerated partial breast irradiation (APBI):** If patient meets eligibility criteria

	Surgery	LN Status	Radiation
No neoadjuvant systemic	BCS + SLNB/ALND	pN0/(i+)[a]	• No radiation
		pN0/(i+)/mic	• APBI • WBI • WBI + RNI[c]
		1-2 LN+	• WBI[b] • WBI + RNI[c]
		≥3 LN+	• WBI + RNI
	Mastectomy + SLNB/ALND	0-2 LNs	• No radiation • PMRT[c]
		≥3 LN+	• PMRT
Neoadjuvant systemic	BCS + SLNB/ALND	ypN0	• WBI • WBI + RNI[d,e]
		yp ≥1 LN+	• WBI + RNI
	Mastectomy + SLNB/ALND	ypN0	• No radiation • PMRT[d,e]
		yp ≥1 LN+	• PMRT

[a]Consider radiation omission (CALGB9343): age ≥70, tumor size ≤3 cm, N0, margin >2 mm, ER+, and willing to undergo hormone therapy.

[b]Patients with LN+ SLNB and no ALND w/ significant risk factors (http://www3.mdanderson.org/app/medcalc/bc_nomogram2), consider modifying tangents to include level 1 and 2 LNs (high tangents).

[c]Consider WBI + RNI/PMRT in patients meeting the following criteria:

- pN1 and ≥**1** of the following: Age ≤40 and upfront surgery, ≥3 LN+ and upfront surgery, cT3N1, ER− and upfront surgery, age <50 and Oncotype DX RS >18, ER− and upfront surgery, and ypN+
- p1-2 LN+, age >40, ER+ and ≥**2** of the following: Luminal B (Ki-67 >20% or Her 2+), grade 3, LVSI, Oncotype DX RS > 18
- pN0/pN0(i+)/pN1mic and ≥**3** of the following: Age ≤40, >1 LN with micromet (0.21-2 mm), T3, central/medial tumor, ER−, grade 3, LVSI, Ki-67 >20% Oncotype DX RS > 18

[d]Consider WBI + RNI/PMRT in patients with ≥cT3N1 or <cT3N1 and ≥1 of the following criteria: Premenopausal, TNBC, greater initial clinical tumor burden, residual tumor in the breast.

[e]Consider omission of RNI/PMRT in patients who are ypT0N0 as part of a clinical trial.

APBI SUITABILITY CRITERIA (N0(i+/i−) TUMORS ONLY)

	Age	Margins	T Stage	DCIS
Suitable (if all criteria match)	≥50	≥2 mm	Tis or T1	(Only if all criteria below are met) • Screen-detected • Low to intermediate grade • ≤2.5 cm • Margin ≥3 mm
Cautionary	• 40-49 if all other criteria for "suitable" are met • ≥50 if ≥1 unsuitable pathology factors exist[a] and otherwise all other criteria for "suitable" are met	<2 mm		≤3 cm and does not meet criteria for "suitable"
Unsuitable[a] (if any criteria match)	• <40 • 40-49 and do not meet criteria for cautionary	Positive		>3 cm

[a]Unsuitable pathology factors: Size 2.1-3 cm, T2, margins <2 mm, limited/focal LVSI, ER−, clinically unifocal with size 2.1-3 cm, invasive lobular histology, pure DCIS ≤ 3 cm if criteria for "suitable" not fully met, extensive invasive component ≤3 cm

ASTRO Consensus Guidelines, Adapted from *Correa et al. Pract Radiat Oncol* 2017.

RADIATION TREATMENT TECHNIQUE

For WBI, see **DCIS** chapter. For chest wall + RNI, see **LABC** chapter.

RADIATION TREATMENT TECHNIQUE FOR APBI

- **Dose:** 38.5 Gy in 10 fractions bid photon-based EBRT (Fig. 45.1)
  34 Gy(RBE) in 10 fractions bid proton-based EBRT (special planning considerations described elsewhere, *Strom et al. Pract Radiol Oncol* 2015)
  Alternative: Using minitangents to treat with APBI per UK IMPORT Low Regimen also acceptable (40.05 Gy/15 fx)
- **Target:** (based on NSABP B-39)

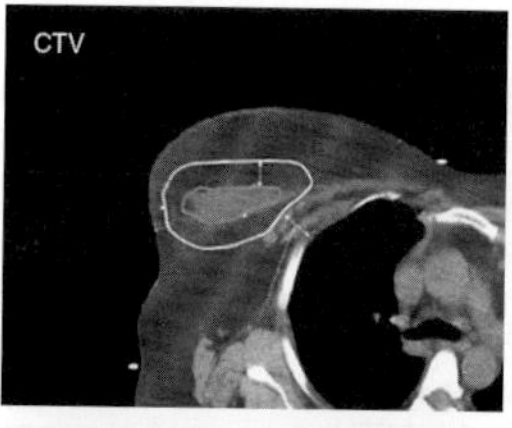

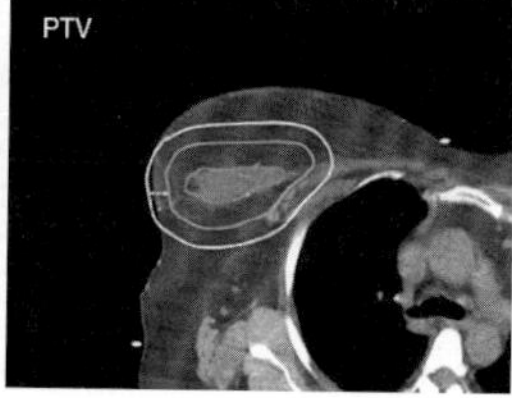

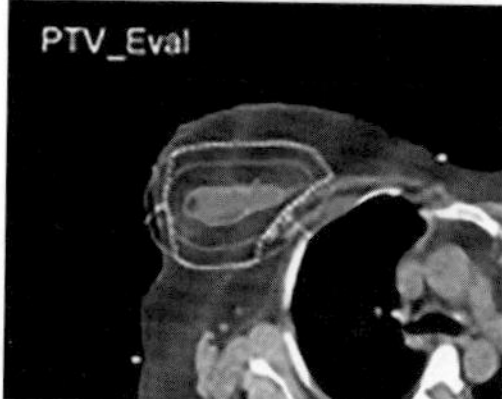

Figure 45.1 External beam APBI volumes. (From NSABP B-39.)

- CTV: Surgical cavity + 15 mm; but limited to 5 mm from skin and excludes chest wall/pectoralis muscles
- PTV: CTV + 10 mm
- PTV_Eval: PTV but limited to 5 mm from skin and excludes chest wall/pectoralis muscles

- **Technique:** 3DCRT: multiple noncoplanar beams
- **SIM:** Supine, upper Vac-Lok device, ipsilateral arm abducted/externally rotated over the head, head turned slightly away (open neck). Use 5- to 15-degree slant board if breast intact or to minimize SCV lung dose. Wire surgical scar. Deep inspiration breath-hold for left-sided tumors to reduce heart/lung doses

Planning Directive for APBI

- PTV_EVAL: ≥90% receives >90% of Rx
- Uninvolved ipsi breast: <35% receives 100% of Rx
- <60% receives <60% of Rx
- Contralateral breast: <3% of Rx dose
- Ipsilateral lung: <15% of volume receives ≤30% of Rx
- Contralateral lung: <15% of volume receives ≤5% of Rx
  - Heart (right breast target): <5% receives ≤5% of Rx
  - Heart (left breast target): <40% receives ≤5% of Rx
- Thyroid: D_{max} is ≤3% of Rx

IGRT (EBRT APBI)

- kV every treatment, align to clips

Side Effect Management/Follow-up

- **Skin care:** Aquaphor → Cool Magic → Mepilex dressings
- **Fatigue:** Encourage exercise and adequate daily protein intake, good sleep hygiene → referral to fatigue clinic
- **Lymphedema:** Referral to physical therapy for education and sleeve fitting → plastic surgery options include LN transfer and lymphatic bypass

Systemic Therapy

See **LABC** chapter.

Surgical Definitions

- **Breast-conserving surgery (BCS) or lumpectomy:** Removal of tumor and surrounding area of breast tissue to ensure negative margins
- **Total or skin-sparing mastectomy:** Complete removal of the breast ± overlying skin
- **Sentinel lymph node biopsy (SLNB):** Conducted in all cLN− patients. Blue dye and/or radioactive tracer injected into the ipsilateral breast to locate one to three sentinel nodes for removal
- **Axillary lymph node dissection (ALND):** Conducted in all patients with invasive disease if cLN+ or cLN− and SLNB+. Adequate if 10 LNs dissected from axillary levels 1-2. Consider extended level 3 or level 2 Rotter node (intrapectoral) dissection if disease identified in these areas. Consider omitting ALND for cLN− and SLNB+ if T1-2 and 1-2 sLN+ when doing lumpectomy and no neoadjuvant therapy (*Guiliano et al. JAMA* 2011).

Notable Trials

Radiation after BCS improves local control and breast cancer deaths

- **EBCTCG meta-analysis** (*Lancet* 2011): RT after BCS decreases any first recurrence at 10 years from 35% to 19.3% ($P < .001$), reduces 15-year risk of BCA death from 25.2% to 21.4% ($P < .001$).

Lumpectomy boost after whole breast radiation

- **EORTC Boost Trial** (*Bartelink et al. Lancet Oncol* 2015): 50 Gy in 25 fractions WBI vs 50 Gy in 25 fractions + 16 Gy boost. Median f/u 17-year IBTR 16.4% vs 12% ($P < .001$). No difference in OS or DMFS.

Omission of RT after BCS is acceptable in low-risk breast cancer patients

- **CALGB 9343** (*Hughes et al. JCO* 2013): Low-risk early breast cancer patients (age ≥70 years, T1 N0, ER+). BCS + observation vs BCS + WBI 45 Gy/25 fx + 14 Gy boost → tamoxifen (TAM) ≥5 years. 10-Year LRFS lower with WBI 98% vs 90% LRFS

($P < .001$). However, the risk of locoregional failure was deemed acceptable with observation.

- **PRIME II** (*Kunkler et al. Lancet Oncol* 2015): Low-risk early breast cancer patients (age ≥65 years, HR+, T1/2 [≤3 cm], N0, grade 3 or LVSI [not both], margins ≥1 mm). BCS + observation vs BCS + WBI 40-50 Gy in 15-25 fractions → hormone ≥5 years. 5-Year IBTR lower with WBI, 1.3% vs 4.1% IBTR ($P < .001$). No difference in OS

Hypofractionation has equivalent efficacy and at least as good cosmesis as conventional fractionated radiation

- **Canada** (*Whelan et al. N Engl J Med* 2010): HF-WBI (42.56 Gy/16 fx) vs CF-WBI (50 Gy/25 fx) in patients with T1/2 N0, margin-negative disease. No boost. 10-Year LR 6.7% vs 6.2% (NS). No difference in OS or DFS. Excellent/good cosmesis in 70% vs 71% (NS)
- **UK START** (*Haviland et al. Lancet Oncol* 2013): Combination of two RCTs, START A and B. HF-WBI (multiple regimens: 40 Gy/15 fx, 41.6 Gy/13 fx, and 39 Gy/13 fx) vs CF-WBI (50 Gy/25 fx) in patients with pT1-3a N0-1, margin-negative disease. 10-Year LR 4%-6% vs 5%-7% (NS). No difference in OS or DFS. Better long-term cosmesis in 40 Gy vs 50 Gy arm (START B)
- **MDACC** (*Shaitelman et al. JAMA Oncol* 2015): HF-WBI (42.56 Gy/16 fx + 10-12.5 Gy/4-5 fx boost) vs CF-WBI (50 Gy/25 fx + 10-14 Gy/5-7 fx boost) in patients with Tis-2 N0-1a disease. Significantly less physician-reported acute toxicity on HF-WBI arm (dermatitis, 36% vs 69%; pruritus, 54% vs 81%; pain, 55% vs 74%; hyperpigmentation, 9% vs 20%; fatigue, 9% vs 17%)

Accelerated partial breast irradiation is associated with good efficacy and cosmesis

- **GEC-ESTRO** (*Strnad et al. Lancet* 2015): Interstitial brachytherapy (32 Gy/8 fx or 30.3 Gy/7 fx bid) vs CF-WBI (50-50.4 Gy/25-28 fx + 10 Gy/5 fx boost) in patients with T1/2 N0 (≤3 cm), margin-negative disease. 5-Year IBTR 1.4% vs 0.9% (NS).
- **RAPID** (*Olivotto et al. JCO* 2013): External APBI (38.5 Gy/10 fx bid) vs WBI (50 Gy/25 fx or 42.56 Gy/16 fx optional 10 Gy boost) in patients with T1/2 N0 (≤3 cm). Increased fibrosis and worse cosmesis in APBI arm at 3 years
- **IMPORT LOW** (*Coles et al. Lancet* 2017): Reduced dose WBI (36 Gy/15 fx with 40 Gy to partial breast) vs PBI (40 Gy/15 fx) vs WBI (40 Gy/15 fx) in patients with pT1-2 (≤3 cm) N0-1, margin ≥ 2 mm disease. 5-Year LR: 0.2% (reduced dose) vs 0.5% (APBI) vs 1.1% (WBI) (NS). Similar to improved cosmesis with APBI and reduced dose compared with WBI

Axillary LN dissection can be omitted in select patients with positive SLNB

- **ACOSOG Z11** (*Guiliano et al. JAMA* 2017): BCS → SLNB +/– ALND in patients with T1/2, cN0, 1 or 2 SN+. 10-Year OS 86.3% vs 83.6% (NS). 10-Year DFS 80.2% vs 78.2% (NS). 46% of SN+ were micromets, and 27.4% of patients treated with ALND had additional positive nodes beyond SLNB.
- **ACOSOG Z11 radiation field analysis** (*Jagsi et al. JCO* 2014): Post hoc analysis of 28.5% evaluable RT records. Of these, 50% received high tangents and 20% had separate regional nodal field.

Regional nodal irradiation (RNI) associated with similar axillary control compared with LN dissection in low-risk patients

- **AMAROS** (*Rutgers et al. Lancet Oncol* 2014): BCS → SLND. If SN+ → axillary RT vs ALND in patients with T1/2 disease. 5-Year axillary recurrence 1.2% vs 0.4%. 5-Year OS 94% vs 94%. 5-Year DFS 87% vs 83%.

Regional nodal irradiation (RNI) associated with improved efficacy in high-risk patients

- **NCIC MA.20** (*Whelan et al. NEJM* 2015): 1832 pts with high-risk (primary >5 cm or >2 cm and <10 ALN removed and either grade 3 histology, ER–, or LVIS) pN0 or pN1-3 s/p BCS + adjuv chemo → WBI vs WBI + RNI. RNI included IMC, SCV, and axillary coverage. Improved 10-year DFS with RNI (82% vs 77%, $P = .01$). No difference in OS between arms (82.8% vs 81.8%, $P = .38$). Increased rates of grade 2+ acute pneumonitis (1.2% vs 0.2%, $P = .01$) and lymphedema (8.4% vs 4.5%, $P = .001$) observed in RNI group

Inclusion of IM nodes in comprehensive PMRT fields may improve efficacy

- **EORTC 22922/10925** (*Poortmans et al. NEJM* 2015): 4004 pts with axillary LAD (~55%) or medial tumors s/p BCS or MRM randomized to PMRT +/– IMC/medial SCV RT. IMC/median SCV RT associated with lower DFS (72.1% vs 69.1%, $P = .04$) and DMFS (78% vs 75%, $P = .02$) at 10 years, trend toward higher OS (82.3% vs 80.7%, $P = .056$). No increased toxicities reported

LOCALLY ADVANCED BREAST CANCER (LABC)

JENNIFER LOGAN • WENDY WOODWARD

Background

- **Definition:** Includes stage III patients (T3N1, N2-3, T4) but can also include stage IIB (T3N0) pts. IBC patients are a subset of LABC (see separate **Inflammatory/Recurrent Breast Cancer** chapter). Stage IV patients are not included.
- **Incidence/prevalence:** LABC accounts for 8%-15% of all detected breast cancers in the United States, with decreased rates in regions of increased screening. Impoverished or minority communities can experience higher rates of LABC and increased mortality.
- **Outcomes:** 5-Year survival rates for stage IIIA and IIIB breast cancers are 52% and 48%, with median survival for stage III at 4.9 years (SEER data).
- **Risk factors:** See **General Breast Cancer** chapter.

Tumor Biology and Characteristics

- **Pathology:** See **ESBC** chapter. Predominant histologies include infiltrating ductal and lobular carcinoma. More favorable histologies, such as tubular or medullary carcinoma, are less common in LABC.
- **Genetics and molecular subtypes:** See **ESBC** and **General Breast Cancer** chapter.

Anatomy/Workup/Staging/Treatment Algorithm

See **ESBC** and **DCIS** chapters.

Radiation Treatment Technique for Comprehensive Breast/Chest Wall Irradiation

- **SIM:** Supine, upper Vac-Lok device, ipsilateral arm abducted/externally rotated over the head, head turned slightly away (open neck). Use 5- to 15-degree slant board if breast intact or to minimize SCV lung dose. Wire surgical scar and treatment borders (optional). Deep inspiration breath-hold for left-sided tumors to reduce heart/lung doses. Aquaplast masks are appropriate for patients who need supraclavicular nodal boosts or who will be treated with protons.
- **Dose:** 50 Gy in 25 fractions → boost to 10-16 Gy in 2 Gy/fx
- **Target:** Entire breast/chest wall and regional nodes (SCV, IMC, undissected cN+)

Comprehensive Breast/CW Treatment Borders for Locally Advanced Breast Cancer: Multi-isocenter Technique *(Example fields may be found at the back of the book insert)*

A general starting point for 3D treatment fields/borders is detailed below. This technique must also include volume-based planning with contouring of appropriate CTVs (ie, chest wall, regional nodal volumes including axillary levels I-III, internal mammary nodes, surgical scars/changes, tissue expander placement, etc.).

- Utilize upfront and cross-sectional imaging for CTV delineation.
- **Field borders are then modified accordingly to encompass these CTVs.**
- Please see the RTOG Breast Cancer Atlas for additional contouring guidelines (https://www.rtog.org/LinkClick.aspx?fileticket=vzJFhPaBipE=)

Tangents:	*Medial and lateral photon tangents*
Superior	Nondivergent field border ~2 cm below humeral head (sagittal) and just below clavicular head (coronal) if not using high tangents
Inferior	2 cm below inframammary fold
Anterior	Flash ipsilateral breast/CW
Posterior	≤2 cm of ipsilateral lung, include pectoralis muscles, chest wall muscles, and ribs
Medial	Sternum (avoid treating contralateral breast, allow IMC field width of at least 4 cm)
Lateral	Midaxilla (cover entire ipsilateral breast/CW)

IMC and medial CW:	*Typically a 15- to 25-degree angled electron field with a mid IMC isocenter. May use upper and lower IMC fields with different electron energies to reduce heart dose*
Superior	Matched to nondivergent superior border of tangent fields
Inferior	Matched on skin rendering to inferior border of medial tangent
Medial	Allow for at least 2 cm on IMC and CW scar, width of at least 4 cm
Lateral	
Posterior	Electron energy chosen such that 90% isodose line covers IMC
SCV/ICV:	*Typically a 15- to 20-degree angled photon field with an SCV isocenter and half beam block*
Superior	At cricoid (if ICV LN+, raise to arytenoids; if SCV LN+, raise to mastoid)
Inferior	Matched to nondivergent superior border of tangent fields
Medial	Angled off spinal cord, pedicles of vertebrae
Lateral	To cover lateral edge of pectoralis muscle. Contour the undissected axilla (including level III) to ensure coverage while also blocking humeral head.
Cone-down Tumor Bed/CW and Involved Node Boost	
BCS boost: At least 2-cm expansion around tumor bed and involved nodes.	
CW boost: Determined clinically using visual inspection and CT imaging of the surgical bed to determine and cover the surgical laps.	
Boosts are usually conducted with appositional electron field(s).	
Resimulate with breast compression device if needed for boost RT planning.	

- **Considerations:** Boost doses: 10 Gy for negative SM; 14 Gy for <2 mm SM; 16 Gy for positive SM (reexcision preferred but if not possible [ie, positive SM at fascia] give higher boost dose). If gross or residual nodes, consider 10 Gy boost with a 2-cm CTV margin. Postmastectomy, utilizing 3-mm bolus every other day for 2 weeks and then PRN to achieve a brisk skin reaction.
- **Technique:** Multi-isocenter technique utilizing photon-based tangent fields matched to AP oblique SCV field and appositional electron IMC field

IGRT/Planning Directive

- **IGRT:** Weekly MV once setup is stable

Planning directive considerations for comprehensive breast/chest wall

- Evaluate each beam separately for adequate coverage
- Entire breast/CW covered by 98% isodose line (IDL)
- All nodal CTV covered by >90% IDL
- Evaluate cold triangle between IMC and tangents
- Continuous coverage of 35 Gy line, most notably at IMC and tangent interface
- Boost target covered by 90% IDL

Dose constraints

- Total lung: V20 < 35%
  V40 < 20%
- Heart: V5 ≤ 40% (≤50% for left-sided tumors)
- Brachial plexus: D_{max} ≤ 66 Gy

Side Effect Management/Follow-up

- Same as **ESBC** chapter.

Systemic Therapy

- See **General Breast Cancer** chapter.

Notable Trials

Neoadjuvant chemotherapy improves outcomes in LABC

- **NSABP B-18** (*Fisher et al. JCO* 1997): Randomized 1523 operable pts to presurgery AC vs postsurgery AC. In preoperative arm, breast tumor size reduced in 80% and nodal reduction in 89%. 73% clinical CR and 44% of those had clinical CR. 12% more lumpectomies performed with pre-op AC. No difference in OS or DFS. OS and DFS trend favoring pre-op AC in women <50 years old (*P* = .06, *P* = .09)

- **NSABP B-27** (*Rastogi et al. JCO* 2008): Randomized 1567 pts to pre-op AC, pre-op AC + Taxotere, or pre-op AC with post-op Taxotere. Pre-op AC + Taxotere showed increased pCR (26% vs 13%, *P* < .001). No difference in DFS or OS

Improved outcomes with PMRT

- **Premenopausal Danish Trial (DBCG 82b)** (*Overgaard et al. NEJM* 1997): Randomized 1708 premenopausal pts with T3/T4 or axillary N+ s/p MRM + ALND to CMF chemo vs CMF + PMRT to 50 Gy/25 fx or 48 Gy/22 fx. PMRT included CW, scar, and regional LN (SCV/ICV/IMC). PMRT improved 10-year DFS from 34% to 48%, 10-year OS from 45% to 54%, and LRR 9% vs 32% (all *P* < .001).
- **Postmenopausal Danish Trial (DBCG 82c)** (*Overgaard et al. Lancet* 1999): Randomized 1375 postmenopausal women <70 years old with T3/T4 or axillary N+ disease s/p MRM + ALND to tamoxifen alone vs tamoxifen + PMRT to 50 Gy/25 fx or 48 Gy/22 fx. PMRT improved 10-year DFS from 24% to 36% (*P* < .001) and 10-year OS 36% to 45% (*P* = .03).
- **Early Breast Cancer Trialists' Collaborative Group (EBCTCG RT meta-analysis)** (*Clarke et al. Lancet* 2005; update *McGale et al. Lancet* 2014): 78 randomized trials of 42 000 women. Subgroups analyzed: N0 s/p BCS, adjuvant RT reduced 5-year LR (22.9% → 6.7%) and 15-year breast cancer mortality (BCM) (31.2% → 26.1%). N+ s/p BCS, adjuvant RT reduced 5-year LR (41.1% → 11%) and 15-year BCM (55%→ 47.9%). N0 s/p MRM, PMRT reduced 5-year LR (6.3% → 2.3%) but increased 15-year BCM (27.7% → 31.3%). N+ s/p MRM, PMRT reduced 5-year LR (22.8% → 5.8%) and 15-year BCM (60.1% → 54.7%). Tamoxifen use for 5 years reduced LR risk by ~50% in ER+ pts. 2014 updates showed no benefit to PMRT in N0 MRM pts but confirmed significant reduction in LR and BCM in pts with 1-3 and ≥4 positive axillary LN.

INFLAMMATORY/RECURRENT BREAST CANCER

JENNIFER LOGAN • WENDY WOODWARD

Background

- **Definition:** Inflammatory breast cancer (IBC) is primarily a clinical diagnosis requiring (1) rapid onset of breast erythema, edema, and/or peau d'orange with or without a palpable mass or skin thickening, (2) <6-month duration of symptoms, (3) erythema occupying at least 1/3 of the breast, and (4) pathologic confirmation of invasive carcinoma. Note: Erythema not classically "red" in all skin tones, and pathologic evidence of lymphatic involvement not required
- **Incidence/prevalence:** IBC accounts for 1%-4% of all detected breast cancer with ~70% presenting with regional disease and 30% with metastatic disease.
- **Outcomes:** Lower than non-IBC. Best reported outcomes with trimodality treatment. Retrospective series suggest presence of dermal lymphatic invasion, lack of breast-feeding, obesity, and triple-negative subtype are negative prognostic indicators.
- **Risk factors:** Bimodal incidence by age. IBC tends to be diagnosed at younger ages with increased prevalence in African American/Hispanic vs white women and is associated with obesity. Pregnancy is not protective. No difference in BRCA status or family history compared to non-IBC.

Tumor Biology and Characteristics

- **Pathology:** Although all subtypes present, there is higher incidence of ER/PR– and Her2 +/– than non-IBC. Luminal A not associated with clearly favorable prognosis. Commonly, dermal lymphatic invasion or tumor emboli are noted in the involved skin but are not required for diagnosis. Emboli-clogged dermal lymphatics are purported cause of erythema and swelling.
- **Molecular/biologic features:** 90% express RhoC (*van Golen et al. Cancer Res* 2000). All E-cadherin positive. IBC tumors can demonstrate increased angiogenic properties such as increased mRNA expression of VEGF and VEGFR, as well as several cytokines (IFN-γ, IL-1, IL-12, bFGF, FGF-2, IL-6, and IL-8). Role for tumor-promoting stromal macrophages demonstrated

Workup

See **General Breast Cancer** chapter.

- **Imaging modifications:** Bilateral breast and bilateral nodal imaging required (*contralateral nodes involved in 10%*). CT of the chest/abdomen/pelvis/neck or PET/CT. Prechemo cross-sectional imaging of involved regional nodes and including the neck helpful in RT planning. Upfront medical photography. Mammogram can be negative except for skin thickening.

Treatment Algorithm

An aggressive trimodality approach is optimal.

- **Algorithm:** Neoadjuvant chemotherapy ± Her2-targeted therapy → non–skin-sparing MRM → PMRT → completion hormone therapy × 5-10 years and/or completion Her2-targeted therapy × 1 year

Radiation Treatment Technique for Comprehensive Chest Wall (CW) Irradiation

- **Dose:** If pCR to neoadjuvant systemic and age > 45 years old: 50 Gy/25 fx + 16 Gy/8 fx boost (QD)
  If <pCR to neoadjuvant systemic or age ≤ 45 years old: 51 Gy/34 fx + 15 Gy/10 fx boost (bid)
- **Target/technique/SIM:** Same as PMRT techniques listed in **LABC** chapter. Critical to use upfront imaging and photographics to increase field size and cover all disease prior to neoadjuvant chemotherapy

Comprehensive CW Treatment Borders for Inflammatory Breast Cancer: Multi-isocenter Technique
*See **LABC** chapter for PMRT field design and details*

Special Considerations: Treatment + Field Design Modifications	
Inflammatory Breast Cancer/T4 Disease/Recurrent	
Radiation fields	• Wider medial margin needed on scar and surgical bed. Compromise contralateral breast if needed for coverage. • Double treat all junctions (~2- to 3-mm field overlap) to ensure skin is fully treated.
Bolus	• IBC cases: 3-mm bolus qod × 2 wk, then prn if treatment daily, or 3-mm bolus bid × 1 wk, qAM × 1 wk, then prn for bid treatment. • Skin is a target. Goal is to achieve brisk erythema/moist desquamation. • Bolus over ICV in the SCV field

Systemic Therapy

- See **General Breast Cancer** chapter for systemic therapy regimens. IBC patients are treated primarily with neoadjuvant systemic therapy.
- Minimal response or progressive disease with neoadjuvant systemic therapy → follow closely and perform MRM before the window of operability is lost given morbidity of local failure. Consider pre-op radiotherapy if margin-negative surgery is unlikely.

Surgical Options and Pathology

- **Non–skin-sparing modified radical mastectomy (MRM):** Complete removal of the breast, overlying skin, and axillary levels I-II. SLNB not effective in IBC. Cannot place tissue expander due to non–skin-sparing procedure
- **Pathology report:** Review ER/PR/Her2 status, tumor grade, tumor size, extent (multifocal?), surgical margin status (either positive, close [0-1.9 mm], or negative [≥2 mm]), extent of response to chemotherapy, presence of dermal lymphatic invasion/tumor emboli

Notable Studies (All Retrospective Single Institution)

Dose and Local Control in IBC (Adapted from *Woodward et al. Int J Radiat Oncol Biol Phys* 2014)

Center	Dose	5-Year LRC (%)	Era	Notes
MDACC (*Bristol et al. Int J Radiat Oncol Biol Phys* 2008)	60-66 Gy, prn bolus (66 Gy bid)	91	1977-2004, N = 125	66 Gy improved LRC for age < 45 y, + margins, and poor CT response
Cleveland (*Rehman et al. Int J Radiat Oncol Biol Phys* 2012)	45-66 Gy, bolus NS ≥60.4 Gy	83 100	2000-2009, N = 104	11/13 pts received bid
Florida (*Liauw et al. Cancer* 2004)	42-60 Gy, qd bolus	78	1982-2001, N = 61	≥60 Gy, MVA $P = .06$
MSKCC (*Damast et al. Int J Radiat Oncol Biol Phys* 2008)	50 Gy, qd bolus	87	1995-2006, N = 107	100% LC @ 60 Gy
Mayo (*Brown et al. Int J Radiat Oncol Biol Phys* 2014)	60-66 Gy, qd bolus	81	2000-2010, N = 49	pCR associated with better LRC
Penn (*Abramowitz et al. Am J Clin Oncol* 2009)	46-50 Gy, qod bolus	88	1986-2006, N = 19	Only pts with dermal lymphatic invasion had LRR
British Columbia Cancer Agency (*Panades et al. J Clin Oncol* 2005)	42.4 Gy (hypofx), bolus NS	63	1980-2000, N = 148	pCR associated with better LRC

Dose escalation/patient selection in IBC

- ***Bristol et al. IJROBP* 2008 (MDACC):** 256 M0 IBC pts treated with trimodality therapy. 192 completed treatment. Demonstrated pts with unknown/close/+ margins, <pCR to NAC, or age < 45 years benefited from dose escalation of PMRT from 60 to 66 Gy. For those that completed all treatment: 5-year LRC 84% vs 51%, 5-year DMFS 47% vs 20%, and 5-year OS 51% vs 24% (all $P < .001$).
- ***Rosso et al. Ann Surg Oncol* 2017 (MDACC)**: Prospective study with 114 nonmetastatic IBC pts receiving trimodality treatment: AC ± carboplatin (for TNBC) ± Her2-directed therapy (for HER2+) → Taxol → MRM → PMRT to >60 Gy → ± hormone therapy. 2-Year LRR 3.2% and 5-year OS 69.1%. Improved DFS in Her2+, clinical stage IIIB, complete or partial radiologic response to NAC, pCR, and lower initial nodal burden.

Aggressive local therapy in metastatic IBC

- ***Akay et al. Cancer* 2014 (MDACC):** 172 stage IV IBC pts. 55% of pts with oligomet IBC. 46% of pts underwent curative primary tumor resection (93% MRM). PMRT involved 51 Gy/34 fx bid + 15 Gy/10 fx CW boost. 5-Year OS 29% and 5-year DPFS 17%. MVA showed improved OS with response to chemotherapy (HR 0.49, $P = .005$) and surgery + PMRT (HR 0.9, $P = .0001$).

Recurrent Breast Cancer

Background

- **Definition:** Recurrences can be local (ipsilateral breast/tumor bed), regional (in nearby lymph nodes), or distant. Contralateral breast disease is not considered recurrent.
- **Outcomes:** Dependent on type/timing, 5-year OS 50% (any recurrence) vs 70% (CW only)
- **Workup:** Similar workup to IBC workup, important to note previous therapies received. Depending on site and timing of recurrence, repeat biopsies are likely. Multidisciplinary evaluation is essential.

Surgical options and systemic therapy

- Dependent on multidisciplinary evaluation and prior therapies received
- Trimodality treatment preferred when possible (*Aebi et al. Lancet Oncol* 2014)

Treatment algorithm

Locoregional recurrence after mastectomy, no prior RT	Evaluation for chemotherapy → surgery → comprehensive RT
Ipsilateral breast recurrence after BCS and prior RT	Mastectomy → no RT[a]
Ipsilateral breast/node recurrence after BCS and prior RT	Mastectomy ± nodal dissection → consideration of nodal irradiation[a]

[a]Careful review of prior records, consideration of reirradiation in extenuating circumstances in which safety may not be compromised.

Considerations for prior RT

General principles: Prior dose recall is 50% at 10 years; flap placement can reduce volume of previously irradiated tissue. If adequate dose for tumor control cannot be given safely, the risk-benefit ratio favors no treatment.

If indications for local recurrence are high and other therapies not feasible, reirradiation may be considered. Greater consideration for radiation techniques that limit reirradiation of ribs and other normal structures (eg, electrons/protons).

Radiation treatment technique for recurrent breast cancer

- **Rationale:** Recurrent disease in the setting of prior therapy as opposed to persistent or inadequately treated disease has had time and pressure to increase resistance. As such, an empiric 10% dose escalation is recommended.
- **Dose:** 54 Gy in 27 fraction → boost of 12 Gy/6 fx (empiric 10% dose escalation)
- **Target/technique/SIM** for locoregional recurrence is similar to PMRT techniques in **LABC** chapter.

PROSTATE CANCER (DEFINITIVE)

DARIO PASALIC • GEOFFREY V. MARTIN • SEUNGTAEK CHOI

Background

- **Incidence/prevalence:** Third most common cancer with 160 000 new cases of prostate cancer per year with 27 000 deaths in the United States in 2017. Most prevalent cancer in men in the United States with lifetime risk estimated to be ~15%
- **Outcomes:** Prostate cancer–specific survival at 10 years with treatment is 99% for low risk (*Hamdy et al. NEJM* 2016), 95% for intermediate risk (*Pisansky et al. JCO* 2015), and 84% for high risk (*Nguyen et al. Cancer* 2013).
- **Demographics:** African American men present with more advanced disease and have shorter progression-free survival than Caucasian counterparts (*Chornokur et al. Prostate* 2011).
- **Risk factors:** Advanced age, African American race, family history, smoking

Tumor Biology and Characteristics

- **Genetics:** 5%-10% familial (*Bratt et al. J Urol* 2002). RR of 2.5 and 3.5 in patients with 1 and 2 first-degree relative(s), respectively (*Johns and Houlston BJU Int* 2003). Associated with *BRCA2* mutations, and increased risk in patients with Lynch syndrome and Fanconi anemia.
- **Pathology:** Majority acinar adenocarcinoma (~95%), but more high-risk variants include sarcomatoid, ductal, squamous, small cell, urothelial (*Humphrey Histopathology* 2011)
- **Imaging:** 1.5 T (with endorectal coil) or 3 T (with/without endorectal coil) multiparametric MRI with contrast: T2 hypointense (Fig. 48.1), contrast enhancing, and DWI restricted.

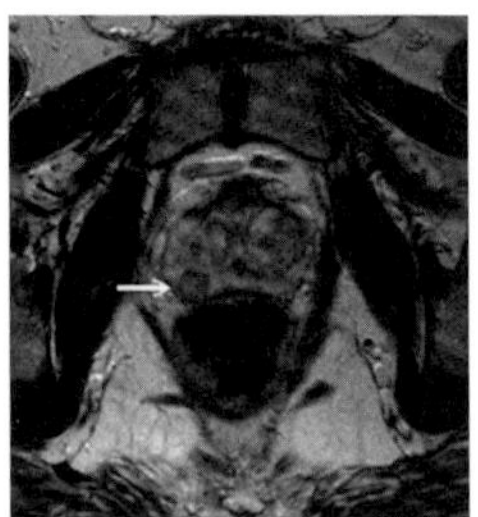
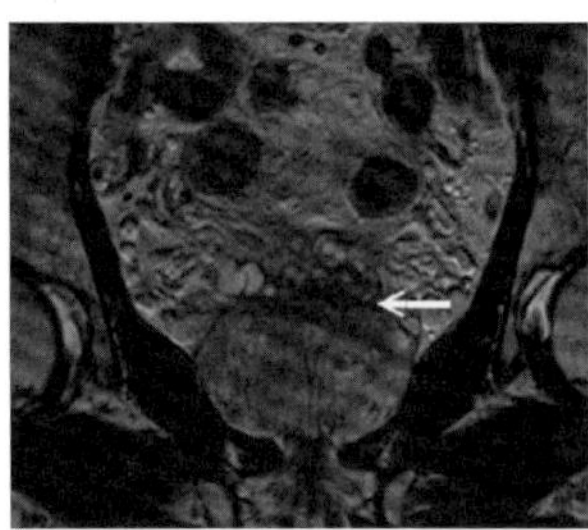

Figure 48.1 Representative MRI T2 sequence identifies dominant lesion appearing as T2 hypointense on axial **(left)** and coronal **(right)** cross-sectional images (*white arrows*). (Images acquired from Medscape.com.)

- **Anatomy:** Prostate bordered by bladder/bladder neck (superiorly), fascia of urogenital diaphragm (inferiorly), attached to pubic symphysis by puboprostatic ligament (anteriorly), separated from rectum by Denonvilliers fascia and attached to the rectum near the prostate apex via the recto-urethralis muscle (posteriorly), and levator ani muscles (laterally)
  - Prostatic lymph node drainage
    - First echelon: Periprostatic, obturator
    - Second echelon: External iliac, internal iliac, presacral, presciatic
    - Third echelon (M1a): Common iliac, inguinal, retroperitoneal

Workup

- **History and physical:** Specific attention to PSA screening history, history of urologic procedures including TURPs, AUA score, SHIM score, history of IBD (ulcerative colitis and Crohn's), collagen vascular disease, and colonoscopy. Digital rectal exam (DRE)
- **Labs:** PSA, testosterone. If treating with hormone therapy: CBC, LFTs
- **Procedures/biopsy:** 10-12 core US-guided biopsy. MRI-guided biopsy if discordant finding between MRI, DRE, and/or US-guided biopsy.
- **Imaging:** MRI of the pelvis/prostate >6 weeks after biopsy. Tc-99m bone scan (positive in 49.5% T3-T4 and 29.9% Gleason ≥ 8) for high risk or GI 4+3 and PSA > 10. Consider baseline DEXA scan prior to start of long-term ADT and colonoscopy prior to start of RT.
  *Imaging (MRI, CT scan, etc.) can only be used to evaluate LN staging and is not used to evaluate primary staging.

Prostate Cancer Staging (AJCC 8th Edition)

T Stage (c = clinical, p = pathologic)[b]		
T1	Clinically inapparent tumor that is not palpable	
T1a	Incidental histologic finding in ≤5% tissue resected	
T1b	Incidental histologic finding in >5% tissue resected	
T1c	Identified by needle biopsy in one or both sides, but not palpable	
T2	Palpable and confined within prostate	
cT2a	Involves ½ of ≤ one side	pT2: Organ confined disease
cT2b	Involves >½ of one side but not both sides	
cT2c	Involves both sides	

T Stage	
T3	Extraprostatic tumor that is not fixed or does not invade adjacent structures
T3a	Extraprostate extension (unilateral or bilateral)
T3b	Invades seminal vesicle(s)
T4	Fixed or invades adjacent structures other than seminal vesicles (eg, external sphincter, rectum, bladder, levator muscles, and/or pelvic wall)
N Stage	
N0	No regional lymph nodes
N1	Involves regional lymph nodes
M Stage	
M0	No distant metastases
M1	Distant metastasis
M1a	Nonregional lymph node(s)[a]
M1b	Bone(s)
M1c	Other site(s) +/– bone disease

Gleason Score	ISUP[c] Grade Group	NCCN Risk Group	
6 (3 + 3)	1	Low	cT1-T2a, GS ≤ 6, PSA < 10
7 (3 + 4)	2	Intermediate	cT2b-c, GS = 7, 10 ≤ PSA < 20
7 (4 + 3)	3		
8	4	High	≥cT3a, GS ≥ 8, PSA ≥ 20
9-10	5		

<table>
<tr><th colspan="8">Summative Stage</th></tr>
<tr><th>T stage</th><th>G1</th><th>G2</th><th>G3</th><th>G4</th><th>G5</th><th>N1</th><th>M1</th></tr>
<tr><td>cT1-2a, pT2 (PSA < 10)</td><td>I</td><td rowspan="3">IIB</td><td colspan="2" rowspan="3">IIC</td><td rowspan="5">IIIC</td><td rowspan="5">IVA</td><td rowspan="5">IVB</td></tr>
<tr><td>cT1-2a, pT2 (10 ≤ PSA < 20)</td><td rowspan="2">IIA</td></tr>
<tr><td>cT2b-c (PSA < 20)</td></tr>
<tr><td>cT1-T2 (PSA ≥ 20)</td><td colspan="4">IIIA</td></tr>
<tr><td>cT3-4</td><td colspan="4">IIIB</td></tr>
</table>

[a]Nonregional LNs refer to common iliacs and superior and inguinals and inferior.

[b]Unless noted, pathologic stage is the same as clinical stage.

[c]ISUP, International Society of Urological Pathology.

Treatment Algorithm

Low risk	• **Active surveillance**
	  • Biopsy, PSA, prostate MRI at baseline (fusion biopsy if discordant finding between MRI and pathology)
	  • PSA, DRE repeated every 6 months
	  • Prostate MRI every 12 months
	  • Consider repeat prostate biopsy at 12 months after diagnosis and yearly thereafter as needed based on clinical/imaging factors
	  • Taken off active surveillance if >10 years life expectancy and GS increases to ≥4 + 3, ≥50% cores positive, or patient preference
	• **EBRT**
	  • No ADT unless needed for prostate shrinkage
	• **Brachytherapy monotherapy** (see **Brachytherapy** chapter)
	  • AUA < 15, no TURP or prostate surgery, no large median lobe, no pubic arch interference (based on axial CT or MRI)
	  • No ADT unless needed for prostate shrinkage to allow brachy eligibility in which case 3-6 months ADT given prior to brachy reassessment
	• **Radical prostatectomy + bilateral pelvic lymph node dissection**

Intermediate risk	• **ADT → EBRT**
	  • Total 6 months of neoadjuvant/concurrent ADT; ADT strongly considered in patients with GS 7 (4 + 3) disease, ≥2 intermediate risk factors, ≥50% cores positive
	  • May consider omitting ADT in patients with moderate to severe comorbidities
	• **Brachytherapy monotherapy**
	  • Only consider in patients with one intermediate risk factor. See low-risk brachytherapy for other criteria.
	• **Radical prostatectomy + bilateral pelvic lymph node dissection**

High risk	• **ADT ± abiraterone → EBRT**
	  • Total 24 months of neoadjuvant/concurrent/adjuvant ADT
	  • Pelvic lymph nodes not routinely treated at MDACC; consider nodal RT if high risk of involvement or suspicious on imaging
	• **ADT → EBRT + brachytherapy boost**
	  • Total 12 months of neoadjuvant/concurrent/adjuvant ADT
	  • Consider nodal RT if high risk of involvement or suspicious on imaging.
	  • Consider brachytherapy boost 2-4 weeks after EBRT
	• **Radical prostatectomy + bilateral pelvic lymph node dissection**

LN+ disease	• **ADT ± abiraterone → EBRT**
	  • Total 24 months of neoadjuvant/concurrent/adjuvant ADT and consider abiraterone + prednisone
	  • Treat pelvic LNs

Radiation Treatment Technique

- **SIM:** Fiducial marker placement (2 carbon for proton; 3 gold for photon) prior to simulation; head first, supine, lower extremity immobilization (Fig. 48.2), bladder full, empty rectum (milk of magnesia day before and enema day of SIM). Endorectal balloon if proton simulation or if sigmoid/small bowel close to radiation field. Isocenter in middle of the prostate
- **Dose:** 78 Gy in 39 fractions (all eligible intact prostate EBRT patients)
  72 Gy in 30 fractions or 60 Gy in 20 fractions (low-intermediate-risk patients, small/medium prostate, AUA < 15, and no recent TURP)
  46 Gy in 23 fractions to pelvic LN, boost radiographically enlarged LN to 54-60 Gy
  44 Gy in 22 fractions followed by brachytherapy boost
    Pd-103 to 90 Gy
    I-125 to 110 Gy

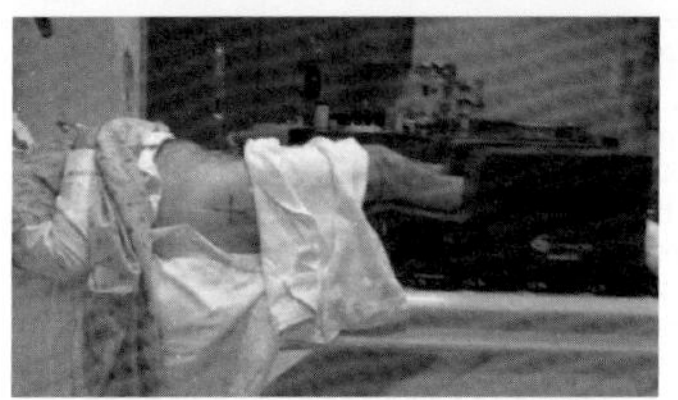

Figure 48.2 Standard setup at simulation for definitive EBRT for prostate cancer. We typically immobilize lower extremity with Medtec© device.

- **Target:** Prostate only (low risk)
  Prostate, proximal 1.5-2 cm of seminal vesicles (intermediate risk)
  Prostate, full seminal vesicles, ± pelvic lymph nodes (high risk)
- **Technique:** IMRT/VMAT; consider protons

CTV for Intact Prostate/Seminal Vesicles	
Low risk	Prostate
Intermediate risk	Prostate + proximal 1.5-2 cm of seminal vesicles (SVs)
High risk	Prostate + entire SV. Consider treating distal SVs to lower dose 54-60 Gy sequential if no MRI evidence of involvement
IMRT PTV = CTV + 0.4 cm posterior, 0.6 cm elsewhere	
Proton PTV = CTV + 0.4 cm posterior, 0.6 cm anterior, 0.6 cm superior/inferior, 1.1 cm lateral	
CTV for Pelvic Lymph Nodes	
Start L4/L5 or L5/S1 (level of distal common iliac and proximal presacral nodes) or vertebral body above any radiographically involved LNs.	
Include subaortic presacral nodes to bottom of S2 or S3 (posterior border of anterior rectum and anterior border ~1 cm anterior to anterior sacral bone; carve out bowel, bladder, bone).	
Stop external iliac nodes at top of femoral heads.	
Stop internal iliac nodes at top of pubic symphysis.	

- **IGRT:** Bladder volume scan prior to each treatment, treat if bladder volume is within 20% of simulation
  Daily kV imaging with alignment to intraprostatic fiducials
  Consider CBCT if fiducial is not available or if anticipated problems with setup.
- **Planning directive (for conventional fractionation at 2 Gy/day):**
  PTV V100 ≥ 98%
  Rectum V80, 70, 60, 40 Gy ≤ 3, 20, 40, 60, respectively (do not have V30 line encompass the entire rectum on a single axial slice)
  Bladder V70Gy ≤ 20% (allow up to ≤30%)
  Femoral heads V45Gy ≤ 10%; V50Gy ≤ 5%; D_{max} < 55 Gy
  Small bowel D_{max} < 50-54 Gy
  Sigmoid D_{max} < 60 Gy
- **Planning directive (for 72 Gy in 30 hypofraction regimen):**
  PTV V100 ≥ 98%
  Rectum 70, 60, 35 Gy ≤ 5, 20, 60, respectively
  Bladder V60 ≤ 20%, respectively
  Femoral heads V50Gy ≤ 5%; V45Gy ≤ 10%; D_{max} < 55 Gy
  Small bowel D_{max} < 50 Gy
  Sigmoid D_{max} < 54 Gy

SURGERY

- Radical prostatectomy either open or minimally invasive, generally robotic. Robotic surgery associated with lower blood loss and decreased hospital stays. Oftentimes combined with pelvic lymph node dissection, especially for some low-risk and all intermediate/high-risk patients.

Chemotherapy/Hormone Therapy

- **Androgen deprivation therapy:** Neoadjuvant/concurrent/adjuvant lupron with 14-30-day course of Casodex. Practice at MDACC includes 6 months with unfavorable intermediate-risk patients receiving EBRT, 24 months in high-risk patients with EBRT and 12 months with EBRT + brachytherapy boost. ADT duration may vary based on response, tolerance, and patient factors.
- **Abiraterone:** Concurrent/adjuvant treatment reasonable to consider for high-risk or LN+ patients, refer to medical oncology for patients with highly unfavorable disease (*James et al. NEJM* 2017). Given with prednisone 5 mg daily
- **Docetaxel:** More evidence is needed; consider referral to medical oncology for patients with highly unfavorable disease (*Vale et al. Lancet Oncol* 2016)

Side Effect Management

- Obstruction: *Decreased flow/hesitancy/frequency.* 1st-line tamsulosin (0.4 mg 30 minutes after dinner up to 2 tablets per evening) → 2nd-line terazosin (1 mg 30 minutes after dinner, can titrate up to 10 mg as tolerated)
- Overactivity: *Urgency/frequency.* 1st-line ibuprofen (400 mg 2 tablets bid prn; avoid in kidney disease) → oxybutynin (5 mg 2-4 times per day)
- Cystitis: *Urgency/frequency + dysuria.* UA + urine culture to r/o UTI. Treat if positive. If negative, 1st-line ibuprofen (400 mg 2 tablets bid prn; avoid in kidney disease) → 2nd-line Pyridium (100-200 mg tid after meals; short course, turns urine orange; avoid in kidney disease)
- Diarrhea: 1st diet modification (low residue, lower fiber, and low dairy) → 2nd-line Imodium titrating to a max of 8 pills/day → 3rd-line alternating Lomotil 2 pills and Imodium 2 pills every 3 hours
- Proctitis: *Rectal pain.* 1st-line cortisone suppository → 2nd-line steroid enemas.

Follow-Up

- History and PSA (get testosterone if on ADT): Every 3-6 months for 2 years then every 6-12 months until year 5, annually thereafter
- Consider DRE every 12 months.
- Minimize instrumentation (eg, colonoscopy, cystoscopy) in first 2 years.

Notable Trials—Low Risk

Treatment options

- PROTECT (*Hamdy et al. NEJM* 2016): Established the role of active surveillance. RCT comparing active surveillance, prostatectomy, or EBRT + ADT in early stage prostate cancer. Most patients Gleason 6 (76%) and T1c (76%). RT was to 74 Gy and patients received 3-6 months of ADT. Median follow-up of 10 years. Treatment with RP or EBRT improved DFS (9% compared to 23% in AS arm), but no difference in prostate cancer–specific survival (99%) and OS (88%) at 10 years. 53% of AS patients received definitive treatment during study period.
- PROTECT QOL (*Donovan et al. NEJM* 2016): QOL surveys for patients on PROTECT trial with 6-year follow-up. Radical prostatectomy associated with worse sexual and incontinence. Radiation associated with worse urinary urgency and bowel symptoms

Notable Trials—Intermediate Risk

Combination ADT + EBRT

- RTOG 94-08 (*Jones et al. NEJM* 2011): Established the role of neoadjuvant ADT in intermediate-risk prostate cancer. RCT comparing EBRT + ADT vs EBRT alone in 1979 patients. Inclusion criteria were T1-T2b, PSA < 20, and 60% Gleason 6 and 27% Gleason 7. RT was 66.6 Gy to prostate, 46.8 Gy to pelvis with 4 months of ADT. Median follow-up of 9.1 years. Treatment with ADT + EBRT improved 10-year OS by 5% (62% with ADT, 57% without), and 10-year disease-specific mortality (4% with ADT, 8% without ADT).
- Harvard (*D'Amico et al. JAMA* 2008): Established the role of adjuvant ADT in intermediate-risk prostate cancer. RCT comparing EBRT + ADT vs EBRT alone in 206 patients. Inclusion criteria was T1-T2b on exam with at least one unfavorable feature of GS

≥ 7, PSA > 10, or T3 on MRI. RT was 70 Gy to prostate only with 6 months of ADT. Median follow-up of 7.6 years. Treatment with ADT + EBRT improved 8-year OS by 13% (74% with ADT, 61% without), and disease-specific mortality (4% with ADT, 13% without ADT).

Notable Trials—High Risk

EBRT + ADT

- SPCG-7 (*Widmark et al. Lancet* 2009): Established the role of RT. Randomized, multicenter to RT + ADT vs ADT-alone. Enrolled cT1b-T2 and grade 2-3, or cT3; 40% with PSA ≥ 20; 19% grade 3; 78% T3. RT was to 70 Gy and patients received 3 months of leuprorelin + flutamide followed by indefinite flutamide. Median follow-up of 7.6 years. RT improved 10-year biochemical-free survival (74.1% vs 25.3%; $p < .001$), disease-specific survival (88.1% vs 76.1%; $p < .001$), and overall survival (70.4% vs 60%; $p = .004$).
- RTOG 8610 (*Roach et al. JCO* 2008): Established the role of neoadjuvant ADT. Randomized phase III trial to RT alone vs RT + neoadjuvant ADT 2 months before RT and concurrent with RT. Enrolled patients with bulky T2-4 tumors +/– lymph node involvement. RT was 65-70 Gy to the prostate and 44-46 Gy to the lymph nodes. Median follow-up 12.5 years. Neoadjuvant ADT improved prostate cancer–specific mortality (23% vs 36%; $p = .01$) and distant metastases (35% vs 47%; $p = .006$).
- EORTC 22863 (*Bolla et al. Lancet* 2002): Established the role of concurrent long-term ADT. Randomized to RT-alone vs RT + concurrent ADT for 3 years. Enrolled patients with T3-4 or T1-2 with Gleason ≥ 7. RT was 70 Gy with whole pelvis to 50 Gy. Median follow-up of 9 years. Three-year ADT improved 5-year overall survival (78% vs 62%; $p = .0002$) and disease-specific survival (94% vs 79%; $p = .0001$).
- RTOG 9202 (*Horwitz et al. JCO* 2008): Confirmed that long-term ADT is better than short-term ADT. Randomized to RT + neoadjuvant ADT for 4 months vs additional 24 months. Enrolled patients with cT2c-T4, PSA < 150. RT was 65-70 Gy (45 Gy to whole pelvis). Median follow-up of 11.3 years. Long-term ADT improved 10-year disease-specific survival (89% vs 84%; $p = .004$) and distant metastases (15% vs 23%; $p < .0001$).

Note: All of the above ADT + EBRT studies were done prior to the era of dose escalation to 78 Gy in 2 Gy/day fractions; therefore there is some question as to the impact of hormones with a higher dose.

EBRT + brachytherapy boost + ADT

- ASCENDE-RT (*Morris et al. IJROBP* 2017): Randomized, multicenter trial that treated patients with EBRT alone vs EBRT + LDR brachytherapy boost. Enrolled intermediate and high-risk patients (~69%); T1c-T3a disease; all patients received 12 months ADT (8 months neoadjuvant ADT). RT was 46 Gy in 23 fractions for all patients, followed by boost to 78 Gy in EBRT alone vs I-125 brachytherapy boost with minimal peripheral dose of 115 Gy. Median follow-up of 6.5 years. EBRT + brachytherapy boost improved biochemical progression-free survival at 7 years (86% vs 75%; $p < .001$).

EBRT to lymph nodes

- RTOG 9413 (*Roach et al. JCO* 2003; update *Lawton et al. IJROBP* 2007): Phase III randomized 2 × 2 factorial design—whole-pelvis RT (WPRT) to 50.4 Gy vs prostate-only RT to 70.2 Gy in 1.8 Gy fractions and neoadjuvant ADT vs adjuvant ADT for 4 months. Included those with PSA < 100 and LN-positive risk >15%; excluded surgical staging. Majority of patients were unfavorable intermediate risk or high risk (>T2c, PSA < 30, GS > 7); all RT was 4-field 3DCRT. Median follow-up of 7 years. No significant difference in PFS between neoadjuvant ADT vs adjuvant ADT or WPRT vs prostate only RT. Criticisms include low hormone therapy duration and RT doses by today's standards, as well as a complex interaction between RT field size and ADT.
- GETUG-01 (*Pommier et al. JCO* 2007; *IJROBP* 2016): Randomized, multicenter trial of prostate RT to 66-70 Gy +/– pelvis to 46 Gy. Inclusion criteria of T1b-T3c, N0M0 with normal bone scan and pelvic CT, surgical staging not allowed. Approximately 50% of patients had <15% risk of lymph node positive disease. Majority of patients (~80%) were high risk and received 4-8 months of neoadjuvant ADT; all RT was 4-field 3D CRT. Median follow-up 11.4 years. No significant difference in PFS or OS between the arms. Criticisms include low hormone therapy duration and RT doses by today's standards, as well as small pelvic field volume.

PROSTATE CANCER (ADJUVANT/ SALVAGE)

DARIO PASALIC • GEOFFREY V. MARTIN • SEUNGTAEK CHOI

BACKGROUND, TUMOR BIOLOGY, AND CHARACTERISTICS

See Definitive Prostate Cancer chapter.

WORKUP FOR PSA RECURRENCE

- **History and physical:** AUA score, SHIM score, IBD (ulcerative colitis and Crohn's), collagen vascular disease, and colonoscopy (within 3-5 years). Initial stage. Type and date of surgery, PSA measurements after surgery. Digital rectal exam. Delay post-op RT until urinary function maximized/stabilized to ≤1 pad/day (typically ≥3 months from the date of surgery).
- **Labs:** PSA, testosterone. If treating with hormone therapy: CBC
- **Procedures/biopsy:** Consider image-guided biopsy if nodule is palpated or visible on imaging.
- **Imaging:** MRI of the pelvis/prostate. Tc-99m bone scan. CT chest and abdomen with contrast. Consider advanced PET imaging modalities.
- **Anatomy:**
  - Prostate fossa: Top of pubic symphysis (superiorly), 1 cm below vesicourethral anastomosis (inferiorly), bladder wall or posterior edge of pubic bone (anteriorly), anterior rectal wall (posteriorly), and pelvic floor muscles/fascia (laterally)
  - SV fossa: Top of the prostate fossa (inferiorly), posterior wall of the bladder (anteriorly) to the anterior rectum wall (posteriorly) up to the remnants of the vas deferens (superiorly)
  - Prostatic lymph node drainage
    - First echelon: Periprostatic, obturator
    - Second echelon: External iliac, internal iliac, presacral, presciatic
    - Third echelon (M1a): Common iliac, inguinal, retroperitoneal

PROSTATE CANCER STAGING *(AJCC 8TH EDITION)*

See Definitive Prostate Cancer chapter.

TREATMENT ALGORITHM

Adjuvant (PSA undetectable)	• EBRT • Indicated for positive margins, SV involvement, and/or ECE • PSA undetectable to be considered adjuvant • ADT not typically given for adjuvant pN0
Salvage (PSA detectable)	• ADT → EBRT • 0.2 ≤ PSA ≤ 0.5 consider 4-6 months ADT[a] • PSA > 0.5 give for 6 months ADT • 6-12 months ADT for clinical and/or radiologic recurrence on imaging
Pathologic lymph node involvement	• ADT → EBRT • ≥12 months ADT for pN1 • If PSA detectable treat fossa as per adjuvant • If PSA detectable treat fossa as per salvage

[a]Factors favoring ADT use include negative margins, Gleason ≥ 8, and short time to PSA recurrence.

RADIATION TREATMENT TECHNIQUE

- **SIM:** Lower extremity immobilization, bladder full, empty rectum (milk of magnesia day before and enema day of SIM), +/− endorectal balloon. Isocenter in the middle of prostate fossa
- **Dose:** SIB 66 Gy in 33 fractions to the prostate fossa (post-op adjuvant). Consider 59.4 Gy in 33 fractions to SV fossa (if pSV−).
  SIB 70 Gy in 35 fractions to the prostate fossa (post-op salvage). Consider 63 Gy in 35 fractions to SV fossa (if pSV−).

Pelvic LN radiation to 46 Gy in 23 fractions. Consider boosting gross LNs to 54-60 Gy. Consider boosting gross disease in the fossa to 72-74 Gy in 35 fractions.

- **Target:** Prostate fossa and SV fossa ± pelvic lymph nodes
- **Technique:** IMRT/VMAT

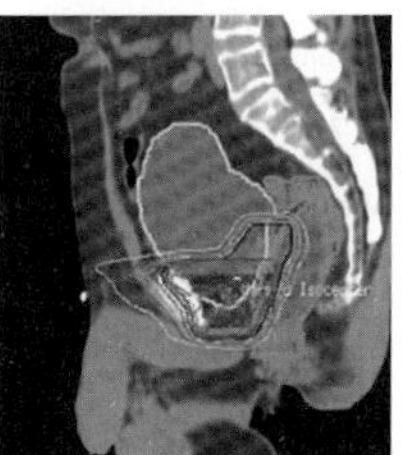

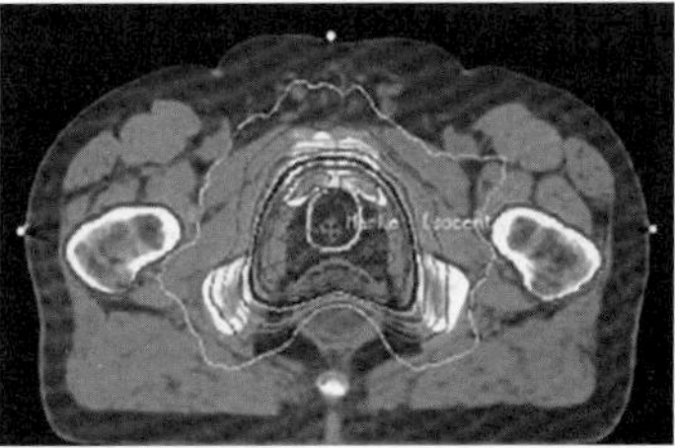

Figure 49.1 Sagittal and axial views showing an RT plan treating the prostate fossa to 70 Gy (*blue colorwash*) and SV fossa (*yellow colorwash*) to 63 Gy. **See color insert.**

CTV for Post-op Prostate/Seminal Vesicle Fossa	
Superior	Level of cut of vas deferens or 3-4 cm above superior symphysis
Inferior	1 cm below vesicourethral anastomosis
Anterior	Pubic symphysis, 1 cm of bladder wall above pubic symphysis
Posterior	Anterior rectal wall, mesorectal fascia
Lateral	Levator ani muscles, sacrogenitopubic fascia
IMRT PTV = CTV + 0.4-0.5 cm posterior, 0.7 cm elsewhere	
CTV for Pelvic Lymph Nodes	
Start L4/L5 or L5/S1 (level of distal common iliac and proximal presacral nodes) or vertebral body above any radiographically involved LNs.	
Include subaortic presacral nodes S2-S3 with posterior border of anterior rectum and anterior border ~1 cm anterior to anterior sacral bone; carve out bowel, bladder, bone.	
Stop external iliac nodes at the top of femoral heads.	
Stop internal iliac nodes at the top of pubic symphysis.	

- **IGRT:** Daily kV imaging with alignment to bone. Consider CBCT if anticipated problems with setup.
- **Planning directive (for conventional fractionation):**
  PTV:V100 ≥ 98%
  Rectum:V70Gy < 20%, V60Gy < 40%, V40Gy < 60%, respectively (do not have V30 line encompass the entire rectum on a single axial slice)
  Bladder:V70Gy ≤ 20%
  Femoral heads: V45Gy ≤ 10%; V50Gy ≤ 5%; D_{max} < 55 Gy
  Small bowel: D_{max} < 50-54 Gy
  Sigmoid: D_{max} < 60 Gy

Chemotherapy/Hormone Therapy

- **Androgen deprivation therapy:** Neoadjuvant/concurrent/adjuvant lupron. Consider 4-6 months for early salvage (0.2 ≥ PSA ≥ 0.5), 6 months for salvage (PSA ≥ 0.5) and ≥12 months for pLN+ disease. Can consider RT without ADT for early salvage PSA < 0.5 especially if positive surgical margin.

Side Effect Management

See Definitive Prostate chapter.

Follow-Up

- History and PSA (get testosterone if on ADT): Every 3-6 months for 2 years, then every 6-12 months until year 5, annually thereafter
- Consider DRE every 12 months.
- Minimize instrumentation (eg, colonoscopy, cystoscopy) in first 2 years.

Notable Studies

Advantage of adjuvant radiation over salvage radiation

- Multi-institutional (*Hwang et al. JAMA Oncol* 2018): Multi-institutional retrospective review in patients with pT3 and/or + margins. Propensity score matching to compare adjuvant (n = 366; PSA < 0.1) vs salvage (n = 366; 0.1 ≥ PSA ≥ 0.5). Adjuvant radiation associated with statistically significant improvement in freedom from biochemical failure (12-year: 69% vs 43%, p < .001), freedom from distant metastases (12-year: 95% vs 85%, p < .03), and overall survival (12-year: 91% vs 79%, p = .01). Sensitivity analysis demonstrated that decreased risk of biochemical failure with adjuvant radiation remained significant unless >56% of patients in adjuvant group were cured by surgery alone.

Benefit of adjuvant/salvage radiation after prostatectomy

- SWOG 8794 (*Thompson et al. J Urol* 2009): Phase III trial randomizing 425 patients with pT3 disease (ECE or SV involvement) with or without positive surgical margins after prostatectomy to adjuvant EBRT 60-64 Gy vs observation. Enrolled patients were 79% adjuvant (PSA undetectable) and 31% salvage (PSA detectable). Treatment with adjuvant radiation improved metastasis-free survival (median: 14.7 vs 12.9 months, p = .016). Overall survival also improved in adjuvant radiation arm (total deaths: 52% vs 41%, p = .023).
- ARO 96-02/AUO 09/95 (*Wiegel et al. J Urol* 2014): Phase III trial randomizing 388 pT3-4N0 (ECE or SVI involvement) with or without positive surgical margins after prostatectomy to adjuvant EBRT 60 Gy vs observation. All patients were treated adjuvant (PSA undetectable). Adjuvant radiation resulted in significantly better PFS (10 years: 35% vs 56%, p < .001). No significant improvement in metastases-free survival or overall survival
- EORTC 22911 (*Bolla et al. Lancet* 2012): Phase III trial randomizing 1005 patients with pT3 (ECE or SVI) or + surgical margins after prostatectomy to adjuvant EBRT 60 Gy (50 Gy followed by 10 Gy conedown boost) vs observation. Enrolled patients were 70% adjuvant (PSA undetectable) and 30% salvage (PSA detectable). Treatment with adjuvant radiation improved biochemical-free survival (10 years: 61% vs 41%, p < .001). Metastasis free and overall survival not different between arms. Any grade late adverse effects more common in EBRT arm (10 years: 71% vs 60%)

Benefit of hormone therapy with salvage radiation

- RTOG 9601 (*Shipley et al. NEJM* 2017): Phase III trial randomizing 760 patients to ADT for 2 years + salvage EBRT after prostatectomy, vs EBRT alone. Inclusion in study was post-op PSA > 0.2, pN0, M0. RT was 64.8 Gy, and ADT was 150-mg bicalutamide daily for 24 months. Median follow-up of 13 years. At 12-year follow-up, treatment with ADT reduced metastases (cumulative incidence: 14.5% vs 23%, p = .005) and prostate cancer death (cumulative incidence: 5.8% vs 13.4%, p < .001). Overall survival also improved in ADT arm (10 years: 76% vs 71%, p = .04). Gynecomastia significantly increased with ADT (cumulative incidence: 70% vs 11%, p < .001).
- GETUG-AFU-16 (*Carrie et al. Lancet Oncol* 2016): Phase III trial randomizing 743 patients. to ADT + salvage EBRT after prostatectomy, vs EBRT alone. Inclusion in study was post-op PSA ≥ 0.2 but <2, pN0, M0. RT was 66 Gy, and ADT was goserelin for 6 months. Median follow-up of 5.2 years. Treatment with ADT improved PFS (5 years: 80% vs 62%, p < .0001) but no difference in OS (5 years: 96% vs 95%)

BLADDER CANCER

RACHIT KUMAR • CHAD TANG

Background

- **Incidence/prevalence:** Fourth most common diagnosed cancer in men and 11th in women in the United States. Approximately 81,000 cases will be diagnosed in 2018 in the United States, with almost 19 000 deaths predicted. Approximately 25% of cases would be muscle invasive.
- **Risk factors:** Tobacco use (urothelial type), industrial exposures (aromatic amines, hair dyes, arsenic), *Schistosoma* infection, and indwelling catheter use (squamous cell type)

Tumor Biology and Characteristics

- **Genetics:** Papillary tumors are frequently seen to have mutations in *FGFR3*, and nonpapillary tumors often have mutated *TP53* and *RB1*.
- **Pathology:** Majority urothelial carcinomas (>90%). Minority squamous cell carcinomas and small cell carcinomas. Consider testing for *PD-L1* based on recent data demonstrating the efficacy of immunotherapeutic agents in the metastatic setting. Common presentation with synchronous primary in the upper urinary tract (ureter and renal pelvis)
- **Imaging:** Direct visualization with cystoscopy and exam under anesthesia often required to assess location and stage. CT urogram can demonstrate three-dimensional lesions. Bladder MRI appearance is T1 hypointense (bladder wall is medium in intensity) and T2 intense.
- **Anatomy:**
  - Situated anterior to the rectum; in men superior to the prostate, in women both superior and anterior to the vagina/uterus
  - Urothelial lining is in the bladder, as well as in the upper GU tract up to the renal pelvis and inferiorly to the urethra. This contributes to the risk of "field cancerization effect" in which the entire GU tract may be subject to the same neoplastic effect seen in the bladder tissue. This necessitates assessment of the entire GU epithelium when bladder cancer is identified.
  - Lymph node drainage:
    - Internal iliac, external iliac, and obturator nodes

Workup

- **History and physical:** History of exposure including aniline dyes, smoking, and bladder parasites. Symptoms including hematuria, bladder cramping, and dysuria
- **Labs:** CBC and basic chemistry panel including alkaline phosphatase.
- **Procedures/biopsy:** Bimanual exam under anesthesia for staging and transurethral resection of bladder tumor (TURBT).
- **Imaging:** While direct visualization using cystoscopy with transurethral resection is required for diagnosis, urine cytology may often initially detect the disease. The extent of disease in the abdomen/pelvis is best established with CT or MRI, though the upper tract may be imaged using an IV pyelogram or retrograde ureteroscopy. Metastatic disease to the chest is generally evaluated with a chest x-ray or CT chest, and a bone scan/PET scan is often used in patients with muscle-invasive disease.

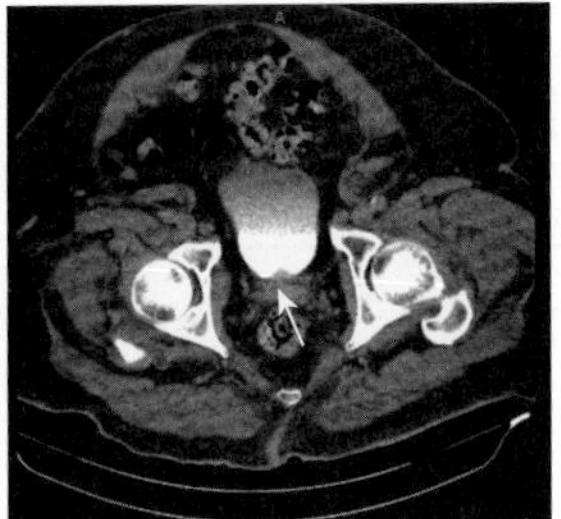

Figure 50.1 Representative CT urogram cross-sectional image from a bladder cancer patient. Mild thickening at the posterior wall of the bladder (*arrow*) represents the primary tumor.

Bladder Cancer Staging (*AJCC 8th edition*)

T Stage		N Stage	
Ta	Noninvasive papillary carcinoma	NX	Lymph node status cannot be assessed
Tis	Carcinoma in situ—"flat" tumor	N0	No lymph node metastasis
T1	Invades the subepithelial connective tissue	N1	Single lymph node metastasis in true pelvis (hypogastric, obturator, external iliac, or presacral node)

T Stage		N Stage	
T2a	Invades the superficial muscularis propria (inner half)	N2	Multiple regional lymph node metastasis in the true pelvis
T2b	Invades the deep muscularis propria (outer half)	N3	Lymph node metastasis to the common iliac lymph node
		M Stage	
T3a	Invades microscopically the perivesical tissue	M0	No distant metastasis
T3b	Invades macroscopically the perivesical tissue	M1	Distant metastasis
T4a	Invades prostatic stroma, uterus, vagina		
T4b	Invades pelvic/abdominal wall		

Summative Stage[a]

	N0	N1	N2	N3	M1
T1	I				
T2a	II				
T2b					
T3a		IIIA	IIIB	IIIB	IVB
T3b	IIIA				
T4a					
T4b	IVA				IVB

[a]Note that major change in staging from *AJCC* 7th to 8th edition is shift from node-positive disease from Stage IV (7th edition) to Stage III (8th edition).

Treatment Algorithm

Stage 0	• Transurethral resection of bladder tumor (TURBT) alone
Stage I	• TURBT + BCG × 6 weeks or intravesicle chemotherapy (if persistent disease >1 year → cystectomy) • Bladder preservation (chemoradiation)
Stage II	• Neoadjuvant chemotherapy → radical cystectomy with prostatectomy (in men) • Partial cystectomy if only involving bladder dome if 2 cm of margin can be achieved • Bladder preservation (chemoradiation)
Stage III	• Neoadjuvant chemotherapy → radical cystectomy with prostatectomy (in men) • Bladder preservation (chemoradiation)
Stage IV	• Systemic therapy, palliative radiation, or best supportive care

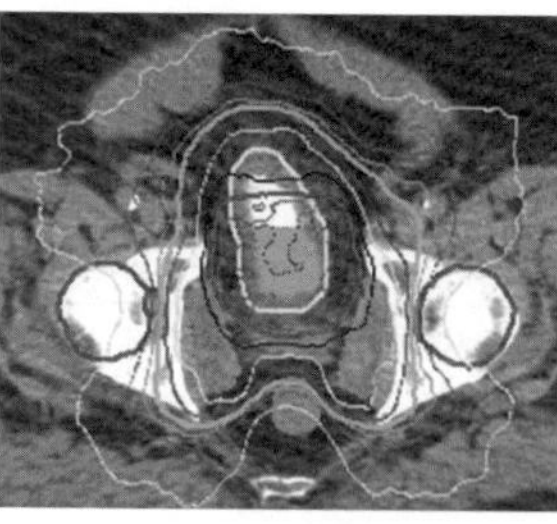

Figure 50.2 IMRT bladder conservation radiation plan treating to 45 Gy (*blue isodose line*) in 25 fractions to LNs and whole bladder followed by a sequential boost to the bladder resection cavity to 64.8 Gy (*red isodose line*) in 26 fractions. **See color insert**.

Radiation Treatment Technique

- **SIM:** Supine, arms on chest. When treating with a bladder boost, two simulations are needed—whole pelvic and whole bladder fields are treated with an empty bladder, and boost fields utilize a full bladder. Empty bowel

- **Dose (acceptable regimes):**
  - Whole pelvis to 45-50.4 Gy in 25-28 fractions at 1.8 Gy/fx → Bladder tumor boost to 60-65 Gy in 1.8-2.0 Gy/fx
  - 64 Gy in 32 fractions to whole bladder
  - 55 Gy in 20 fractions to whole bladder
- **Target:** Whole pelvis CTV fields: Bladder, prostate, internal iliac, external iliac, obturator, and presacral nodes
  LN PTV: LN CTV + 0.7 cm setup margin
  Bladder PTV: Bladder + 1.5 cm PTV setup margin
  Include prostatic urethra for men.
- **Boost target:** Initial TURBT area or known bladder tumor with 2-cm mucosal margin
  Considerations: Midcourse cystoscopy to evaluate response is optional and is normally conducted between the initial pelvic RT field and initiation of radiation boost.
- **Technique:** 3DCRT or IMRT; IMRT may be necessary to help reduce small bowel dose.

Initial fields (whole pelvis): 45-50.4 Gy in 25-28 fractions	
GTV	Visible tumor using multimodality evaluation (cystoscopy with bladder mapping + imaging)
CTV	Entire bladder, prostatic urethra (males), and draining nodes (obturator, internal iliac, and external iliac) up to S2-3
PTV	2-cm margin on bladder with 7-mm margin on nodal fields with CT planning, organ/nodal contouring, and daily imaging
Tumor/tumor bed boost (whole pelvis): 18-20 Gy in 10-11 fractions	
Cover tumor/tumor bed as identified by bladder mapping, if 3DCRT, then tumor + 1-1.5 cm margin	

- **IGRT:** Daily US bladder + daily kV or CBCT at least weekly + daily kV, consider more frequent CBCT if difficulty with bladder filling.
- **Planning directive (for 1.8-2 Gy/day fractionation):**
  Spinal cord D_{max} < 45 Gy
  Femoral heads V45 < 20%
  Small bowel V50 < 10 cc, D_{max} < 54 Gy
  Bowel "bag" V45 < 195 cc

Surgery

- **Transurethral resection of bladder tumor (TURBT):** Cystoscopically guided tumor resection with the goal of resecting all visible tumor with negative margins. Random biopsies should be performed to identify multifocal disease or carcinoma in situ. Ideally, the surgeon should perform a thorough mapping of the bladder to assist in radiation planning.
- **Cystectomy:** Resection of the bladder and prostate. If ileal conduit (neobladder) is created, surgeon should ensure that urethral margin is negative.
- **Lymphadenectomy:** Surgeons should perform bilateral pelvic lymphadenectomy at the same as an surgery with the goal of disease cure. Completion of a pelvic lymphadenectomy (specifically external iliac, internal iliac, and obturator lymph nodes) has demonstrated improvements in disease-specific survival and pelvic recurrence risk.

Chemotherapy

- **Concurrent:** Cisplatin weekly (30-40 mg/m^2) or every 3 weeks (100 mg/m^2). Alternatively, 5FU and MMC can be utilized. Acceptable single agents include 5FU, cisplatin, or gemcitabine.
- **Adjuvant/neoadjuvant:** Multiagent cisplatin-based chemotherapy should be utilized, most frequently. Regimes generally feature gemcitabine and cisplatin.

Side Effect Management

- **Nausea:** 1st-line Zofran (8 mg q8h prn) → 2nd-line Compazine (10 mg q6h prn) → ABH (lorazepam 0.34 mg, diphenhydramine 25 mg, and haloperidol 1.5 mg) 1 capsule q6h
- **Diarrhea:** 1st-line Imodium titrating to a max of 8 pills/day → 2nd-line alternating Lomotil 2 pills and Imodium 2 pills every 3 hours
- **Cystitis:** *Urgency/frequency and dysuria.* UA to r/o UTI. Treat if positive. Hyoscyamine (0.125 mg q4-6h prn, do not take more than 12 pills in a day)
- **Obstruction:** *Decreased flow/hesitancy/frequency.* 1st-line Tamsulosin (0.4 mg 30 minutes after dinner up to 2 tablets per evening) → 2nd-line Terazosin (1 mg 30 minutes after dinner, can titrate up to 10 mg as tolerated)

- **Proctitis:** *Diarrhea/abdominal pain.* 1st-line alternating Lomotil and Imodium (as above) → 2nd-line steroid enemas.

Follow-Up

- History/physical with urine cytology and cystoscopy every 3 months × 1 year, then every 6 months × 2 years, then annually
- CT abdomen/pelvis every 6-12 months for 2-3 years, then annually
- Vaginal dilators for women

Notable Papers

Improvement in survival with neoadjuvant chemotherapy prior to cystectomy

- **SWOG8710:** Phase III trial randomizing 317 patients with muscle-invasive bladder cancer to radical cystectomy or neoadjuvant chemotherapy followed by radical cystectomy. Chemotherapy was methotrexate, vinblastine, doxorubicin, and cisplatin (MVAC). Neoadjuvant chemotherapy associated with a trend in OS improvement (median: 46 vs 77 months, $p = .06$) and with significantly higher rate of no residual disease (38% vs 15%, $p < .001$).

Improvement in bladder preservation outcomes with concurrent chemo

- **BC2001:** Phase III trial 2:2 randomization of 360 patients with muscle-invasive bladder cancer to (1) definitive radiation + concurrent chemotherapy or radiation alone and (2) whole bladder or reduced high-dose volume radiation therapy (RHDVRT). Radiation dose was either 55 Gy in 20 fractions or 64 Gy in 32 fractions. Concurrent chemotherapy was 5FU and MMC.
  - **Chemoradiation vs radiation alone** (*James et al. NEJM* 2013): Chemoradiation improved locoregional DFS (2 years: 67% vs 54%, $p = .03$). No significant difference in OS (5 years: 48% vs 35%, $p = .16$). Grade 3-4 adverse events more common with chemoradiation during treatment (36% vs 27.5%, $p = .07$).
  - **Whole bladder vs RHDVRT** (*Huddart IJROBP* 2013): No difference in overall survival (38% vs 44%) or locoregional failure (61% vs 64%). No difference in bladder capacity reduction or grade 3-4 toxicities.

Retrospective review of outcomes and toxicities with bladder preservation

- **MGH long-term outcomes-bladder preservation** (*Giacolone Eur Urol* 2017): Retrospective review of 472 patients with T2-4 bladder cancer treated with bladder preservation from 1986 to 2013 with a median FU of 7.21 years. Risk of salvage cystectomy at 5 years was 29%. 5-Year OS was 57%, and DSS with bladder intact was 66%.
- **Pooled analysis of RTOG bladder-preservation trials** (*Mak JCO* 2014): Retrospective review of 468 patients with muscle-invasive bladder cancer included on five prospective phase II RTOG trials (8802, 9506, 9706, 9906, and 0233). The 5- and 10-year OS rates were 57% and 36%, respectively, and 5- and 10-year DSS were 71% and 65%, respectively.
- **Late pelvic toxicities related to bladder-preservation trials** (*Efstathiou JCO* 2009): Compiled toxicity related to RTOG bladder-sparing trials: 8903, 9506, 9706, 9906 after a median follow-up of 5.4 years. Late grade 3 pelvic toxicities: 7%, late grade 3 GU toxicities: 5.7%, and late grade 3+ GI toxicities: 1.9%. There were no late grade 4 or 5 toxicities noted.

TESTICULAR CANCER

GEOFFREY V. MARTIN • SEUNGTAEK CHOI

Background

- **Incidence/prevalence:** 8000-9000 new cases of testicular cancer per year. Incidence of testicular germ cell tumors increasing in the past two decades. Overall 1% of tumors in males
- **Outcomes:** 5-Year survival in patients with testicular cancer is 98%.
- **Demographics:** Most common solid malignancy in males between ages 15 and 35
- **Risk factors:** Family history, cryptorchidism, testicular dysgenesis, Klinefelter syndrome

Tumor Biology and Characteristics

- **Pathology:** 95% of testicular tumors are germ cell tumors (GCTs), classified as seminoma or nonseminoma. Nonseminomatous tumors consist of varied histologies including embryonal, choriocarcinoma, yolk sac, tumor, and teratomas. Non-GCTs include lymphoma and sex cord–stromal tumors.
- **Serum markers:**
  - **Seminomas:** Mild elevation of β-HCG can be observed (~100 IU/L). Alpha-fetoprotein rarely elevated. LDH may be elevated and is associated with prognosis but is a nonspecific marker.
  - **Nonseminomatous tumors:** Moderate to extreme elevation of β-HCG observed (>10 000 IU/L) in 10%-20% of early-stage tumors and 40% of late-stage tumors. Moderate to extreme elevation of alpha-fetoprotein (>10 000 ng/mL), often associated with a yolk sac component. LDH may be elevated and is associated with prognosis but is a nonspecific marker.
- **Imaging:** Hypoechoic mass on testicular transscrotal ultrasound

Workup

- **History and physical:** History and examination including testicular. Discussion of sperm banking.
- **Labs:** AFP, β-HCG, LDH, chemistry panel, and CBC. Repeat AFP, β-HCG, and LDH after orchiectomy for staging purposes
- **Procedures/biopsy:** Radical inguinal orchiectomy, consider inguinal biopsy of contralateral testes if indicated. **Note:** Avoid transscrotal procedures as this may alter lymphatic drainage.
- **Imaging:** Testicular ultrasound, CT abdomen/pelvis, chest imaging (chest x-ray or CT of chest)
- **Anatomy:**
  - Testicle surrounded by fibrous tunica layer (tunica vaginalis: outer layer, tunica albuginea: inner layer). Each testicle divided into lobules with multiple seminiferous tubules. Seminiferous tubules drain into the rete testis, which is attached to the spermatic cord via epididymis, which empties into the vas deferens and then the urethra at the prostate. Blood-testis barrier established by tight junctions between Sertoli cells
  - Testicle/scrotum lymph node drainage
    - Testes: Retroperitoneal/para-aortic nodes
    - Scrotum: Inguinal lymph nodes

Testicular Cancer Staging (AJCC 8th Edition)

T Stage (Pathologically Determined)		M Stage	
pT1	Tumor limited to testis with absence of LVI. Can involve rete testis	M0	No distant metastases
pT1a	≤3 cm in size	M1	Distant metastasis
pT1b	>3 cm in size	M1a	Nonretroperitoneal nodal or pulmonary metastasis
pT2	Hilar soft tissue, epididymal invasion, or any vascular invasion	M1b	Nonpulmonary visceral metastasis
		Serum Tumor Markers (LDH, hCG, AFP)	
pT3	Contiguous invasion into spermatic cord from testis	Sx	Markers not available/not performed
		S0	Markers within normal limits
pT4	Invasion into scrotum	S1	LDH < 1.5 ULN and β-hCG < 5000 IU/L and AFP < 1000 ng/mL
		S2	1.5 ≤ LDH < 10 ULN or 5000 ≤ β-hCG < 50 000 IU/L or 1000 ≤ AFP < 10 000 ng/mL
		S3	LDH > 10 ULN or β-hCG > 50 000 IU/L or AFP > 10 000 ng/mL

pN Stage		cN Stage	
pN0	No regional lymph nodes	cN0	No regional lymph nodes
pN1	≤5 lymph positive lymph nodes all ≤2 cm in size	cN1	Single lymph node ≤2 cm in size or multiple with none >2 cm
pN2	Single lymph node 2-5 cm, >5 enlarged lymph nodes all ≤5 cm in size, or extranodal extension	cN2	Single lymph node 2-5 cm in size or multiple with the largest measuring 2-5 cm
pN3	Lymph node size > 5 cm	cN3	Lymph node size > 5 cm

<table>
<tr><th colspan="7">Summative Stage</th></tr>
<tr><th></th><th>N0</th><th>N1</th><th>N2</th><th>N3</th><th>M1a</th><th>M1b</th></tr>
<tr><td>pT1, S0</td><td>IA</td><td rowspan="3">IIA</td><td rowspan="3">IIB</td><td rowspan="3">IIC</td><td rowspan="5">IIIC</td><td rowspan="5">IIIC</td></tr>
<tr><td>pT2-T4, S0</td><td>IB</td></tr>
<tr><td>Any pT, S1</td><td rowspan="3">IS</td></tr>
<tr><td>Any pT, S2</td><td colspan="3">IIIB</td></tr>
<tr><td>Any pT, S3</td><td colspan="3">IIIC</td></tr>
</table>

Treatment Algorithm—Pure Seminoma

All algorithms describe treatment after an initial radical inguinal orchiectomy, preferably a high ligation of the spermatic cord.

Stage IA-IB	• Surveillance (preferred for pT1-T3) • Single-agent carboplatin (AUC = 7 × 1-2 cycles) • EBRT (para-aortic nodes only)
Stage IIA	• EBRT (para-aortic and ipsilateral iliac nodes: "Dogleg") • BEP chemotherapy ×3 cycles or EP ×4 cycles
Stage IIB	• BEP ×3 cycles or EP ×4 cycles (primary chemotherapy preferred) • EBRT in nonbulky (≤3 cm) to include para-aortic and ipsilateral iliac lymph nodes)
Stage IIC, III	• BEP ×3-4 cycles or EP ×4 cycles

Treatment Algorithm—Nonseminoma

All algorithms describe treatment after an initial radical inguinal orchiectomy, preferably a high ligation of the spermatic cord.

Stage IA	• Surveillance (preferred) • Nerve sparing retroperitoneal lymph node dissection (RPLND) → postoperative chemotherapy (BEP/EP) for pN2/N3 otherwise surveillance • BEP ×1 cycle
Stage IB	• Surveillance • Nerve-sparing RPLND → postoperative chemotherapy (BEP/EP) for pN2/N3 otherwise surveillance • BEP ×1 cycle

Stage IIA	• Markers negative
	  • Nerve-sparing RPLND → postoperative chemotherapy (BEP/EP) for pN2/N3 otherwise surveillance
	  • BEP ×3 cycles or EP ×4 cycles → RPLND if negative markers and ≥1 cm residual mass otherwise surveillance after chemo
	• Persistent marker elevation
	  • BEP ×3 cycles or EP ×4 cycles → RPLND if negative markers and ≥1 cm residual mass otherwise surveillance after chemo

Stage IIB-III	• BEP ×3 cycles or EP/VIP ×4 cycles → surgical resection of significant masses otherwise surveillance after chemo

Radiation Treatment Technique—Seminoma

- **SIM:** Head first, supine, Med-Tec lower extremities, clamshell contralateral testis
- **Dose:** 20 Gy in 10 fractions to at-risk lymphatics (para-aortic, ipsilateral iliacs) in stage I-II seminoma
  30 Gy in 15 fractions for stage IIA seminoma to gross nodes
  36 Gy in 18 fractions for stage IIB seminoma to gross nodes
- **Target:** Para-aortic lymph nodes in all patients being treated (Fig. 51.1)
  Add ipsilateral iliac lymph nodes (common, internal, external) for "dogleg" field in stage II
  Boost gross nodes with 2-cm margin to block edge for stage II (Fig. 51.2)
- **Technique:** AP/PA with photons or single PA beam with protons
- **IGRT:** Weekly MV ports, consider daily kV as needed.

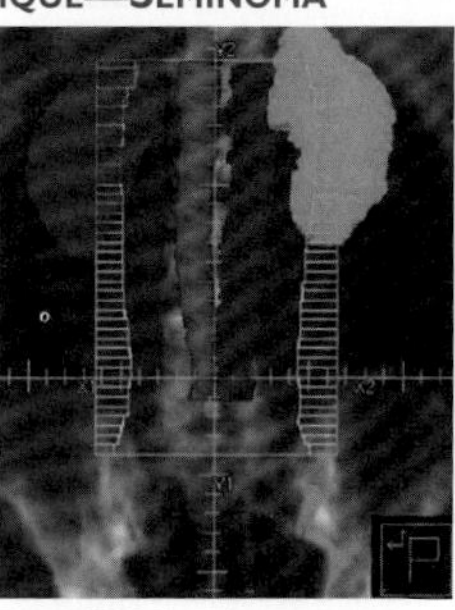

Figure 51.1 Example para-aortic radiation plan utilized to treat stage I patients (*Wilder et al. IJROBP* 2012).

Field borders—dogleg (ie, para-aortic and ipsilateral iliacs)	
Superior	Bottom of T11
Inferior	Para-aortic (medial)—bottom of L5 Ipsilateral iliac (lateral)—superior acetabulum
Medial	Tip of contralateral transverse process
Lateral	Tip of ipsilateral transverse process and cover ipsilateral renal hilum

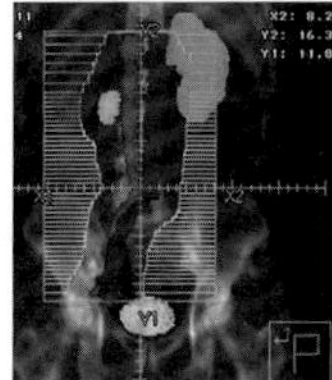

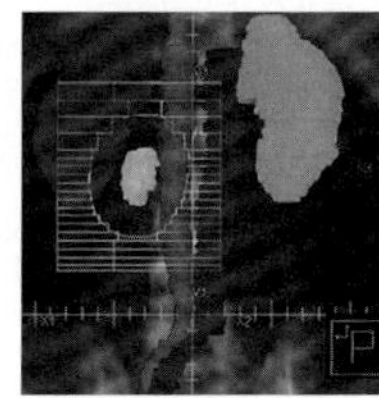

Figure 51.2 Example para-aortic and ipsilateral iliac LN field for a stage II seminoma showing the initial field **(left panel)** and subsequent sequential nodal boost **(right panel)** (*Wilder et al. IJROBP* 2012).

- **Planning directive:**
  Kidney V20 < 33%

Surgery

- Transinguinal orchiectomy with high ligation of spermatic cord is therapeutic, establishes diagnosis, and establishes T stage.
- Nerve-sparing retroperitoneal lymph node dissection used in treatment of some stage IIB or higher seminoma patients and in select nonseminoma tumors.

Chemotherapy

- **BEP:** Etoposide 100 mg/m^2, cisplatin 20 mg/m^2, bleomycin 30 units every 21 days
- **EP:** Etoposide 100 mg/m^2, cisplatin 20 mg/m^2 every 21 days
- **VIP:** Etoposide 75 mg/m^2, cisplatin 20 mg/m^2, ifosfamide 1200 mg/m^2 every 21 days with mesna 240 mg/m^2 prior to ifosfamide

Side Effect Management

- Nausea: For prophylaxis, 4-8 mg PO 1-2 hours prior to each fraction of RT. For treatment, 8 mg po q8h until 1-2 days after RT completion

Follow-Up

After definitive treatment with adjuvant radiation, chemotherapy, and/or LN dissection

- History and physical: Every 6 months for years 1-2, then yearly
- CT of chest/abdomen/pelvis with contrast yearly for 1-3 years after treatment, then as indicated. Can substitute CT of abdomen/pelvis with chest x-ray
- For nonseminoma, obtain serum markers on the same schedule as history/physical exams.

Active surveillance after orchiectomy without adjuvant therapy

- History and physical: Every 2 months for year 1, every 3 months for year 2, and every 4-6 months for years 3-5. Annually after year 5
- CT of chest/abdomen/pelvis with contrast every 4-6 months for years 1-2 and every 6-12 months for years 3-4. Annually thereafter. Can substitute CT of abdomen/pelvis with chest x-ray
- For nonseminoma, obtain serum markers on the same schedule as history/physical exams.

Notable Trials—Seminoma

Stage I seminoma

- MRC TE19/EORTC 30982 (*Oliver et al. JCO* 2011): Established the noninferiority of adjuvant carboplatin compared to adjuvant radiotherapy in stage I seminoma. Total of 1477 stage I patients randomized to single-dose carboplatin (AUC 7 × 1 dose) or radiotherapy to 20 Gy. Most patients (87%) received para-aortic field only. Overall relapse-free survival was the same between arms at 95%-96% at 5 years. Contralateral seminoma was more common in radiotherapy-only arm (5-year incidence: 1.2% vs 0.2%, $p = .03$).
- MRC TE10 (*Mead et al. JNCI* 2011): Established para-aortic only field as equivalent to dogleg. Total of 478 stage I patients randomized to the para-aortic vs dogleg field. Radiation dose was 30 Gy in 15 fractions. No difference in 5-year recurrence-free survival (96% in both arms). Only four pelvic relapses in para-aortic arm, no pelvic relapses in dogleg arm.
- MRC TE18 (*Mead et al. JNCI* 2011): Established the dose of radiation in stage I seminoma. Total of 1094 patients randomized to 20 Gy in 10 fractions vs 30 Gy in 15 fractions para-aortic fields (included dogleg for prior inguinopelvic or scrotal surgery). No difference in 5-year recurrence-free survival (for 20 and 30 Gy: 95% and 97%). All but one relapse occurred within 3 years of treatment.

PENILE CANCER

SHALINI MONINGI • CURTIS A. PETTAWAY • KAREN ELIZABETH HOFFMAN

Background

- **Incidence/prevalence:** Rare cancer, 0.4%-0.6% of all malignant neoplasms in men
- **Outcomes:** 5-Year survival is 50%.
- **Demographics:** Higher incidence in Asia, Africa, and South America. Most commonly seen in ages between 50 and 70 years
- **Risk factors:** Increasing age, phimosis, balanitis, chronic inflammation, penile trauma, lack of neonatal circumcision, lichen sclerosus, STDs (particularly HPV types 16 and 18 and HIV), and tobacco use

Tumor Biology and Characteristics

- **Genetics:** Overall about 50% associated with HPV infection, but this varies with histology; oncogenic HPV types (ie, 16, 18, others) result in E6 and E7 suppression of p53 and Rb, respectively.

- **Pathology:** Majority are squamous cell carcinomas (95%).
- **Anatomy**
  - **Penile shaft:** Consists of skin, subepithelial tissues, corpus cavernosum, and corpora spongiosum, which surrounds the urethra
  - **Head of penis (glans penis):** Primarily consists of an expansion of the corpora spongiosum. Urethral meatus located at the tip. The corona is the proximal rounded surface, which is the junction between the penile shaft and glans.
  - **Lymph node drainage:** Superficial inguinal nodes → Deep inguinal nodes → External/internal iliac nodes

Workup

- **History and physical:** Exposure history and examination of the penis and inguinal LNs
- **Labs:** CBC and chemistry panel including calcium
- **Procedures/biopsy:** Punch, excisional, or incisional biopsy of primary lesion. Percutaneous LN biopsy of palpated LNs. If planning for definitive radiation (eg, brachytherapy or external beam), circumcision should always precede RT to prevent radiation-related complications.
- **Imaging:** If palpable inguinal adenopathy then CT or MRI of abdomen and pelvis to evaluate pelvic/inguinal LNs. If no palpable adenopathy routinely CT or MRI utilized for ≥T1b primary tumor, obese patients, and those with prior inguinal surgery

Penile Cancer Staging *(AJCC 8th edition)*

T Stage	
Tis	Carcinoma *in situ (penile intraepithelial neoplasia [PeIN])*
T1	Glans: Tumor invades lamina propria Foreskin: Tumor invades dermis, lamina propria, or dartos fascia Shaft: Tumor invades connective tissue between epidermis and corpora regardless of location
T1a	Tumor is without lymphovascular invasion or perineural invasion and is not high grade
T1b	Tumor exhibits lymphovascular invasion or is poorly differentiated (grade 3-4)
T2	Tumor invades corpus spongiosum with or without urethral invasion
T3	Tumor invades corpus cavernosum with or without urethral invasion
T4	Tumor invades adjacent structures (eg, scrotum, prostate, pubic bone)

N Stage			
c/pN0	No regional lymph nodes involved		
cN1	Palpable mobile unilateral inguinal lymph node	pN1	≤2 unilateral inguinal metastases, no ENE
N2	Palpable mobile ≥2 unilateral inguinal LN or bilateral inguinal LN	pN2	≥3 unilateral inguinal metastases or bilateral metastases
N3	Palpable fixed inguinal nodal mass or unilateral/ bilateral pelvic LNs	pN3	ENE of inguinal LN metastases or pelvic LN metastases

M Stage	
M1	Distant metastasis

	N0	N1	N2	N3	M1
T1a	I	IIIA	IIIB	IV	IV
T1b	IIA	IIIA	IIIB	IV	IV
T2	IIA	IIIA	IIIB	IV	IV
T3	IIB	IIIA	IIIB	IV	IV
T4	IV	IV	IV	IV	IV

TisN0M0 is stage 0is and TaN0M0 is stage 0a

Treatment of the Primary

Most patients are treated with partial or complete penectomy. Limited excisions and laser ablation are appropriate for lower-stage lesions to accomplish organ preservation.

Surgery

- Penile organ-sparing approaches:
  - Wide local excision (WLE): Consider for Tis, Ta, T1, and select T2 lesions involving the distal glans penis only.
  - Mohs surgery: An alternative to WLE in some select patient cases
  - Glansectomy: Consider in patients with glans-only tumors; clinical Ta, T1, and select T2 tumors.
- Penectomy: Partial or total penectomy. Partial penectomy is sufficient for most tumors as they arise distally. Consider total penectomy for large tumors when the remaining phallus would not provide sufficient length to stand and void.

Radiation therapy for the primary penile tumor may also permit organ preservation.

Interstitial brachytherapy

- **Indication:** Tumor ≤4 cm, no deep shaft invasion (<1 cm), ideally confined to the glans, but minor extension across the coronal sulcus is acceptable.
- **Dose:** PDR/LDR: 60 Gy over 5 days, ~50 cGy/hour
  HDR: 3 Gy bid ×5 days
- **Toxicity:** Meatal stenosis (8%-25%; especially >50 Gy); tissue necrosis (<20%)

Definitive external beam RT

- **Indication:** T1-2N0
- **Dose:** Shaft: 45-50 Gy
  10-20 Gy boost to primary disease + 2 cm margin
  Consider concurrent cisplatin-containing regime.
- **Target:** GTV, penile shaft
- **Technique:** 6 MV photons utilized for larger lesions to treat the full thickness. Electrons can be considered for superficial lesions.
- **SIM:** Arms on chest holding a bar, frog leg, lower Vac-Loc, rice, wax, or lucite block technique to provide full bolus to penile skin surface (Fig. 52.1). Reproducible setup can be challenging.

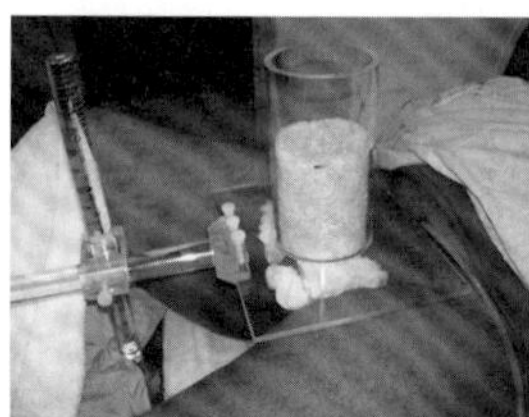

Figure 52.1 Simulation setup for a man receiving primary external beam radiation therapy for penile cancer. Setup shows Vac-Loc device immobilization into a frog-leg position. Rice bolus utilized to ensure dose coverage to the penis surface.

Regional Lymph Node Management

- No palpable or visible nodes pTstage ≥T1b: Dynamic sentinel lymph node biopsy or superficial inguinal dissection.
- Biopsy proven nodal disease(mobile <4 cm): Complete ipsilateral inguinal node dissection and modified contralateral dissection → pelvic lymph node dissection for extranodal metastasis, or >2 inguinal node metastases or bilateral positive inguinal nodes.
- Among patients with bulky inguinal metastases, inguinal and pelvic lymph node dissection, chemotherapy, and radiotherapy may be indicated. External beam RT can be used as neoadjuvant treatment to downsize unresectable LNs, definitive treatment instead of LN dissection, as adjuvant treatment after LN dissection for patients at high risk of recurrence, or as palliative treatment. The optimal integration of chemotherapy, chemoradiation, and surgery is being studied in the ongoing International Penile Advanced Cancer Trial (InPACT; NCT02305654).

External beam RT for LN management

- **SIM:** Arms on chest holding a bar, frog leg, and lower Vac-Loc. Consider bolus for superficial LN coverage in thin men.

- **Indication:** Adjuvant radiation considered for N3 disease, ≥3 LNs involved, bilateral positive nodes or ECE
- **Dose:** 60-70 Gy to gross nodes or sites of ECE
  45-50.4 Gy to at-risk inguinal/pelvic node basins and the prepubic fat (Fig. 52.2)
  Concurrent chemotherapy preferred utilizing a cisplatin-containing regime
- **Technique:** 6× photons delivered by VMAT

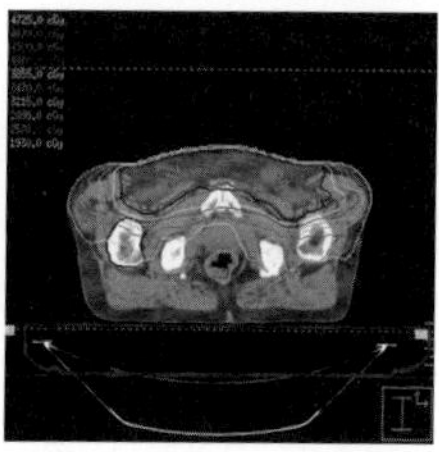

Figure 52.2 Example of neoadjuvant treatment of inguinal LNs and prepubic fat.

Follow-Up

- History/physical: Every 3 months for years 1-2, every 6-12 months for years 3-5, and yearly after year 5. CT or MRI of the abdomen/pelvis for LN+ and CT or x-ray chest for N2-3 disease.

Notable Data

Outcomes after definitive organ preservation surgery for invasive penile cancer

- *Philippou et al. J Urol* 2012: Reported on 179 patients having undergone a variety of organ-sparing procedures, including glansectomy, excisions, and distal corporectomy. With a mean follow-up of 43 months, the incidence of local, regional, or distant recurrence was 8.9% (16 patients), 10.6%(19 patients), and 5% (9 patients), respectively. The 5-year overall local recurrence-free survival rate was 86.3%. It is important to note that local relapse did not affect disease-specific survival as patients who recurred could often be salvaged with additional local therapy.

Outcomes after definitive external beam radiation

- Lausanne (*Ozsahin et al. IJROBP* 2006): Retrospective review of 60 patients treated with surgery ± postoperative RT or definitive RT. Among patients treated with penile preservation therapy, the 5- and 10-year rates of surviving with an intact penis were 43% and 26%, respectively. Locoregional relapse occurred in 56% treated with organ-sparing technique. No difference in survival between treatments

Outcomes after definitive brachytherapy

- Princess Margaret (*Crook et al. World J Urol* 2009): Retrospective review of 67 patients with T1-T3 penile cancer who were treated with definitive EBRT or brachytherapy. Local control rate was 87%, and 5-year penile preservation rate was 88%. Ten-year OS was 59%, and cause-specific survival was 83.6%. Late soft tissue necrosis and urethral stenosis rates were 12% and 9%, respectively.

Adjuvant lymph node radiation

- MDACC (*Reddy et al. BJU Int* 2017): Retrospective review of 182 patients who underwent lymph node dissection for penile squamous cell carcinoma. On multivariate analysis, clinical N3 (HR = 3.53, P = .001), ≥3 pathologically involved lymph nodes (HR = 3.78, P < .001) and ECE (HR = 3.32, P < .001) associated with worse recurrence-free survival. These data suggest that patients with these pathologic features may benefit from adjuvant therapies including chemoradiation. This is being prospectively evaluated in the ongoing International Penile Advanced Cancer Trial (InPACT; NCT02305654).

CERVICAL CANCER

SHANE R. STECKLEIN • PATRICIA J. EIFEL

BACKGROUND

- **Incidence/prevalence:** Uncommon in developed countries, and incidence continues to decrease. Third most common gynecologic cancer in the United States (12 578 diagnoses, 4115 deaths in 2014 [CDC]). 80% of cases occur in developing countries; 3rd most common cancer and 2nd most frequent cause of cancer-related death in women worldwide
- **Outcomes:** 5-Year survival across all stages is estimated at 67% (SEER data).
- **Demographics:** Lifetime risk 1 in 167 (0.6%). In the United States, incidence in Hispanic and African-American women is higher than that in non-Hispanic white women.
- **Risk factors:** Infection with high-risk human papillomavirus (HPV; virotypes 16, 18, 31, 33), immunosuppression, smoking, multiparity, early age at coitarche, multiple sexual partners.

TUMOR BIOLOGY AND CHARACTERISTICS

- **Pathology:** 75%-80% are squamous carcinomas, and about 20% are adenocarcinomas; rare subtypes include neuroendocrine (small cell, large cell, low-grade carcinoid-like). Nearly all squamous and adenocarcinomas are positive for HPV DNA and stain positively for p16; neuroendocrine cancers are positive for CD56, chromogranin A, synaptophysin.
- **Imaging:** PET-CT most accurate for detection of nodal metastasis. MRI pelvis useful for establishing extent of primary cervical disease; tumor best visualized on T2-weighted images with intravaginal gel (Fig. 53.1). Lung and liver are the most common sites of metastatic disease.

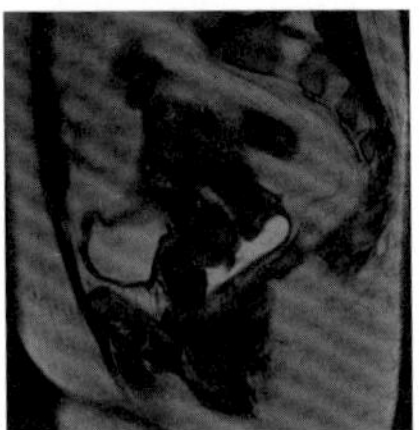

Figure 53.1 MRI T2 sequence in sagittal axis for a patient with a newly diagnosed 3-cm cervical adenocarcinoma of the anterior lip. Note the hyperintense signal in the vagina indicating presence of intravaginal gel, which allows for improved contrast and detection of cervical tissue.

ANATOMY

- Cervix is located at the caudal portion of the uterus. Composed of muscle covered by stratified squamous epithelium (ectocervix) or simple columnar epithelium (endocervix).
- Length of endocervical canal is ~2 cm.
- Lymph node drainage:
  - External iliac → common iliac → para-aortic
  - Obturator and internal iliac → common iliac → para-aortic
  - Presacral → para-aortic
  - Tumors that involve the uterine fundus can spread directly to the para-aortic lymph nodes via lymphatics along the gonadal veins.
  - Inguinal lymph nodes, if tumor involves distal 1/3 of vagina
  - Perirectal lymph nodes, if tumor invades the rectovaginal septum, cul-de-sac, or rectum

WORKUP

- **History and physical:** Presentation may include postcoital bleeding, irregular or heavy vaginal bleeding, vaginal discharge, and lower back or pelvic pain. May be asymptomatic and detected during routine gynecologic examination. Conduct complete pelvic examination including bimanual examination and placement of fiducial markers at caudal extent of vaginal disease.

- **Screening:** Women aged 21-65 should be screened with (Papanicolau ["Pap"] smear) every year. Consider lengthening screening interval to every 5 years with combination Pap smear and HPV testing for women aged ≥30 (USPTF grade A recommendation).
- **Labs:** CBC, CMP, and LFTs. Consider HIV testing and pregnancy test.
- **Procedures/biopsy:** Cervical biopsy and cone biopsy as indicated. For advanced stages (stage ≥IB2), consider examination under anesthesia, cystoscopy, and/or proctoscopy as indicated.
- **Imaging:** PET/CT. Pelvic MRI with intravaginal water-based gel. Chest imaging with chest x-ray or CT chest

CERVICAL CANCER STAGING *(FIGO 2009)*

Note: FIGO cervical cancer staging is based on clinical examination and does not include most advanced imaging modalities or any surgical findings. It allows the following diagnostic tests to determine stage: physical examination, colposcopy, endocervical curettage, cystoscopy, proctoscopy, intravenous urography, or CT/MRI to evaluate for urinary tract obstruction only. Plain chest radiograph and skeletal radiograph to evaluate for metastases.

T Stage	
IA1	Microscopic tumor, confined to cervix, ≤3 mm depth, ≤7 mm lateral spread
IA2	Microscopic tumor, confined to cervix, 3-5 mm depth, ≤7 mm lateral spread
IB1	Microscopic tumor >IA2, or clinically visible lesion ≤4 cm
IB2	Clinically visible lesion >4 cm
IIA	Involvement of upper 2/3 of the vagina
IIB	Involvement of parametria
IIIA	Involvement of distal 1/3 of the vagina
IIIB	Extension to the pelvic sidewall, hydronephrosis, or nonfunctioning kidney
IVA	Spread of tumor to adjacent pelvic organs
IVB	Spread of tumor to distant organs

TREATMENT ALGORITHM

Stage IA1	Simple (type I) hysterectomy[a]
Stage IA2–IB1	Modified radical (type II) hysterectomy with pelvic lymphadenectomy[a]
Stage IB2–IVA	Definitive chemoradiation
Stage IVB	Chemotherapy or best supportive care. Consider definitive therapy for patients with oligometastatic disease.

[a]Motivated women with tumors ≤2 cm may be a candidate for fertility-sparing approaches, which include cone biopsy (stages IA1 and IA2) ± LN dissection or radical trachelectomy (stage IB1) ± LN dissection.

- **Indications for postoperative chemoradiotherapy (Peters criteria [GOG 109]):**
  - Positive margin, positive nodes, positive parametria
- **Indications for postoperative radiotherapy (simplified Sedlis criteria [GOG 92]):**
  - At least two of three: Tumor size >4 cm, deep (>1/3) cervical stromal invasion, LVSI

RADIATION TREATMENT TECHNIQUE

- **SIM:** Supine, lower Vac-Lok (add upper Vac-Lok if treating extended fields), arms on chest (above head if treating extended fields). If treating with IMRT acquire scans with full and empty bladder. Scan from midlumbar spine to midfemur (extend scan superiorly to T10 if treating extended fields). Place isocenter midline, midplane, ~2 cm superior to femoral heads.
- **Dose:**
  - Overall goal is HR-CTV D90 to ≥87 Gy (EQD_2) (EMBRACE), gross lymph nodes and parametrial involvement to ≥60 Gy (EQD_2), and subclinical nodal volumes to 43-45 Gy (EQD_2).
  - External beam: 45 Gy in 25 fractions at 1.8 Gy/fx (consider 43.2 Gy in 24 fractions at 1.8 Gy/fx for clinically node-negative patients). Boost grossly involved lymph nodes and parametrial disease using sequential or simultaneous integrated boost.
  - Brachytherapy:
    - HDR: 6 Gy × 5 fractions ($EQD_{2,\,\alpha/\beta=10}$ = 40 Gy)

- LDR/PDR: Generally ~18-22 Gy × 2 fractions, respecting normal tissue constraints
- Details regarding brachytherapy doses and volumes. See **Brachytherapy** chapter.

- **Targets:**
  - Definitive radiotherapy
    - External beam: Uterus and cervix (generate uterocervix ITV), uterosacral and cardinal ligaments, parametria, obturator, internal iliac, external iliac, presacral, common iliac, ± para-aortic lymph nodes.
    - Brachytherapy: HR-CTV, defined as the entire cervix and any gross disease at the time of applicator placement; also any vagina or uterine body initially involved with disease
  - Postoperative radiotherapy
    - External beam: Vaginal cuff ITV, remnants of the parametria, obturator, internal iliac, external iliac, presacral, common iliac, ± para-aortic lymph nodes (Fig. 53.2)
    - Brachytherapy (if indicated): Vaginal cuff and target proximal ~2 cm of the vagina

Considerations: If tumor involves distal 1/3 of the vagina, cover inguinal lymph nodes. If disease invades posteriorly into the rectovaginal septum, cul-de-sac, or rectum, cover the perirectal lymph nodes.

- **Technique:** 4-field 3DCRT (AP/PA and opposed laterals). Use IMRT in posthysterectomy setting or if covering inguinal or para-aortic lymph nodes.

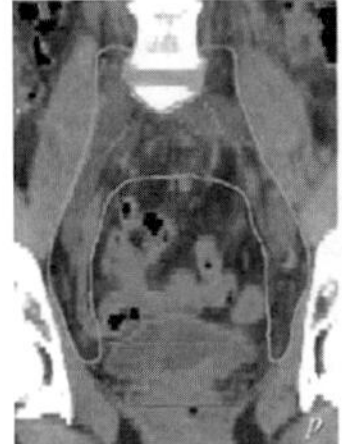

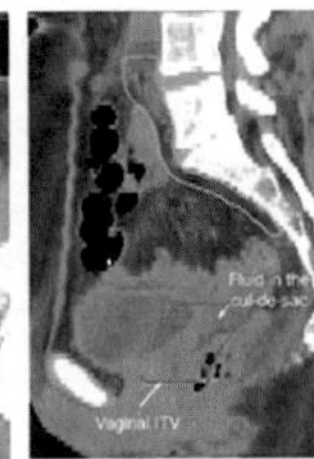

Figure 53.2 *Aqua blue* contour line in coronal **(left)** and sagittal **(right)** planes representing target lymph nodes in a postoperative cervical cancer case that was treated with IMRT. Note the vaginal ITV in *turquoise*. **See color insert**. *(Adapted from Eifel and Klopp. Gynecologic Radiation Oncology, a practical guide. Wolters Kluwer, 2016.)*

3DCRT Fields (Fig. 53.3)	
Superior	Bifurcation of the aorta (do not use bony anatomy, usually occurs L3-L5); extend to top of T12 (or 1.5-2 cm superior to most superior grossly involved para-aortic lymph node) if treating extended para fields.
Inferior	Bottom of obturator foramen or 3 cm below tumor
Anterior	Anterior edge of the pubic symphysis
Posterior	Cover entire sacrum to level of S3/S4 interspace
Lateral	2 cm lateral to pelvic brim

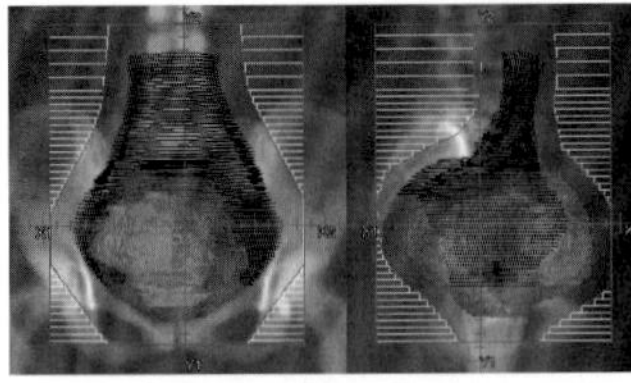

Figure 53.3 Standard AP **(left panel)** and lateral **(right panel)** fields. The imaging shows the contoured uterocervix ITV (*grey*), and nodal CTV (*black*).

- **IGRT:** Weekly kV imaging for 3DCRT, daily kV imaging for IMRT
- **Dose constraints (external beam only)**
  Bladder V45 Gy < 50%
  Rectum V45 Gy < 80%
  Femoral heads V40 < 15%

Kidney (each) V20 < 33%, V15 < 50%
Small bowel V40 < 30%
Duodenum V55 < 15 cc, V60 < 2 cc
Spinal cord <45 Gy max

- **Dose constraints (brachytherapy; doses include external beam contribution)**
  HR CTV D90% > 87 Gy
  Bladder D2cc < 80 Gy
  Sigmoid D2cc < 75 Gy
  Rectum D2cc < 70 Gy

Chemotherapy

- **Concurrent:** Cisplatin (40 mg/m^2 once weekly) for 5-6 cycles

Side Effect Management

- Diarrhea: Imodium titrating to a maximum of 8 pills/day; schedule Imodium if diarrhea persists on prn dosing → may consider alternating Lomotil and Imodium or recommending 1-2 pills before meals and at bedtime → 3rd-line tincture of opium. Rule out other causes of diarrhea, especially if presentation is early (eg, *Clostridium difficile*).
- Cystitis: UA with culture and sensitivity to rule out UTI. Treat if positive. Pyridium for noninfectious radiation cystitis
- Nausea: 1st-line Zofran (8 mg q8h prn) → 2nd-line Compazine (10 mg q6h prn) → 3rd-line Emend (aprepitant) → 4th-line ABH (lorazepam 0.34 mg, diphenhydramine 25 mg, and haloperidol 1.5 mg) 1 capsule q6h.

Follow-Up

- H&P 1 month after completing radiotherapy, PET-CT 3 months thereafter. Interval H&P every 3-6 months for 2 years, every 6-12 months for 3-5 years, and then annually
- Cervical/vaginal cytology as recommended for detection of lower genital tract neoplasia
- Imaging of para-aortic nodes for patients with positive pelvic nodes who were treated with pelvic RT may be performed to detect salvageable para-aortic recurrences. Additional imaging can be performed based on symptoms or examination findings suggestive of recurrence.
- Vaginal dilators or intercourse 2-3 times per week starting 2-3 weeks after completing radiotherapy to mitigate vaginal stenosis.

Notable Trials

Surgery vs Radiotherapy

- Milan (*Landoni et al. Lancet* 1997): 343 stage IB-IIA patients randomized to radical hysterectomy vs definitive radiotherapy. Improved 5-year PFS (66% vs 47%, p = .02) and OS (70% vs 59%, p = .05) in surgery arm for adenocarcinoma, but no difference in PFS (76% vs 78%) or OS (84% vs 88%) for squamous cell carcinoma. 63% of surgery patients received adjuvant radiotherapy for high-risk features. Toxicity (mainly urinary) 28% for surgery vs 12% for radiotherapy (p = .0004).

Concurrent chemoradiation

- RTOG 90-01 (*Morris et al. NEJM* 1999; *Eifel et al. JCO* 2004): Stage IIB-IVA patients comparing extended-field radiation therapy (EFRT) vs pelvic radiotherapy with concurrent cisplatin and 5-fluorouracil (CRT). 51% reduction in disease recurrence with CRT. 8-Year OS 67% for CRT vs 41% for EFRT (p < .0001). Additional contemporary chemoradiation trials include GOG-120 (*Rose et al. NEJM* 1999), GOG-123 (*Keys et al. NEJM* 1999), GOG-85 (*Whitney et al. JCO* 1999), SWOG 87-97 (*Peters et al. JCO* 2000), and NCIC (*Pearcey et al. JCO* 2002).

IMRT for posthysterectomy radiotherapy

- NRG-RTOG 12-03 (*Klopp et al. JCO* 2018): Randomized trial of patients with cervical or endometrial cancer with an indication for postoperative radiotherapy comparing 3D CRT vs IMRT. Significant reduction in acute (5 week) bowel and urinary toxicity and improved quality of life and sense of physical well-being with IMRT. At the end of radiation, IMRT was associated with significantly less diarrhea (52% vs 34%, p = .01) and less use of antidiarrheal medications (20% vs 8%, p = .04).

Additional guidance: Eifel PJ, Klopp AH. *Gynecologic Radiation Oncology: A Practical Guide*. Wolters Kluwer; 2016.

ENDOMETRIAL CANCER

BHAVANA S. VANGARA CHAPMAN • ANN H. KLOPP

BACKGROUND

- **Incidence/prevalence:** Most common gynecologic cancer in developed countries (53 028 diagnoses and 9727 deaths in the United States in 2014 [CDC]), second most common gynecologic cancer in developing countries, and second most common cause of gynecologic cancer deaths; overall incidence is increasing
- **Outcomes:** 5-Year survival across all endometrial histologies and stages is estimated at 81% (SEER).
- **Demographics:** Lifetime risk 2.8%. Generally, postmenopausal women of 55-85 years old, Caucasian > African American, but African American women have higher mortality rates than other racial groups.
- **Risk factors:** Unopposed estrogen (obesity, PCOS, nulliparity, early menarche, late menopause, tamoxifen), Lynch syndrome (consider genetic testing if <50 years old with family history of colorectal cancer +/– endometrial cancer)

TUMOR BIOLOGY AND CHARACTERISTICS

- **Pathology/genetics:**
  - Endometrial:
    - **Type 1:** Endometrioid (75%-80%), mucinous (1%-5%); genomic perturbations in *PTEN*, *KRAS*, *PIK3CA*, *PAX2*, and *CTNNB1* (β-catenin). May be associated with microsatellite instability (MSI)
    - **Type 2:** Nonendometrioid (10%-15%); serous, clear cell, carcinosarcoma (previously malignant mixed müllerian tumor [MMMT]), squamous cell, and undifferentiated); genomic perturbations in *TP53*, *ERBB2* (HER2), *CDKN2A* (p16), and *CDH1* (E-cadherin) and may overexpress EGFR or HER2
  - Uterine sarcoma (5%): Leiomyosarcoma, endometrial stromal sarcoma, and adenosarcoma
- **Imaging:** Typical presentation of early-stage disease is a thickened endometrium.

ANATOMY

- 1-2 cm muscular uterine wall composed of inner endometrium (epithelial origin), myometrium (mesenchymal origin), and outer serosa (mesenchymal origin)
- Cranial to caudal: *Fundus* is the dome superior to the fallopian tubes; *body*; and *internal os* is the constriction in the middle of the uterus above the cervix
- Determining uterine position and degree of flexion is important when sounding for intracavitary brachytherapy.
- Lymph node drainage:
  - Endometrium has few lymphatics, but subserosa has rich lymphatics, so depth of invasion (DOI) is related to nodal metastases (GOG 33, *Creasman et al. Cancer* 1987).
  - Fundus can drain directly to para-aortics via lymphatics along gonadal vessels and inguinal nodes via round ligament.
  - Fundus and upper body: Hypogastric route
    - Junctional interiliac nodes → common iliac → para-aortic
  - Middle and lower body, internal os: Lateral route to parametrial LNs, then
    - External iliac → common iliac → para-aortic
    - Obturator and internal iliac → common iliac → para-aortic
    - Presacral → para-aortic

WORKUP

- **History and physical:** Presentation includes vaginal bleeding (classically postmenopause), pelvic pain, and/or dyspareunia. May be asymptomatic and detected during routine gynecologic exam. Conduct complete pelvic examination including bimanual examination and rectovaginal exam.
- **Labs:** CBC, CMP, CA125, and LFTs. Consider pregnancy test.
- **Procedures/biopsy:** Endometrial sampling/biopsy under hysteroscopy, and consider dilation and curettage if unable to obtain adequate biopsy. Patients are surgically staged via hysterectomy.
- **Imaging:** Preoperative CXR only for early-stage, low-grade endometrioid endometrial cancer; CT C/A/P or PET-CT if FIGO G3, high-risk histology/sarcoma, or suspect extrauterine disease; MRI pelvis if gross cervical or vaginal involvement

Grade and Staging

Note: FIGO uterine cancer staging relies on evaluation of the surgical pathology.

FIGO Grade	
G1	<5% nonsquamous or nonmorular solid growth pattern
G2	5%-50% nonsquamous or nonmorular solid growth pattern
G3	>50% nonsquamous or nonmorular solid growth pattern; serous, clear cell, carcinosarcoma, undifferentiated histologies

Endometrial Cancer FIGO Staging (2009)[a]	
IA	Limited to endometrium or invades <1/2 of myometrium
IB	Invades ≥1/2 of myometrium
II	Invades cervical stroma but does not extend beyond uterus
IIIA	Invades serosa and/or adnexa (direct extension or metastasis)
IIIB	Vaginal involvement (direct extension or metastasis) or parametrial involvement
IIIC1	Metastasis to pelvic lymph nodes
IIIC2	Metastasis to para-aortic lymph nodes ± pelvic lymph nodes
IVA	Invades bladder and/or bowel mucosa
IVB	Distant metastases including inguinal lymph nodes and/or peritoneum

[a]*Includes carcinosarcoma.*

Treatment Algorithm

Operable Endometrioid: TAH/BSO and Lymph Node Evaluation			
	Grade 1	Grade 2	Grade 3
IA	Observe	Observe or VBT[a]	VBT
IB	VBT	VBT ± WPRT[a]	WPRT + VBT ± chemo[a]
II	WPRT + VBT		WPRT ± VBT ± chemo[a]
IIIA	Adjuvant chemotherapy ± WPRT with concurrent chemotherapy ± VBT[a]		
IIIB	WPRT with concurrent chemotherapy ± VBT[b] ± adjuvant chemotherapy		
IIIC1	WPRT with concurrent chemotherapy ± VBT + adjuvant chemotherapy		
IIIC2	EFRT with concurrent chemotherapy ± VBT + adjuvant chemotherapy		
IVA	Chemotherapy ± WPRT/EFRT + concurrent chemotherapy ± VBT boost[a]		

[a]Consider risk factors: Age >60 years, DOI, LVSI, large tumor, lower uterine involvement, cervical glandular involvement; EBRT for inadequate LND or >20% risk on Mayo Clinic nomogram (*Alhilli et al. Gyn Oncol* 2013).

[b]May require interstitial brachytherapy if patient had thick or extensive disease at presentation.

VBT, vaginal brachytherapy; WPRT, whole pelvic radiation therapy; EFRT, extended-field radiation therapy.

Other Treatment Considerations

- **Extensive cervical involvement:** Pre-op WPRT/EFRT + ICRT → surgery vs radical hysterectomy if negative margins can be achieved.
- **Vaginal involvement:** Pre-op WPRT/EFRT + intracavitary brachytherapy (ICRT) → surgery vs definitive chemoRT. If distal vaginal involved, need to include inguinal nodes.
- **Adnexal involvement:** Chemotherapy with RT recommended based on relative risk factors for local recurrence.
- **Inoperable:** WPRT/EFRT + ICRT (like cervical cancer with HR-CTV including endometrial target) with consideration of chemotherapy
- **Uterine sarcoma:** Generally simple hysterectomy and BSO, consider ovarian preservation in young patients with early-stage disease; role of chemotherapy and radiation is limited.
- **Other unfavorable histologies (eg, serous carcinoma):** Consider the addition of concurrent chemotherapy and adjuvant chemotherapy if not otherwise planned due to stage.

Radiation Treatment Technique

- **SIM:** Supine, arms on chest holding A-bar (above head holding T-bar for EFRT), lower Vac-Lok (add upper Vac-Lok for EFRT), legs straight. Scan full and empty bladder to identify an ITV, from T12 to midfemur (from T10 for EFRT). Isocenter midline, midplane, ~2 cm superior to femoral heads
- **Dose (Fig. 54.1):**
  - EBRT: 45-50.4 Gy in 25-28 fractions at 1.8 Gy/fx. Boost grossly involved lymph nodes to 60-66 Gy. 40 Gy in 2 Gy/fx for patients receiving EBRT without chemotherapy.
  - HDR VBT for prophylaxis: 6 Gy × 5 fractions prescribed to the vaginal surface ($EQD_{2,\alpha/\beta=10}$ = 40 Gy) for VBT alone, 5 Gy × 2 fractions ($EQD_{2,\alpha/\beta=10}$ = 12.5 Gy) with WPRT/EFRT to 45 Gy
- **Targets:**
  - Postoperative radiotherapy
    - EBRT: Vaginal cuff ITV generated with full and empty bladder; nodal CTV including common iliac, external iliac, and internal iliac (hypogastric and obturator), presacral if cervical involvement ± para-aortic nodes
      - If disease involves distal 1/3 of the vagina, cover medial inguinal lymph nodes.
      - If disease invades posteriorly to rectovaginal septum, cul-de-sac, or rectum, cover the perirectal lymph nodes. For significant rectal gas on sim scan, extend vaginal ITV to cover rectum.
    - VBT: Vaginal cuff and proximal ~2 cm of the vagina
    - See **Brachytherapy Chapter** for more details regarding brachytherapy.
- **Technique:** IMRT (Fig. 54.1) (NRG-RTOG 1203; *Klopp et al.* unpublished).

Anatomic References for Field Borders	
Superior	**WBRT:** Bifurcation of the aorta **EFRT:** Extend to top of T12 (or 1.5-2 cm superior to most superior grossly involved para-aortic lymph node)
Inferior	Bottom of obturator foramen or 3 cm of the upper half of the vagina
Anterior	Anterior edge of pubic symphysis
Posterior	Entire sacrum to level of S2-S3; S3-S4 interspace for cervical stromal involvement
Lateral	2 cm lateral to pelvic brim

- **IGRT:** Weekly CBCT or CT-on-rails, daily kV imaging
- **Dose constraints:**

EBRT	EBRT + Brachy for Intact Uterus
Bladder V45 Gy < 50%	Bladder D2cc < 80 Gy[a]
Rectum V45 Gy < 80%	Sigmoid D2cc < 70 Gy[a]
Small bowel V40 < 30%	Rectum D2cc < 70 Gy[a]
Duodenum V55 < 15 cc, V60 < 2 cc	
Kidney (each) V20 < 33%, V15 < 50%	
Femoral heads V40 < 15%	
Spinal cord <45 Gy	

[a]*Cumulative EQD_2, including EBRT.*

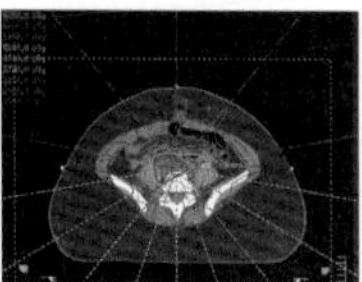
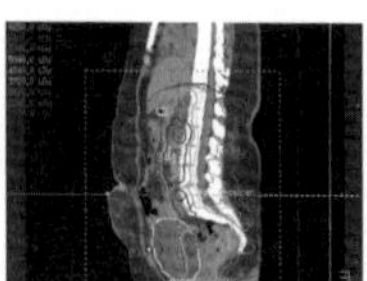
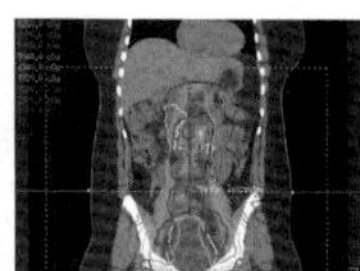

Figure 54.1 Extended-field IMRT (EFRT) plan. *Blue isodose line* representing 50.4 Gy is seen covering nodal CTV and vaginal ITV (*red colorwash*). **See color insert.**

Chemotherapy

- **Concurrent:** Cisplatin (40 mg/m^2 once weekly) for 5-6 cycles. Consider weekly paclitaxel for serous carcinoma (50 mg/m^2 once weekly).
- **Adjuvant:** Carboplatin (AUC 5-6 mg · min/mL) and paclitaxel (175 mg/m^2) for 3-4 cycles

Side Effect Management

See **Cervical Cancer** chapter

Follow-Up

- Physical examination, CT A/P, and CXR q3mo for 2 years, q6mo for 3 years, then annually thereafter
- Vaginal dilators or intercourse 2-3 times per week starting 2-3 weeks after completing radiotherapy to mitigate vaginal stenosis

Notable Trials

Observation vs WPRT: PORTEC 1* (*Creutzberg Lancet* 2000; *Creutzberg IJROBP* 2011): Randomized 714 patients with stage IB (G2-3) and IC (G1-2) endometrial cancer s/p TAH/BSO and no LND randomized to observation vs WPRT (46 Gy/23 fx). 15-Year LRR rates were 6% vs 16% in the WPRT and observation arms, respectively (p < .0001). 15-Year OS was not significantly different between groups.

WPRT vs VBT: PORTEC 2* (*Nout Lancet* 2010): Noninferiority RCT with 427 stage I-IIA high-intermediate-risk endometrial cancer s/p TAH-BSO randomized to WPRT (46 Gy/23 fx) vs VBT. 5-Year vaginal recurrence was not different between groups (p = .74). No difference in LRR (vaginal and/or pelvic recurrence), distant metastases, OS, or DFS between arms. G1-2 gastrointestinal toxicity was lower in the VBT group at the completion of RT (13% vs 54%).

Whole abdominal radiation therapy (WART) vs chemotherapy: GOG 122* (*Randall et al. JCO* 2006): RCT with 396 patients with stage III-IV endometrial carcinoma s/p TAH/BSO randomized to WART (30 Gy/10 fx + 15 Gy boost) vs doxorubicin/cisplatin × 7 cycles + cisplatin × 1 cycle. Improved 5-year PFS (50% vs 38%, p = .007) and OS (55% vs 42%, p = .004) in the chemotherapy arm. G3-4 hematologic toxicities worse with chemotherapy arm (88% vs 14%). Criticisms include stage-adjusted statistical analysis and inclusion of patients with gross residual disease treated to insufficient doses.

Concurrent chemoradiation + chemotherapy: RTOG 9708* (*Greven et al. Gyn Oncol* 2006): Phase II study with 46 G2-3 endometrial cancer with high-risk features s/p TAH/BSO who underwent concurrent chemoradiation (45 Gy/25 fx with cisplatin) + VBT + cisplatin/paclitaxel after completion of RT. 4-Year pelvic, regional, and distant recurrence rates were 2%, 2%, and 19%, respectively. 4-Year OS and DFS rates were 85% and 81%, respectively. G3 and G4 toxicities occurred in 16% and 5% of the cohort, respectively.

Chemotherapy vs chemoradiation: NSGO-EC-9501/EORTC-55991 and MaNGO ILIADE-III* (*Hogberg et al. Eur J Cancer* 2010): Pooled analysis of two RCTs of 540 patients with stage I-III endometrial cancer with high-risk features s/p TAH/BSO ± LND randomized to adjuvant RT ± sequential chemotherapy. In combined analysis, 5-year PFS was improved in the chemoradiation arm (78% vs 69%, p = .009) and OS trended toward significance.

Radiation vs concurrent chemoradiation: PORTEC-3 (*de Boer et al. Lancet Oncol* 2018): RCT of 686 patients with IA-IIIC endometrial cancer with high-risk features s/p TAH or TLH ± BSO ± LND randomized to WPRT (48.6 Gy/27 fx) ± VBT vs concurrent WPRT and cisplatin ± VBT + concurrent carboplatin + adjuvant carboplatin/paclitaxel. Improvement with addition of chemotherapy in 5-year failure-free survival (76% vs 69%, p = .022). No difference in 5-year OS between groups (82% vs 77%, p = .11). Grade 3 or worse adverse events occurred in 60% of patients receiving chemoradiation vs 12% who received radiation (p < .001).

WPRT vs VBT + chemotherapy: GOG 249 (*Randall et al. ASTRO abstract* 2017): Phase III RCT of 601 patients with high-risk early-stage I-II endometrial, serous, or clear cell endometrial cancer s/p TAH or TLH ± BSO ± LND who underwent WPRT ± VBT vs VBT + chemotherapy. Preliminary results showed no difference in recurrence-free survival, distant failure, or OS. Acute and late toxicities and pelvic/PA-nodal failure rates were greater in the VBT + chemotherapy arm.

Uterine sarcoma and carcinosarcoma—observation vs RT: EORTC 55874* (*Reed et al. Eur J Cancer* 2008): Phase III RCT of 224 patients with stage I-II high-grade uterine sarcoma and carcinosarcoma s/p TAH/BSO randomized to observation vs WPRT 50.4 Gy/28 fx. LRR was reduced in the adjuvant RT arm (22% vs 40%, p = .004) but PFS and OS were no different. On subtype analysis, RT improved LC in carcinosarcomas, but not in leiomyosarcomas.

*Studies used 1988 FIGO staging

Additional guidance: Eifel PJ, Klopp AH. *Gynecologic Radiation Oncology: A Practical Guide*. Wolters Kluwer; 2016.

VAGINAL CANCER

SHANE R. STECKLEIN • ANUJA JHINGRAN

Background

- **Incidence/prevalence:** Least common of all gynecologic cancers (<3000 vaginal cancers diagnosed each year in the United States)
- **Outcomes:** 5-Year survival across all stages is estimated at 60%-70% (SEER data).
- **Risk factors:** Infection with high-risk human papillomavirus (HPV; detected in 75% of vaginal cancers), immunosuppression, early age at coitarche, multiple sexual partners, smoking, increasing age

Tumor Biology and Characteristics

- **Pathology:** 80%-90% of all vaginal cancers are squamous. Adenocarcinomas classically associated with in utero exposure to diethylstilbestrol (DES), but DES-associated adenocarcinomas are now exceedingly rare. Vaginal adenocarcinoma associated with higher risk of in-field failure and higher risk of distant metastasis. Other rare subtypes include neuroendocrine cancers and melanoma.

Anatomy

- The average vaginal length is 7-10 cm. Most vaginal cancers arise in the upper vagina.
- Lymph node drainage:
  - Proximal vaginal cancers share the same pattern of spread as cervical cancers:
    - External iliac → common iliac → paraaortic
    - Obturator and internal iliac → common iliac → paraaortic
    - Presacral → paraaortic
  - Distal vaginal cancers may spread through the inguinal lymph nodes similar to vulvar cancers.
  - Invasion of the rectovaginal septum, cul-de-sac, or rectum warrants coverage of the perirectal lymph nodes.

Workup

- **History and physical:** Presentation includes postcoital bleeding, irregular or heavy vaginal bleeding, vaginal discharge, pelvic pain, painful/frequent urination.
- **Labs:** CBC, CMP. Consider pregnancy test.
- **Procedures/biopsy:** Lesion biopsy. Examination under anesthesia (EUA) with fiducial placement is critical prior to initiating treatment to delineate extent and location of initial disease to facilitate boost planning.
- **Imaging:** CT abdomen and pelvis and PET-CT (most sensitive) to evaluate for inguinal, pelvic, and paraaortic lymphadenopathy. The vagina is poorly visualized on CT; pelvic MRI with intravaginal gel is the modality of choice for imaging the primary tumor.

Vaginal Cancer Staging *(FIGO 2012)*

Note: FIGO vaginal cancer staging is based on clinical exam, which does not include many imaging modalities or surgical findings. It allows the following diagnostic tests to determine stage: physical exam, proctoscopy, and cystoscopy. Plain chest radiograph and skeletal radiograph to evaluate for metastases.

Clinical Stage	
I	Tumor limited to the vaginal wall
II	Tumor involves the subvaginal tissue but does not extend to the pelvic sidewall.
III	Tumor extends to the pelvic sidewall and/or presence of pelvic and/or inguinal lymph node metastasis.
IVA	Tumor invades bladder and/or rectal mucosa and/or directly extends beyond the true pelvis.
IVB	Spread to distant organs

Treatment Algorithm

Stage I	Primary surgical resection may be considered, but is rarely used.
Stage I-IVA	Definitive radiotherapy or chemoradiotherapy
Stage IVB	Chemotherapy or best supportive care. Consider definitive therapy for patients with oligometastatic disease.

Radiation Treatment Technique

- **SIM:** Supine, frog-leg (if treating inguinal lymph nodes), lower Vac-Lok (add upper Vac-Lok if treating extended fields), arms on chest (above head if treating extended fields). Acquire scans with full and empty bladder. Scan from mid–lumbar spine to mid-femur (extend scan superiorly to T10 if treating extended fields). Place isocenter mid-line, mid-plane, ~2 cm superior to femoral heads.
- **Dose:** If feasible, goal is to treat the tumor with 1- to 2-cm margin to a cumulative dose of 75-90 Gy (EQD_2) using a combination of external beam radiotherapy and interstitial (or intracavitary if original tumor was <7 mm thick) brachytherapy. For some apical lesions where brachytherapy cannot be used, external beam boost to cumulative dose of ~66 Gy may be employed.
- **Targets:** Vagina and paravaginal tissues (ITV), with at least 3-cm distal margin on gross disease, obturator, internal iliac, external iliac, presacral, common iliac, ± inguinal, ± paraaortic lymph nodes.
- **Technique:** IMRT/VMAT, to reduce dose to the central pelvis
- **IGRT:** Daily kV imaging

Chemotherapy

- **Concurrent:** Cisplatin (40 mg/m^2 once weekly) for 5-6 cycles; use is extrapolated from cervical cancer data.

Side Effect Management

- Dermatitis: Aquaphor for radiation dermatitis, hydrogel for areas of moist desquamation. Important to encourage hygiene early in treatment course to prevent bacterial and fungal infection; Domeboro Sitz bath 2-3 times daily. If erythema and pain are out of proportion to expected dermatitis, suspect fungal overgrowth and treat empirically with fluconazole.
- Diarrhea: 1st line Imodium titrating to a max of 8 pills/day; schedule Imodium if refractory on prn dosing → 2nd line alternating Lomotil 2 pills and Imodium 2 pills every 3 hours → 3rd line tincture of opium
- Cystitis: UA with culture and sensitivity to rule out UTI. Treat if positive. Pyridium for noninfectious radiation cystitis
- Nausea: 1st line Zofran (8 mg q8h prn) → 2nd line Compazine (10 mg q6h prn) → 3rd line Emend (aprepitant) → 4th line ABH (lorazepam 0.34 mg, diphenhydramine 25 mg, and haloperidol 1.5 mg) 1 capsule q6h

Follow-Up

- Vaginal dilators or intercourse 2-3 times per week after the vagina has healed to mitigate vaginal stenosis
- Interval H&P every 3-6 months for 2 years, then every 6-12 months for 3-5 years, then annually
- Cervical/vaginal cytology as recommended for detection of lower genital tract neoplasia
- Imaging based on symptoms or examination findings suggestive of recurrence

Notable Trials and Papers

NCDB analysis (*Rajagopalan et al. PRO* 2015): Health research database with 1530 women. Concerning decline in utilization of brachytherapy boost for vaginal cancer, decreasing from 87.7% in 2004 to 68.6% in 2011. Corresponding increase in IMRT external beam boost.

MDACC experience with vaginal SCC (*Frank et al. IJROBP* 2005): Retrospective review of 193 patients with vaginal squamous cell carcinoma treated with definitive radiation. Excellent outcomes using external beam radiotherapy and brachytherapy with 5-year disease-specific survival 85% (stage I), 78% (stage II), and 58% (stage III-IVA). Low rate of 5-year major complications: 4% (stage I), 9% (stage II), and 21% (stage III-IVA)

MDACC experience with vaginal adenocarcinoma (non-DES associated) (*Frank et al. Gynecol Oncol* 2007): Retrospective review of 26 patients with non–DES-associated vaginal adenocarcinoma treated with external beam followed by brachytherapy (77%) or external beam alone (23%). 5-Year survival 34% for adenocarcinoma compared to 58% for SCC. Adenocarcinoma associated with worse pelvic control and higher risk of distant metastasis.

Additional guidance: Eifel and Klopp. *Gynecologic Radiation Oncology: A Practical Guide*. Wolters Kluwer; 2016.

VULVAR CANCER

SHANE R. STECKLEIN • ANUJA JHINGRAN

Background

- **Incidence/prevalence:** <6000 vulvar cancers diagnosed each year in the United States
- **Outcomes:** 5-Year survival across all stages estimated at 72% (SEER data)
- **Risk factors:** Prior infection with high-risk human papillomavirus (HPV; detected in 50% of vulvar cancers), immunosuppression, smoking, increasing age, chronic inflammation (eg, lichen sclerosis).

Tumor Biology and Characteristics

- **Pathology:** 90% of all vulvar cancers are squamous. Adenocarcinoma accounts for the majority of the remaining epithelial neoplasms. Other rare subtypes include neuroendocrine cancers and melanoma.

Anatomy

- Vulvar cancers can arise from the prepuce, clitoris, labia majora, labia minora, urethral opening, Bartholin and Skene glands (more likely to be adenocarcinoma), or perineum.
- Lymph node drainage:
  - Inguinal → external iliac → common iliac → paraaortic
  - Locally advanced tumors that involve the anus, rectum, or rectovaginal septum may also spread through the internal iliac, presacral, and perirectal lymph nodes.

Workup

- **History and physical:** Presentation includes vulvar bleeding, pruritus, discharge, dysuria, vulvar mass, or pain.
- **Labs:** CBC, CMP. Consider pregnancy test.
- **Procedures/biopsy:** Lesion biopsy and/or radical local excision.
- **Imaging:** CT abdomen and pelvis and PET-CT (most sensitive) to evaluate for inguinal, pelvic, and paraaortic lymphadenopathy. The vulva is poorly visualized on CT; pelvic MRI is the modality of choice for imaging the primary tumor.

Vulvar Cancer Staging (*FIGO* 2012)

Note: FIGO vulvar cancer staging is a hybrid of a clinical and surgical staging approach, which includes physical examination, imaging studies, and evaluation of the surgical pathology.

Clinical Stage	
IA	Tumor is ≤2.0 cm, confined to the vulva or perineum and with stromal invasion ≤1.0 mm
IB	Tumor is >2.0 cm or with stromal invasion >1.0 mm but remains confined to the vulva or perineum
II	Tumor of any size with extension to adjacent perineal structures (lower 1/3 of urethra, lower 1/3 of vagina, or anus)
IIIA	(i) One lymph node metastasis ≥5 mm or (ii) 1-2 lymph node metastases <5 mm
IIIB	(i) Two or more lymph node metastases ≥5 mm or (ii) three or more lymph node metastases <5 mm
IIIC	Positive nodes with extracapsular spread
IVA	(i) Tumor invades the upper urethral and/or vaginal mucosa, bladder mucosa, rectal mucosa, or tumor is fixed to the pelvic bone or (ii) fixed or ulcerated inguinofemoral lymph nodes
IVB	Any distant metastasis, including pelvic lymph nodes

Treatment Algorithm

Surgery	• Surgical resection with margins of 1-2 cm • Reexcision preferred for positive margins • Inguinal lymph node assessment (unilateral or bilateral, depending on lateralization of primary) if >1.0 mm invasion present at biopsy • Positive sentinel lymph nodes can be managed with adjuvant radiotherapy ± chemotherapy or inguinofemoral lymph node dissection. • Inguinofemoral lymph node dissection is the standard of care for patients with clinically positive groins.
Radiotherapy	• Adjuvant radiotherapy to LNs indicated if one of the followings (Homesley Criteria): >1 positive lymph nodes or ≥1 node with extracapsular extension (ECE) • Adjuvant radiotherapy to resection bed and vulva indicated if positive margins in whom additional surgery is not feasible. Strongly consider for additional risk factors including LVSI, negative but close (<8 mm fixed or <1 cm fresh) margins, tumor size >4 cm, and >5 mm depth of invasion. • Definitive radiotherapy can be employed for patients with unresectable primary or nodal disease.

Radiation Treatment Technique

- **SIM:** Supine, frog-leg, lower Vac-Lok (add upper Vac-Lok if treating extended fields), arms on chest (above head if treating extended fields). Scan from mid–lumbar spine to mid-femur (extend scan superiorly to T10 if treating extended fields). Place isocenter mid-line, mid-plane, ~2 cm superior to femoral heads.
- **Dose prescribed to volume at risk:**

Adjuvant treatment:

Vulva	Margins >5 mm	45-50 Gy
	Margins >1-2 mm but ≤5 mm	50-54 Gy
	Margins <1-2 mm	54-56 Gy
	Positive margins or gross residual disease	≥60 Gy
Nodes	Microscopic disease, no ECE	45-50 Gy
	Enlarged nodes, but no ECE	50-56 Gy
	ECE	60-66 Gy
	Gross residual disease	60-70 Gy

Definitive treatment:

Vulva	Unresectable primary lesion	60-66 Gy
Nodes	Suspicious nodes <1 cm	56-60 Gy
	Suspicious nodes 1-2 cm	60-66 Gy
	Suspicious nodes >2 cm	64-70 Gy
	Bulky or fixed nodes	66-70 Gy

- Initial external beam treatment: 45 Gy in 25 fractions at 1.8 Gy/fx (consider simultaneous integrated boost to gross disease and/or high-risk clinical target volume(s) to 50-52.5 Gy).
- Boosts: Sequentially boost gross disease and/or high-risk clinical target volume(s) to target dose(s) using external beam treatment at 1.8-2.0 Gy/fx.

- **Targets:**
  - Adjuvant treatment:
    - For close/positive margins: Vulva and tumor bed with at least 2 cm of vagina proximal to operative bed.
    - For positive nodes: Inguinofemoral and pelvic* nodes ± paraaortic lymph nodes.
  - Definitive treatment:
    - Vulva, inguinofemoral and pelvic* nodes (see below) ± paraaortic lymph nodes.

*For negative inguinal lymph nodes, nodal target should extend to the bottom of the sacroiliac (SI) joint or the bifurcation of the common iliac; for positive inguinal lymph nodes but negative pelvic lymph nodes, nodal target should extend to the mid-SI joint; for positive pelvic lymph nodes, upper field border is the aortic bifurcation. For patients with common iliac nodes, the low paraaortic nodes can be treated. If definitive radiotherapy is considered for patients with positive paraaortic nodes, the entire paraaortic nodal CTV should be treated.

- **Technique:** IMRT/VMAT, to reduce dose to the central pelvis and mons pubis. TLDs at first fraction(s) to ensure adequate dose (Fig. 56.1)
- **IGRT:** Daily kV imaging
- **Dose constraints (external beam)**
  Bladder V45 Gy < 50%
  Rectum V45 Gy < 80%
  Femoral heads V40 < 15%
  Kidney (each) V20 < 33%, V15 < 50%
  Small bowel V40 < 30%
  Duodenum V55 < 15 cc, V60 < 2 cc
  Spinal cord <45 Gy max

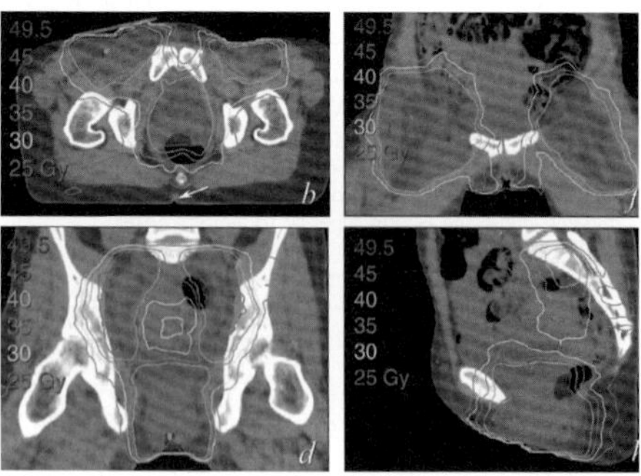

Figure 56.1 Representative treatment plan illustrating coverage of classical CTV (*red colorwash*) and PTV (*purple colorwash*) volumes for a vulvar cancer patient undergoing IMRT. **See color insert.** (Adapted from Eifel and Klopp, *Gynecologic Radiation Oncology: A Practical Guide*.)

Chemotherapy

- **Concurrent:** Cisplatin (40 mg/m^2 once weekly) for 5-6 cycles, extrapolated from cervical cancer data.

Side Effect Management

See **Vaginal Cancer** chapter.

Follow-Up

- Vaginal dilators or intercourse 2-3 times per week after the vulva has healed to mitigate vaginal stenosis.
- Interval H&P every 3-6 months for 2 years, then every 6-12 months for 3-5 years, then annually. Cervical/vaginal cytology as recommended for detection of lower genital tract neoplasia.
- Imaging based on symptoms or examination findings suggestive of recurrence.

Notable Trials and Papers

Adjuvant radiotherapy for positive inguinal lymph nodes: GOG-37 (*Homesley Obstet Gynecol* 1986): Randomized trial of 114 patients with positive groin nodes after radical vulvectomy and bilateral inguinofemoral lymphadenectomy randomized to pelvic node resection or adjuvant groin radiotherapy to 45-50 Gy in 5-6.5 weeks. 2-Year overall survival 68% for radiotherapy group vs 54% for pelvic node resection group (p = .03)

Groin dissection vs radiotherapy for N0-N1 patients: GOG-88 (*Stehman et al. IJROBP* 1992): Randomized trial of 58 (prematurely closed) patients with clinically N0-N1 vulvar squamous cell carcinoma randomized to groin dissection or groin radiotherapy to 50 Gy in 25 fractions prescribed to 3 cm below skin. Groin relapse observed in 18.5% of radiotherapy patients vs 0% in dissection patients (p = .03). Numerous criticism of this trial including preliminary closure of trial and inadequate depth of prescribed dose.

Sentinel lymph node (SLN) metastasis size and risk of additional non-SLNs: GROINSS-V (*Oonk et al. Lancet Oncol* 2010): 403 patients with T1-T4 (<4 cm) vulvar SCC underwent SLN biopsy followed by inguinofemoral lymphadenectomy if SLN was positive. Disease identified in 135 (33%) of patients, of which 115 (85%) underwent lymphadenectomy. Risk of non-SLN metastasis increased with increasing size of SLN metastasis. All patients with SLN metastasis should have additional groin treatment. Prognosis significantly worse in patients with SLN metastasis >2 mm (69.5% vs 94.4%, p = .001)

Contouring atlas: RTOG (*Gaffney et al. IJROBP* 2016): Consensus guidelines for contouring and treatment of vulvar cancer.

Additional guidance: Eifel and Klopp, *Gynecologic Radiation Oncology: A Practical Guide*. Wolters Kluwer; 2016.

OVARIAN CANCER

SHANE R. STECKLEIN • LILIE L. LIN

Background

- **Incidence/prevalence:** 2nd most common gynecologic cancer and 5th most common cause of cancer-related death in women in the United States (22 440 diagnoses, 14 080 deaths in expected in 2017 [ACS]).
- **Outcomes:** 5-Year survival across all stages estimated at 47% (SEER data)
- **Demographics:** Lifetime risk 1 in 77 (1.3%)
- **Risk factors:** Age; family history of breast, ovarian, or colorectal cancers; familial cancer syndromes (hereditary breast and ovarian cancer syndrome, *PTEN* hamartoma syndrome, hereditary nonpolyposis colorectal cancer, Peutz-Jeghers syndrome) obesity; nulliparity; or first pregnancy after age 35

Tumor Biology and Characteristics

- **Pathology:** Epithelial ovarian cancers (EOC) constitute 85%-90% of all ovarian cancers and include primary malignancies of the fallopian tube and primary peritoneal cancer. Type I ovarian cancers include low-grade serous, endometrioid, and mucinous subtypes and often exhibit mutations in *KRAS*, *BRAF*, or *PTEN* (*Singer et al. JNCI* 2015). Type II ovarian cancers are predominately high-grade serous carcinoma (70% of all ovarian cancers), which are associated with *TP53* mutation (*Ahmed et al. J Pathol* 2010), but also include undifferentiated carcinomas and carcinosarcomas. 10%-15% of ovarian tumors are borderline tumors or germ cell tumors.

- **Genetics:** Inherited deleterious mutations in *BRCA1* and *BRCA2* result in ~40% and 15% lifetime risks of ovarian cancer, respectively. Overall, 18%-24% of ovarian cancer patients carry inherited mutations in *BRCA1*, *BRCA2*, *BARD1*, *BRIP1*, *CHEK2*, *MRE11A*, *MSH2*, *MSH6*, *NBN*, *PALB2*, *PMS2*, *RAD50*, *RAD51C*, *RAD51D*, or *TP53* (*Walsh et al. PNAS* 2011; *Norquist et al. JAMA Oncol* 2016). Tumors with mutations in *BRCA* or other homologous recombination pathway genes are hypersensitive to platinum-based chemotherapy and poly(ADP)ribose polymerase (PARP) inhibitors.

Anatomy

- Ovaries lie near the uterine horns at the opening of the fallopian tubes and are connected to the lateral surface of the uterus via the utero-ovarian ligament.
- Lymphatic drainage from the ovaries and fallopian tubes primarily follows the gonadal vessels, and first echelon drainage is the paraaortic and aortocaval nodes. Rarely, ovarian cancers can drain along the round ligament to the inguinal lymph nodes.
- Intraperitoneal dissemination is the primary mechanism of ovarian cancer spread.

Workup

- **History and physical:** Presentation includes bloating, pelvic or abdominal pain, early satiety, and urinary frequency. Genetic risk evaluation for all patients
- **Labs:** CBC, CMP, LFTs, CA125. Consider pregnancy test.
- **Procedures/biopsy:** Biopsy and/or peritoneal cytology as needed
- **Imaging:** Ultrasound, CT or MRI abdomen/pelvis, and/or PET. Chest x-ray or CT chest to evaluate lungs

Ovarian Cancer Staging (*FIGO* 2014)

FIGO Stage	
IA	Tumor limited to one ovary, with intact capsule, no tumor on surface, negative washings
IB	Tumor involves both ovaries, otherwise like stage IA
IC1	Tumor limited to one or both ovaries with surgical spill
IC2	Tumor limited to one or both ovaries with capsule rupture before surgery or tumor on ovarian surface
IC3	Tumor limited to one or both ovaries with malignant cells in ascites or peritoneal washings
IIA	Extension or implant on the uterus and/or fallopian tubes
IIB	Extension to other pelvic intraperitoneal tissues
IIIA1	Positive retroperitoneal lymph nodes (IIIA1(i) $\leq$ 10 mm, IIIA1(ii) > 10 mm)
IIIA2	Microscopic extrapelvic (above the brim) peritoneal involvement with or without positive retroperitoneal lymph nodes
IIIB	Macroscopic extrapelvic peritoneal involvement $\leq$2 cm with or without positive retroperitoneal lymph nodes; includes extension to capsule of liver and/or spleen
IIIC	Like IIIB, but extrapelvic peritoneal involvement is >2 cm
IVA	Pleural effusion with positive cytology
IVB	Hepatic and/or splenic parenchymal metastasis or metastasis to extra-abdominal organs or lymph nodes (including inguinal lymph nodes)

Treatment Algorithm

Stage IA or IB, fertility desired	Unilateral (IA) or bilateral (IB) salpingo-oophorectomy with comprehensive surgical staging
IA-IV, surgically resectable, fertility not desired	Total abdominal hysterectomy, bilateral salpingo-oophorectomy, and comprehensive surgical staging and debulking as needed
Bulky stage III-IV or poor surgical candidate	Consider neoadjuvant chemotherapy with or without interval debulking and total abdominal hysterectomy and bilateral salpingo-oophorectomy.

CHEMOTHERAPY

- Adjuvant platinum/taxane chemotherapy is employed for all high-grade ovarian cancers. Patients with stage I disease get 3-6 cycles, while 6 cycles are recommended for patients with stage II-IV disease.
- Neoadjuvant chemotherapy may be used in patients with bulky or unresectable disease.
- Intraperitoneal chemotherapy is often recommended for patients with stage II-IV disease who have undergone optimal debulking surgery.
- At relapse, major determinant of response to additional therapy and outcome is interval between last platinum chemotherapy and disease recurrence.
  - >6 months = Platinum sensitive, consider additional platinum-based chemotherapy.
  - $\leq$6 months = Platinum resistant, move to second-line chemotherapy (docetaxel, etoposide, gemcitabine, liposomal doxorubicin [Doxil], topotecan ± bevacizumab).

RADIATION TREATMENT TECHNIQUE

- Radiotherapy is seldom used in the 1st-line treatment of ovarian cancer.
- Prior studies of whole abdominal radiotherapy (WART) showed some efficacy in the curative treatment of ovarian cancer; due to toxicity, technical challenges, and subsequent improvements in chemotherapy, WART has not been widely adopted.
- The major use of radiotherapy for ovarian cancer is in palliation of recurrent or metastatic disease.
- Definitive radiotherapy is warranted in select patients with confined postchemotherapy local or nodal recurrences. Radiotherapy may be particularly effective in patients with clear cell *(Hoskins et al. JCO 2012)*, mucinous, or endometrioid histology. It is less effective and rarely used for borderline or low-grade serous tumors.
  - GTV should be treated to 60-66 Gy(EQD$_2$).
  - CTV that includes regions of possible adjacent soft tissue infiltration and adjacent regional lymph nodes should be treated to 45-50 Gy(EQD$_2$).
  - 3DCRT or IMRT may be used, depending on location, anatomy, and proximity of critical structures.

NOTABLE TRIALS AND PAPERS

WART vs pelvic radiotherapy and chemotherapy: Princess Margaret *(Dembo et al. Cancer Treat Rep 1979)*: Prospective trial randomizing 231 patients with stage IB-III ovarian cancer treated postoperatively with WART vs pelvic radiotherapy and chlorambucil chemotherapy. Recurrence-free survival was 64% in the WART group vs 40% in the pelvic radiotherapy and chlorambucil group.

Benefit of radiotherapy in clear cell ovarian cancer: British Columbia Cancer Agency *(Hoskins et al. JCO 2012)*: Retrospective review of 241 patients with stage I or II clear cell ovarian cancer receiving adjuvant chemotherapy or chemoradiotherapy (WART). On subset analysis, postoperative radiation improved 5-year DFS in patients with stage IC (excluding rupture alone) and stage II disease by 20%.

Radiotherapy for locoregionally recurrent ovarian cancer: MD Anderson *(Brown et al. Gynecol Oncol 2013)*: Retrospective review of 102 patients with localized nodal and extranodal recurrences treated with definitive involved-field radiotherapy (IFRT) to $\geq$45 Gy. 5-Year in-field disease control was 71%. RT is associated with excellent local control, protracted disease-free intervals, and cures in appropriately selected patients.

SOFT TISSUE SARCOMA

KAITLIN CHRISTOPHERSON • B. ASHLEIGH GUADAGNOLO

BACKGROUND

- **Incidence/prevalence:** Heterogeneous group of solid tumors of mesenchymal cell origin. Rare, 12,000 cases diagnosed annually in the United States. Account for 1% of adult cancers. Relatively high rates of distant failure
- **Outcomes:** Disease-specific survival ~60% at 10 years. Prognostic factors for survival: **grade**, size, site, LN involvement, age (older worse). Prognostic factors for local recurrence: **positive margin**, locally recurrent disease, head and neck location, retroperitoneal location, older age
- **Demographics:** Median age at diagnosis is 45-55 years.
- **Risk factors:** Can be associated with genetic syndromes like Li-Fraumeni, tuberous sclerosis, FAP, NF type 1. Prior exposure to ionizing radiation. Majority of cases have no clear predisposing exposure. Injuries have not been associated with an increased risk for developing sarcomas.

TUMOR BIOLOGY AND CHARACTERISTICS

- **Histologic subtypes:** Over 20 major categories of STS with >60 histologic subtypes. Most common histologies include undifferentiated pleomorphic sarcoma (UPS), liposarcoma, synovial sarcoma, and leiomyosarcoma.
- **Pathology:** Core biopsy is ideal. Excisional biopsy should be avoided. Important for expert sarcoma pathology review due to rarity and diversity of tumors. Grade is prognostic for DM and OS. Look for signature translocations (ie, synovial sarcoma t(X;18) SS18-SSX1/SSX2, or myxoid liposarcoma t(12;16)). *MDM2* amplification in well-differentiated liposarcoma and dedifferentiated liposarcoma is used to distinguish from benign adipose tumors and poorly differentiated sarcomas (which are negative for amplification).
- **Imaging:** Mixed appearances. Generally on MRI: T1 tumor is isointense, T2 tumor is hyperintense.

ANATOMY

- Can occur anywhere, most common location lower extremity ≫ upper extremity = superficial trunk = retroperitoneal > head and neck
- LN involvement in <5% of all cases. More common (15%) in "CARE" tumors, clear cell, (cutaneous) angiosarcoma, rhabdomyosarcoma, and epithelioid sarcoma

WORKUP

- **History and physical:** Focus on personal/family history of cancer; refer to genetics when appropriate.
- **Procedures/biopsy:** Core needle or incisional biopsy
- **Imaging:** MRI with gadolinium for primary extremity and superficial trunk lesions. CT with contrast for head and neck and retroperitoneal primaries. CT chest for staging. For **retroperitoneal sites**, obtain renal perfusion scan to assess differential renal function prior to RT or surgery.

SOFT TISSUE SARCOMA CELL CANCER STAGING *(AJCC 8TH EDITION)*

T Stage		N Stage	
T1	Tumor ≤5 cm in greatest dimension	N0	No regional nodes
T2	Tumor >5 cm but ≤10 cm in greatest dimension	N1	Regional lymph node metastasis
T3	Tumor >10 cm but ≤15 cm in greatest dimension		
T4	Tumor >15 cm in greatest dimension	**M Stage**	
		M0	No distant metastasis
		M1	Distant metastasis

<table>
<tr><th colspan="6">Overall Stage</th></tr>
<tr><th></th><th>G1</th><th>G2</th><th>G3</th><th>N1 or M1</th><td rowspan="5">Grade is determined by a score of total differentiation, necrosis, and mitotic count and is incorporated into staging as indicated to the left.</td></tr>
<tr><td>T1</td><td>IA</td><td colspan="2">II</td><td rowspan="4">IV</td></tr>
<tr><td>T2</td><td rowspan="3">IB</td><td colspan="2">IIIA</td></tr>
<tr><td>T3</td><td colspan="2" rowspan="2">IIIB</td></tr>
<tr><td>T4</td></tr>
</table>

Treatment Algorithm

Stage I	Surgery alone, WLE (limb sparing if extremity). If R0, can observe. Consider ability to get negative margins, and what salvage surgery would entail.
Stage II-III	Favor preoperative RT followed by surgery. If upfront surgery is done, recommend post-op RT. Consider neoadj chemotherapy if high grade and stage T2-T4.
Stage IV	Chemotherapy and supportive care

Radiation Treatment Technique

- **SIM:** Depending on anatomic location. Supine position preferred, prone may be needed. For post-op cases, wire the scar or the entire field to help with target delineation. Do not specifically target drain sites.
  Lower extremity: Vac-Lok for involved extremity. CT scan done feet first. Can elevate noninvolved leg to isolate if needed
  Upper extremity: Upper Vac-Lok. Arm position depends on location of primary. May need bolus
  Distal extremities: Can consider custom cushion +/– aquaplast mask to help with immobilization
  Head and Neck: Prior to SIM, consider dental evaluation/need for stent. Aquaplast mask
- **Dose: Pre-op:** 50 Gy at 2 Gy/fx
  Post-op: 60 Gy at 2 Gy/fx for R0 resection, with field size reduction after 50 Gy. Boost to 64-68 Gy for positive margin.
  (Despite higher boost dose, LR is higher for R1/2 resection; in other words, higher radiation dose does not make up for lack of R0 resection.)
  Considerations: If IMRT preferable for postoperative cases, can also consider a simultaneous-integrated boost technique where GTV (post-op bed) treated to 59.92 Gy in 28 fractions (2.14 Gy/fx) and CTV 50.4 cGy in 28 fractions (1.8 Gy/fx). See Figure 58.1.
- **Target: Pre-op:** GTV + 4 cm longitudinally sup/inf along fascial planes and 1.5 cm radially to yield CTV (*Haas et al. IJROBP* 2012).
  Post-op: Virtual GTV = Post-op bed
  CTV50 as above (4 cm sup/inf, 1.5 cm radially off of vGTV)
  Cone down to CTV60-68 (vGTV + 2 cm sup/inf, 1.5 cm radially).

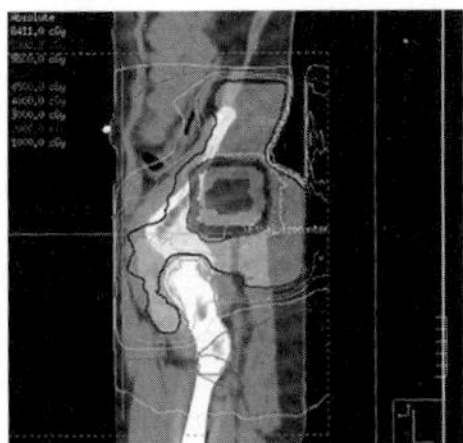
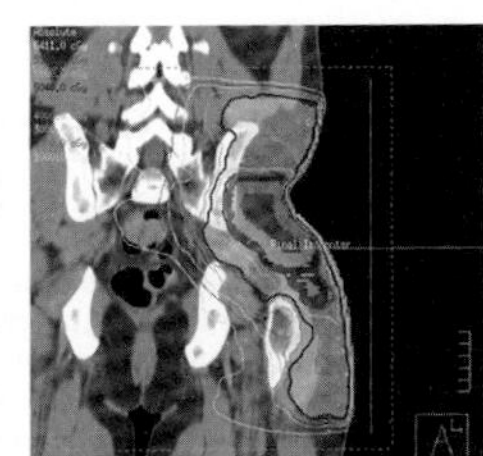

Figure 58.1 Representative sagittal and coronal (L → R) images of an IMRT treatment plan for a 40-year-old male being treated with adjuvant RT following R0 resection of a grade III PNET of the left lower extremity. Using IMRT in this case allowed for reduced dose to the left femoral head/proximal femur. The *red isodose line* represents 59.92 Gy (covering GTV) and *blue* represents 50.40 Gy (covering CTV). **See color insert.**

Considerations: CTV expansions can be increased in areas of difficult surgical access or for superficial spreading histologies. CTVs can be trimmed/carved out of bone if not involved. Do not cover elective nodes for any histology other than alveolar rhabdomyosarcoma in select cases. PTV expansions typically 0.5-1 cm depending on daily imaging techniques

- **Technique: 3DCRT:** We prefer 3D planning in extremities. Consider parallel opposed fields (with nondivergent deep border to spare bone/joint). Other beam arrangements (wedge-pair, obliques, etc.) may be used as well. Asymmetric beam weighting can be used if tumor is not centrally located.

  IMRT: Consider more conformal radiation techniques for proximal lower extremities, thoracic, pelvic, retroperitoneal, head and neck sites (Fig. 58.1).

Adult Extraosseous Ewing Sarcoma: A Different Clinical Entity
Small round blue cell tumor. Very rare. More common in children.
Translocation t(11;22) or t(21;22) in 95% of cases
Upfront intensive chemotherapy for everyone.
Local tumor can be treated with surgery or definitive RT depending on location. Can also use combined modality
RT Doses • Definitive: 60 Gy • Pre-op: 50 Gy • Post-op: 60 Gy
Adult Rhabdomyosarcoma Sarcoma: A Different Clinical Entity
Adults with RMS do worse than pediatric patients.
Alveolar, embryonal, and pleomorphic subtypes
Unclear if pediatric RT doses are sufficient. Normally escalate dose to >50 Gy, upward to 60 Gy respecting adjacent normal tissue tolerance. Dose similar to other STS in adults.

- **IGRT:** Related to modality used and site of body.
  Daily kV typically used. (For 3D planning: consider rotating collimator parallel with long bone for set-up and kV alignment.)
- **Planning directive (for conventional fractionation):**
  Spare 1-cm strip of limb circumference/skin
  Avoid treating entire limb circumference >45 Gy
  Avoid treating entire femur circumference to ≥50 Gy
  Spare ½ cross section of weight-bearing bone; V40 < 64%
  Block part of the joint cavity; V45 < 50%
  Avoid >45 Gy to 50% of major tendons (ie, patellar/Achilles)

Surgery

- Mainstay of treatment for soft tissue sarcomas
- Wide local excision with goal of widely negative margin (goal = 2-cm normal tissue around tumor, unless tumor abuts natural barrier to spread like bone, nerve).
- In unirradiated patients with R1 or R2 resection, consider additional surgery or re-excision prior to RT or pre-op RT to 50 Gy followed by re-excision.

Chemotherapy

- Controversial, as studies have failed to show OS benefit
- We consider neoadjuvant chemotherapy for patients with high-grade, large (>5 cm) tumors. Neoadjuvant chemotherapy is preferred over adjuvant as due to a 20%-30% response rate to chemotherapy, thus intact measurable disease is important. Typically assess response following 2-4 cycles.
- Standard starting chemotherapy regimen involves Adriamycin/ifosfamide for most STS. Other agents commonly used include doxorubicin, gemcitabine, and docetaxel. Targeted therapy with pazopanib (TKI) and trabectedin (targets FUS-CHOP transcription) can be considered as both are FDA approved for advanced STS cases. Can also consider enrolling on trials with other targeted agents (MDM2 inhibitors, immunotherapy)

Side Effect Management

- Skin care: First-line emollients. Can add Domeboro soaks thereafter. If having further grade 2+ skin toxicity, consider Mepilex. For grade 3 dermatitis, consider Silvadene cream (on weekends or after RT has been completed entirely). Have a low threshold for considering infection/antibiotics in setting of fungating tumors.

Local Recurrences

- In a radiation-naive patient with local recurrence of STS, treat with preoperative radiation (50 Gy) followed by surgery if feasible.
- Generally avoid reirradiation, as complications following reirradiation have been reported as high as 80% and reirradiation has not been shown to improve local control for tumors that have been previously irradiated.

Notable Papers

Limb-sparing surgery (LSS) + RT results in similar OS and DFS

- *Rosenberg et al. Ann Surg* 1982: Prospective RCT, (2:1) LSS + post-op RT vs amputation. All points received post-op chemo with Adriamycin and Cytoxan followed by high-dose MTX. RT dose 45-50 Gy between joints, shrinking field boost to 60-70 Gy. Local failure 15% (LSS + RT) vs 0% (amputation) (*P* = .06). OS and DFS for LSS + RT 83%/71% vs amputation 88%/78% (*P* = NS). Conclusion: LSS + RT effective for most points. R1 resection increases risk of LR.

Preoperative radiation results in less long-term fibrosis than postoperative radiation

- *O'Sullivan et al. Lancet* 2002: 2-Arm prospective RCT. 190 patients randomized to pre-op RT 50 Gy in 2 Gy fractions, (plus post-op boost 16-20 Gy if + surgical margin), vs post-op RT 50 Gy, with cone down to 66-70 Gy. Primary endpoint wound complications (≤120 days post-op) higher in pre-op (35% vs 17%, *P* = .01). No difference in LC, PFS, DM. + Surgical margin predicts LF. Size and grade prognostic for RFS and OS.
- *Davis et al. Radiother Oncol* 2005: Analyzed 129 patients from O'Sullivan trial (above). Analysis of function 2 years after treatment. Grade 2+ fibrosis was lower in pre-op arm 31% vs post-op arm 48% (*P* = .07). Edema and joint stiffness also less in pre-op 18% vs 23% (NS). On multivariate analysis, field size was a significant predictor for fibrosis and stiffness. No significant difference in function reported by points or MDs. Conclusion: Post-op RT tends to result in more fibrosis.

Consensus papers

- RT for extremity STS (*Haas et al. Int J Radiat Oncol Biol Phys* 2012). Review of data in regard to RT for extremity STS and the implications for local control, survival, and complications. Pre- and postoperative RT discussed with consensus recommendations for target volumes.
- Treatment guidelines for preoperative RT for retroperitoneal sarcoma (*Baldini et al. Int J Radiat Oncol Biol Phys* 2015). Expert panel of 15 academic radiation oncologists and systematic review of published data regarding pre-op RT for RPS. Role of RT for RPS is not established. Awaiting EORTC STRASS trial. Outlines patient selection and recommended volumes from available data

MELANOMA

KAITLIN CHRISTOPHERSON • B. ASHLEIGH GUADAGNOLO

Background

- **Incidence/prevalence:** Aggressive skin cancer. Accounts for 1% of all skin cancers in the United States. Incidence is ~87 000 new cases annually, with 10 000 deaths annually. Incidence increasing over past three decades
- **Outcomes:** 5-Year survival for localized melanomas varies with depth/thickness but can be upward of 90% for lesions with <1 mm depth. With presence of regional adenopathy, survival at 5 years is 60%. With the presence of DM, survival at 5 years is ~10%-20%.

- **Demographics:** Median age at diagnosis is 60. Caucasians ≫ Hispanics > African Americans. For patients <50 years old, more common in women. For patients >50 years old, more common in men
- **Risk factors:** Ultraviolet (UV) exposure, family history, history of multiple atypical moles or dysplastic nevi. Increased risk among immunocompromised patients. History of Xeroderma pigmentosum

Tumor Biology and Characteristics

- **Histologic subtypes:** Superficial spreading (70% of cases, arise from pigmented dysplastic nevus), lentigo maligna, nodular, acral lentiginous, and desmoplastic (more likely to be neurotropic, may be amelanotic)
- **Pathology:** Cell of origin is melanocyte. Pathology report should include: Breslow thickness, ulceration, primary tumor mitotic rate, resection margins, microsatellitosis, Clark level, and presence of desmoplasia. Molecular genetic testing should be considered to test for BRAF mutational status if nodal or metastatic involvement at presentation, or clinical trial is considered.
- **Imaging:** Stage 0-II routine imaging not recommended unless there are focal symptoms. Stage III (SNLB+), consider baseline CT C/A/P. Stage III (cN+, in-transit mets, or microsatellitosis), at minimum CT of primary body compartment. Consider brain MRI and PET/CT for stage IIIC-IV.

Anatomy

- Can occur anywhere on skin, predominantly on sun exposed areas. Most common locations in males are the back followed by head/neck. Most common locations in females are the extremities and trunk.

Clark Levels (Now Superseded by Depth of Invasion)	
Level 1	Confined to epidermis
Level 2	Invasion of papillary dermis
Level 3	Invasion of junction of the papillary and reticular dermis
Level 4	Invasion into reticular dermis
Level 5	Invasion into the subcutaneous fat

Workup

- **History and physical:** Focused and complete skin examination of the skin and regional lymph nodes w/ assessment of melanoma risk factors
- **Procedures/biopsy:** Optimally, an excisional biopsy is preferred for any suspicious, pigmented lesion with 1-3 mm negative margins. Consider full-thickness punch biopsy if in difficult area (distal digit, face, palms) vs excisional biopsy. Avoid shave biopsies as they give no information on depth.
- **Imaging/labs:** Not recommended for stage 0, IA, IB, and II. Can consider nodal basin ultrasound prior to SLNB in patients with stage I/II disease with equivocal LN physical exam. For stage III-IV or recurrent disease, obtain C/A/P CT imaging w/ contrast or whole-body FDG PET/CT. Obtain MRI brain w/ contrast if clinically indicated.

Melanoma Staging *(AJCC 8th Edition)*

T Stage		N Stage	
Tis	Carcinoma in situ	Nx	Regional LN not assessed
		N1	One tumor-involved node or in-transit, satellite, and/or microsatellite (i/s/m) metastases with no tumor-involved nodes
T1a	Melanoma ≤0.8 mm in thickness without ulceration	N1 a/b/c	A: 1 Clinically occult tumor-involved node detected by SNLB with no i/s/m B: 1 Clinically detected tumor-involved node with no i/s/m C: Presence of i/s/m metastases with no regional lymph node disease
T1b	Melanoma ≤0.8 mm with ulceration, or any melanoma 0.8-1.0 mm		

T Stage		N Stage	
T2 (a/b[a])	Melanoma 1.01-2.0 mm	N2	Metastases in 2-3 regional lymph nodes or i/s/m metastases with 1 tumor-involved node
T3 (a/b[a])	Melanoma 2.01-4.0 mm	N2 a/b/c	A: clinically occult nodes with no i/s/m B: clinically detected nodes (at least 1) with no i/s/m C: i/s/m mets with 1 tumor-involved node
		N3	Metastases in 4 regional lymph nodes or i/s/m metastases with ≥2 tumor-involved nodes, or any number of matted nodes with or without i/s/m
T4 (a/b[a])	Melanomas >4.0 mm	N3 a/b/c	A: clinically occult nodes with no i/s/m B: clinically detected nodes (at least 1) with no i/s/m C: i/s/m metastases with ≥2 tumor-involved nodes, or any number of matted nodes with or without i/s/m mets

M Stage	
M1a	Metastasis to distant skin, subcutaneous tissue or lymph node(s)
M1b	Metastasis to lung
M1c	Metastasis to all other non-CNS distant sites
M1d	Metastasis to CNS

Summative Stage (Clinical)

	N0	N+	M+
Tis	0	III	IV
ST1a	IA		
T1b, T2a	IB		
T2b, T3a	IIA		
T3b, T4a	IIB		
T4b	IIC		

[a]T2-T4 tumors: "a," without ulceration; "b," with ulceration.

Treatment Algorithm

Primary site management	Surgical resection, wide local excision +/− adjuvant RT to primary site (see factors for adjuvant RT to primary site below)
cN0 nodal management	T0-stage IB (T1b): Discuss and consider SNLB. SNLB not required. Stage IB (T2a) or II: Discuss and offer SNLB
Clinically occult, pN+, nodal management	Clinically occult/detected by SNLB: Can offer completion dissection vs regional nodal surveillance. Can consider adjuvant systemic agent
Clinically detected, cN+, nodal management	Complete therapeutic lymph node dissection. Consider adjuvant radiotherapy to the nodal basin for patients at high risk of regional relapse. Can consider adjuvant systemic agent (see factors for adjuvant RT to nodal site below)

Radiation Treatment Technique

- **SIM: Primary:** Radiopaque wire to outline scar or entire primary site. If using electrons, patient positioning important to allow for en face beam arrangement. Consider lateral penumbra when shaping field around CTV.
- **Dose:** 30 Gy in 6 Gy/fx, given twice weekly over 2.5 weeks. Alternative TROG regimen: 48 Gy in 2.4 Gy/fx for 20 fractions
- **Target: Primary:** Primary site/Scar + 1.5 cm margin = CTV

Factors for Adjuvant RT to Primary Site: Typically Look for 2 or More[a]
Desmoplastic histology ([a]do not need a second factor for this indication)
Breslow thickness ≥4 mm
Head and neck location
Ulceration
Satellitosis
Isolated locally recurrent disease

[a]Whether perineural invasion of small- and medium-sized nerves is a risk factor for local recurrence remains and matter of debate. Invasion of large caliber or named nerves should be considered a high-risk factor for local recurrence, and adjuvant RT is thus indicated.

Factors for Adjuvant RT to Nodal Site: For cN+ Patients	Lymphedema Risk
Cervical location (any 1 indication): ECE, ≥2 cm, ≥2 LNs positive	10%
Axillary location (any 1 indication): ECE, ≥3 cm, ≥4 LNs positive	15%
Groin location	30%
BMI < 25 kg/m^2 (any 2 indications): ECE, ≥3 cm, ≥4 LNs positive	
BMI ≥ 25 kg/m^2: discuss systemic therapy options, RT complications may outweigh regional control benefits in this anatomic location	
For any site, consider radiation if recurrent disease in a previously dissected nodal basin	

Nodal: Involved nodal region if high risk features. Do not electively treat LNs.
Head and neck: ipsilateral neck levels I-V, including supraclav fossa. (High facial/scalp primary: include pre/post auricular [superficial] parotid.)
Axilla: Ipsilateral levels I-III. Unless there is bulky or high disease, we usually do not include supraclavicular field.
Groin: Need 2 or more high-risk factors and BMI < 25 kg/m^2 to consider treating groin. Do no electively cover pelvic nodes.

- **Technique:** 3DCRT when possible.
  Primary: Consider electrons to achieve adequate dose to the surface. Bolus often needed for primary tumor. Electrons dosed to D_{max}. May normalize to 100%-105% to prevent hot spots >30 Gy. Consider skin collimation when appropriate.
  Nodal: 3D electrons or photons depending on site.
  For head and neck primaries with need for skin collimation and electrons: draw/wire field and cut out field on mask. If near areas of air gap (ie, ear) consider TX-151 bolus.
  Nodal:
  1. Head and Neck: Open neck (to allow for appositional electrons) can use tissue equivalent bolus to pull dose more superficial and out of critical structures like larynx and temporal lobe.
  2. Axillary: Head away and arm akimbo or, if patient able, can flex at elbow and extend arm superiorly to open axilla. Avoid skin folds in axilla and low neck if possible. Typically AP/PA photon beams
  3. Groin: Slight frog leg position/decrease skin fold. In thin patient can consider appositional electrons
- **IGRT:** Daily kV for hypofractionated schedule. MD verifies kV prior to first fraction. If electrons, see set up on table prior to first fraction to verify setup.
- **Planning directive:** For 30 Gy in 5 fractions: evaluate the 24 Gy line on all axial slices. 24 Gy line should be off of any critical structure (brain, eye, brachial plexus, spinal cord, bowel). Evaluate 27 Gy isodose line for target coverage, as opposed to the 30 Gy line (Fig. 59.1). For 48 Gy in 20 fractions regimen: Max dose to brain and spinal cord <40 Gy.

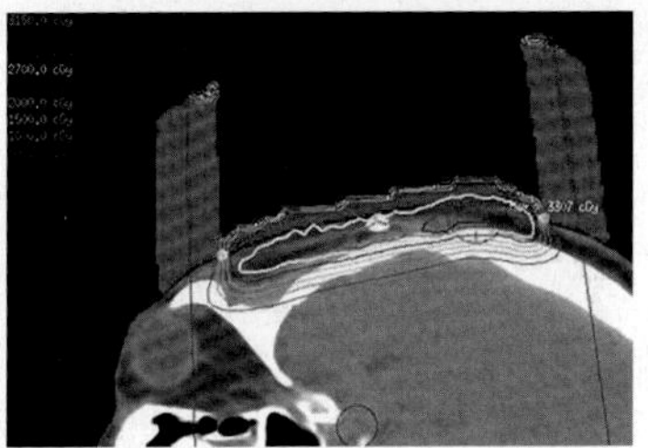

Figure 59.1 Sample RT treatment plan for a patient with a melanoma of the scalp. This patient was treated postoperatively with electrons to the tumor bed to a total dose of 30 Gy in 5 fractions. Note the 27 Gy isodose line in *yellow*, which is used to evaluate target coverage. 30 Gy hotspots are seen in *red*. **See color insert**.

SURGERY

- Primary: Wide local excision with goal of negative margin. Adequate margin is determined by depth of primary.

Primary Tumor Depth	Margin Recommended
In situ	0.5-1 cm
<1.0 mm	1 cm
1.01-2.0 mm	1-2 cm
>2.0 mm	2 cm

- cN0+/– Sentinel lymph node biopsy. SLNB must be done prior to WLE as to not alter the drainage to the sentinel basin. If SLNB+, consider completion LN dissection.
- cN+: Complete involved/regional nodal basin dissection. For certain head and neck primaries, this will involve superficial parotidectomy.

CHEMOTHERAPY

- Interferon-alpha historically used and still considered appropriate. Patients may have fatigue, low blood counts, and a flulike syndrome as side effects.
- Dabrafenib/trametinib for patients with tumors harboring BRAF V600 activating mutations can be used in select patients as adjuvant therapy or for treatment of metastases (*Long et al. Lancet* 2015).
- Immunotherapy (combination nivolumab and ipilimumab) used first line if no actionable BRAF mutation. Side effects include rash, dermatitis, and increased risk of developing autoimmune conditions.

SIDE EFFECT MANAGEMENT

- Side effects may not be present during RT if using 30 Gy in 5 fractions hypofractionated regimen. Advise patients that acute side effects may appear 1-2 weeks after completion of radiotherapy.
- Skin Care: First-line emollients. Can add domeboro soaks. If having further grade 2+ skin toxicity, consider mepilex. Grade 3 dermatitis, consider silvadene cream (on weekends or after RT has been completed entirely).

FOLLOW-UP

- Depending on initial stage, complete skin and regional nodal examination every 3-6 months for 2 years. (More frequent follow-ups for higher-stage patients.) Can space to every 3-12 months after
- For patients with initial stage IIB-III melanoma, consider labs and CT c/a/p or PET/CT to detect asymptomatic recurrence the first 3 years.

NOTABLE PAPERS

Primary site adjuvant radiation

- Review, RT for malignant melanoma (*Ballo and Ang Surg Clin North Am* 2003). Adjuvant radiotherapy improves the local-regional control rate in certain patients with primary melanoma in difficult surgical locations or with high-risk pathologic features. Impact of RT on OS/DM is yet to be determined.

- *Guadagnolo et al. Cancer* 2014: Retrospective review of 130 patients with desmoplastic melanoma treated with surgery alone (45%) or with adjuvant post-op RT (55%). Median follow-up 6.6 years. Surgery-alone patients; 24% developed local recurrence vs 7% for patients treated with PORT (on MVA, use of PORT significantly associated with improved LC, $P < .05$).

Adjuvant nodal RT decreases lymph node relapse in high-risk patients

- **TROG 02.01** (*Burmeister et al. Lancet Oncol* 2012; *Henderson et al. Lancet Oncol* 2015): RCT for 250 patients, cN+ s/p LAD with one of following inclusion criteria: ≥1 parotid node, ≥2 cervical/axillary nodes, ≥3 inguinal nodes, ECE, ≥3 cm cervical node, or ≥4 cm inguinal or axillary node randomized to adjuvant 48 Gy in 20 fractions vs observation of dissected lymph node field and scar. Adjuvant RT decreased lymph node field relapses by ~50%, No impact on RFS or OS. Grade 3-4 toxicities after adjuvant RT in head and neck, axilla, and groin were 8%, 21%, and 29%, respectively. Rate of grade 2-4 toxicities numerically but not statistically higher in RT arm: 68% vs 58% (NS). Measured limb volume ratio over 5 years in both arms; for lower extremities increase in mean volume ratio was higher in pts receiving RT 15% vs 7% in observation group ($P = .014$).

Immediate completion lymph node dissection decreases regional failures, but does not increase melanoma-specific survival

- **MSLT-II** (*Faries et al. NEJM* 2017): RCT of 1934 patients with positive sentinel lymph node biopsy randomized to completion dissection vs "nodal observation" with ultrasound. Primary end point was melanoma-specific survival. Immediate completion lymph node dissection increased the rate of regional disease control (3 year: 92% vs 77%, $P < .001$), but does not increase melanoma-specific survival (3 year: 86% vs 86%, $P = .42$). Lymphedema was higher in LN dissection group (24% vs 6%, $P < .001$).

Adjuvant RT for high-risk nodal metastases

- *Guadagnolo et al. Lancet Oncol* 2009: Review paper. Regional recurrence rates improved with nodal irradiation. Risk of complications differ with anatomic location of nodal basin involved. Additional details about fields and planning.

RT field extent for axillary metastases

- *Beadle et al. IJROBP* 2009: Retrospective review of 200 patients treated with PORT, 48% treated axilla only, and 52% treated extended field including supraclavicular fossa. Median follow-up 59 months. Axillary control rates 89% for axilla only vs 86% for extended field (NS). Treatment with extended field resulted in more treatment-related complications on MVA.

NON-MELANOMA SKIN CANCER

ANNA LIKHACHEVA

Background

- **Incidence/prevalence:** Non-melanoma skin cancers (NMSCs) include basal cell carcinoma and squamous cell carcinoma, which together constitute the most common malignancy worldwide. The highest worldwide incidence is in Australia. Approximately 3.5 million new cases are diagnosed each year in the United States. Incidence is rising. Lifetime risk is 1 in 5.
- **Risk factors:** Cumulative exposure to UV light, increasing age, Fitzpatrick skin types 1-4, immunosuppression (HIV and organ transplant), human papillomavirus (HPV), and certain syndromes or genetic disorders (basal cell nevus syndrome [Gorlin syndrome], xeroderma pigmentosum, epidermolysis bullosa, or oculocutaneous albinism).

Tumor Biology and Special Consideration

- **Prevention:** Reduction in sun exposure and oral nicotinamide (vitamin B_3) (*Chen et al. N Engl J Med* 2015)
- **Pathology:** BCC (~80%) and SCC (~20%) make up the majority of NMSC. Minority are neuroendocrine, sweat gland, mesenchymal tumors, or lymphomas.
- **Pathologic risk factors** are listed in the table below.

Anatomy

- Predominately occurs on sun-exposed areas. Skin layers are epidermis → papillary dermis → reticular dermis → subcutaneous tissues.

Workup

- **History and physical:** Focused and complete examination of the skin as many may have additional cancers and are at increased risk of developing melanoma.
- **Procedures/biopsy:** Shave/punch/excisional biopsies may be used for diagnosis. Skin biopsy should include the deep reticular dermis if suspicion is high for invasion.
- **Imaging:** The majority of NMSCs can be successfully managed without formal imaging. Consider CT if bony invasion and MRI if orbital involvement or perineural spread depending on presenting symptoms and exam. If there is concern for lymph node spread, it is reasonable to obtain a PET/CT scan.

Table 60.1 Risk Factors for Recurrence for Basal Cell Carcinoma (BCC) and Recurrence/Metastasis for Squamous Cell Carcinomas (SCC)

	Low Risk	**High Risk**
Location/size[a]	L < 20 mm M < 10 mm	L > 20 mm M ≥ 10 mm H
Borders	Well-defined	Poorly defined
Primary vs recurrent	Primary	Recurrent
Immunosuppression	(−)	(+)
Site of prior RT	(−)	(+)
PNI[b] or LVSI	(−)	(+)
Pathology	G1 (SCC) Nodular superficial (BCC)	G2-3 (SCC) Aggressive growth pattern (BCC)
Depth, thickness, or Clark level	<2 mm or I, II, III (SCC)	≥2 mm or IV, V (SCC)

[a]H (mask area), M (cheek, forehead, scalp, neck, pretibial), L (trunk and extremities).
[b]PNI is defined as involvement of large-caliber nerves with a diameter of >0.1 mm.

Table 60.2 Skin Cancer Staging (*AJCC* 8th edition)

T Stage		**N Stage (Same as Clinical N Category for p16-Neg Oropharynx Ca)**	
Tis	Carcinoma in situ	N1	Single ipsilateral lymph node, ≤3 cm and ENE (−)
T1	Tumor <2 cm in greatest dimension	N2a	Single ipsilateral lymph node, >3 cm but not >6 cm and ENE (−)
T2	Tumor ≥2 cm and <4 cm in greatest dimension	N2b	Multiple ipsilateral lymph node, none >6 cm and ENE (−)
T3	Tumor ≥4 cm in greatest dimension and/or perineal invasion and/or deep invasion and/or minor bone erosion	N2c	Bilateral or contralateral lymph nodes, none >6 cm and ENE (−)
		N3a	Metastasis in a lymph node >6 cm in greatest dimension and ENE (−)
T4a	Tumor with gross cortical bone/marrow invasion	N3b	Clinically overt ENE (+)
		M Stage	
T4b	Tumor with skull base invasion and/or skull base foramen involvement	M0	Metastasis to 1 distal organ
		M1	Metastasis to ≥1 distal organ

Summative Stage

	N0	N1	N2-3	M1
T1	I	III	IV	IV
T2	II	III	IV	IV
T3	III	III	IV	IV
T4	IV	IV	IV	IV

Treatment Algorithm

Definitive RT is recommended for nonsurgical candidates and clinical instances where skin cancer is located in cosmetically sensitive areas or where surgery might result in a functional deficit.

T1/T2 operable	Surgical resection (WLE, Mohs, or electrodesiccation for low risk)
T1/T2 inoperable	Definitive RT
cN0 but risk >15% (eg, G3, PNI)	Elective dissection Elective RT
cN+ or pN+	Therapeutic dissection Radical RT
Post-op	RT for high risk or positive margins. May be supplemented by chemotherapy in select patients
M1	Chemotherapy, clinical trial, or best supportive care

Radiation Treatment Technique

- **SIM:** CT simulation–based treatment planning is recommended for IMRT, history of adjacent RT, or in anticipation of future retreatment. Clinical setup is reasonable for orthovoltage, fixed geometry electronic brachytherapy, and palliation. Wire CTV. Skin collimation for field size <4 cm or for protection of adjacent uninvolved sensitive structures. Bolus to bring dose to the surface.
- **Dose:**
  Definitive RT:
  - For most lesions and optimal cosmesis: 66 Gy/33 fx (2 Gy/fx) or 55 Gy/20 fx (2.5 Gy/fx) delivered daily; 44 Gy/10 fx (4.4 Gy/fx) delivered 4 times a week
  - For <2-cm lesions or palliation of large lesions: 50 Gy/15 fx (3.3 Gy/fx); 40 Gy/10 fx (4 Gy/fx), 35 Gy/5 fx (7 Gy/fx) delivered daily
  - Skin surface brachytherapy: 40 Gy/8 fx (5 Gy/fx); 44 Gy/10 fx (4.4 Gy/fx) delivered twice or 3 times per week, at least 48 hours apart

  Adjuvant RT to primary site:
  - 60 Gy/30 fx (2 Gy/fx) or 50 Gy/20 fx (2.5 Gy/fx) delivered daily
  - Consider 66 Gy/33 fx if positive margins

  Adjuvant RT to regional nodes:
  - 66 Gy (2 Gy/fx) for ECE or gross residual adenopathy
  - 60 Gy (2 Gy/fx) for no ECE/no residual adenopathy to the involved neck
  - 50 Gy (2 Gy/fx) to the undissected neck
- **Target:**
  Definitive RT:
  - CTV = Primary tumor with 0.5- to 2-cm margin. CTV margin varies based on tumor histology, risk factors, location, and mode of therapy.

  Adjuvant RT to primary site:
  - CTV = Primary tumor bed with 1- to 2-cm margin +/– ipsilateral parotid and neck nodes, +/– trigeminal or facial nerve pathways
  - CTV boost = Primary tumor bed with 0.5- to 1-cm margin
- **Technique:** Electron beam therapy, orthovoltage, brachytherapy, and IMRT in special circumstances, that is, total scalp and neurotropic spread along CN
- **Planning directive (for conventional fractionation):** Electron beam doses are prescribed to 90% of D_{max}. Orthovoltage x-ray doses are specified at D_{max} (skin surface). For normal tissue tolerance, refer to Head and Neck section for planning directive tolerances.

Surgery

- Wide local excision (WLE): Requires the removal of healthy skin; it results in a larger wound.
- Mohs micrographic surgery: Specialized technique for removal of skin cancer. Allows precise microscopic control of the margins by utilizing tangentially cut frozen section histology.
- Curettage and electrodessication (C&E): Commonly performed procedure to remove low-risk BCC and SCC by scraping off the lesion with a curette followed by cauterization. Not recommended for high-risk NMSC.

Systemic Therapy

- Vismodegib (Erivedge) and sonidegib (Odomzo) are inhibitors of the sonic hedgehog pathway and FDA approved for adult patients with advanced BCC. Common side effects are GI upset, muscle spasms, fatigue, alopecia, and dysgeusia.
- Topical 5FU (Efudex) is approved for treatment of actinic keratosis (AK) and superficial BCC.
- Concurrent: Chemoradiation with platinum agents can be considered for patient with high-risk features.

Side Effect Management

- Radiation dermatitis: Bland emollient application and sterile nonadherent dressings to keep site clean and moist.

Follow-up

- BCC: H&P, complete skin exam q6-12mo for life
- SCC localized: H&P q3-12mo for 2 years, then q6-12mo for 3 years, and then q1y for life
- SCC regional: H&P q1-3mo for year 1, then q2-4mo for year 2, then q4-6mo for years 3-5, and then q6-12mo for life

Notable Papers

Adjuvant RT in node + head and neck SCC

- *Veness et al. Laryngoscope* 2005: 167 patients were treated with curative intent at Westmead Hospital, Sydney. Patients underwent surgery (21/167; 13%) or surgery and adjuvant radiotherapy (146/167; 87%). The majority (98/167; 59%) of metastatic nodes were located in the parotid and/or cervical nodes. The remaining 69 (41%) had metastatic cervical nodes (levels I-V). Patients undergoing a combined treatment had a lower rate of locoregional recurrence (20% vs 43%) and a significantly better 5-year disease-free survival rate (73% vs 54%; $P = .004$) compared to surgery alone.

Elective neck management for SCC metastatic to parotid

- *Herman et al. Eur Arch Otorhinolaryngol* 2015: Retrospective review of 107 patients with SCC metastatic to parotid lymph nodes planned for post-op RT. All patients with cN0 cervical nodes. 42 patients with elective neck dissection + RT vs 65 patients with RT alone. Regional control excellent, no difference between surgery + RT vs RT alone. Concluding 50-60 Gy to cN0 neck is a suitable alternative to neck dissection.

Recommendations for CTV margins in RT planning for NMSC

- *Khan et al. Radiother Oncol* 2012: Prospective study measuring the distance of microscopic tumor extension from the gross lesion after excision. The microscopic tumor extent correlated with the size of gross lesion and histology. CTV recommendations are made to provide at least a 95% chance of covering microscopic disease: 10 mm for BCC <2 cm, 13 mm for BCC >2 cm, 11 mm for SCC <2 cm, and 14 mm for SCC >2 cm.

Efficacy of hypofractionation with electrons for epithelial skin cancers

- *van Hezewijk et al. Radiother Oncol* 2010: Retrospective review of 434 NMSCs (332 BCC, 102 SCC) evaluated after the use of 54 Gy in 18 fractions or 44 Gy in 10 fractions. No significant difference between fraction schedules for LRC. 3-year LC for BCC ~97% and 93%-97% for SCC. Electron beam hypofractionation is safe and effective for NMSC.

MERKEL CELL CARCINOMA

KAITLIN CHRISTOPHERSON • B. ASHLEIGH GUADAGNOLO • ANDREW J. BISHOP

Background

- **Incidence/prevalence:** Rare aggressive skin cancer with neuroendocrine differentiation. Cell of origin is Merkel cell mechanoreceptor bound to the ends of sensory nerve fibers in the skin. 1500 cases are diagnosed annually in the United States. Incidence has been increasing over the last three decades. Higher incidence rates are reported in Australia and New Zealand.

- **Outcomes:** 5-Year survival across all stages is variable. Stage I patients have estimated 5-year OS, 60%-80%; stage II, 50%-60%; and stage III, 25%-45%. High rate of recurrence (local recurrence 25%-30%, regional recurrence 50%-60%, distant recurrence 30%-36%). Worst prognosis of all skin cancers.
- **Demographics:** Median age at diagnosis is 75; majority of patients are older than 50. More common in males (2:1 male to female incidence). 90% of cases occur in Caucasians.
- **Risk factors:** Immunosuppression (increases risk 10× that of general population). UV exposure. Merkel cell polyomavirus (MCPyV) is detected in over 75% of cases.

Tumor Biology and Characteristics

- **Histologic subtypes:** Small cell, intermediate cell, and trabecular (best prognosis).
- **Pathology:** MCC typically presents as a dermal mass with rare involvement of the epidermis. It is a small, round blue cell tumor. Staining with immunopanel including CK20 (typically positive in paranuclear "dotlike" pattern), CK7, and TTF-1 (both typically negative) is important to rule out metastatic SCLC. Additional IHC staining for neuroendocrine markers can be done for equivocal lesions (ie, chromogranin, synaptophysin, CD56). MCPyV can be detected via IHC.
- **Genetics:** Associated with mutations in *RB1* and *TP53*, especially in MCPyV-negative tumors.

Anatomy

- Can occur anywhere on skin, predominantly on sun-exposed areas. Most common location is the skin of the head and neck > upper extremities > lower extremities > trunk.

Workup

- **History and physical:** Focused and complete skin examination of the skin and regional lymph nodes.
- **Procedures/biopsy:** Core biopsy is preferred.
- **Imaging:** PET/CT has emerged as important study for staging. Consider CT C/A/P with brain MRI, particularly if PET/CT is unavailable.

Merkel Cell Cancer TNM *(AJCC 8th edition)*

T Stage		**N Stage**	
Tis	Carcinoma in situ	N1	Metastasis in regional lymph node(s)
T1	Maximal clinical tumor diameter ≤2 cm	N1a(sn)	Clinically occult regional lymph node metastasis identified only by sentinel node biopsy
T2	Maximal clinical tumor diameter >2 but ≤5 cm	N1a	Clinically occult regional lymph node metastasis following lymph node dissection
T3	Maximal clinical tumor diameter >5 cm	N1b	Clinically and/or radiologically detected regional lymph node metastasis
		N2	In-transit metastasis without lymph node metastasis
		N3	In-transit metastasis with lymph node metastasis
		M Stage	
T4a	Primary tumor invades bone, muscle, fascia, or cartilage	M1a	Metastasis to distant skin, subcutaneous tissue, or lymph node(s)
		M1b	Metastasis to lung
		M1c	Metastasis to all other distant sites

<table>
<tr><th colspan="7">Summative Pathologic Stage</th></tr>
<tr><th></th><th>N0</th><th>N1a(sn) or N1</th><th>N1b</th><th>N2</th><th>N3</th><th>M1</th></tr>
<tr><td>T0</td><td rowspan="2">0</td><td rowspan="6">IIIA</td><td>IIIA</td><td colspan="2" rowspan="6">IIIB</td><td rowspan="6">IV</td></tr>
<tr><td>Tis</td><td rowspan="5">IIIB</td></tr>
<tr><td>T1</td><td>I</td></tr>
<tr><td>T2</td><td rowspan="2">IIA</td></tr>
<tr><td>T3</td></tr>
<tr><td>T4</td><td>IIB</td></tr>
</table>

Treatment Algorithm

Primary site	Surgical resection, wide local excision, or Mohs +/– adjuvant RT to primary site[a]
cN0 nodal management	SLNB for staging. If SLN positive → clinical trial, multidisciplinary discussion. Consider nodal dissection and/or RT to nodal basin
cN+ or pN+	Surgical resection consisting of WLE with nodal dissection +/– adjuvant RT to primary site/nodal basin

[a]Consider observation following WLE if small tumor (<1 cm), without LVSI, and no history of immunosuppression.

Radiation Treatment Technique

- **SIM:** Depending on anatomic location. Bolus is necessary to ensure that superficial dose is adequate for the skin primary.
  For head and neck location: Aquaplast mask, wire scar or primary site, draw field, and cut out field on mask if using electrons. Consider skin collimation. If near the ear, consider the use of TX-151 bolus.
- **Dose: Primary:**
  Tumor >2 cm, R0 resection → 50-56 Gy at 2 Gy/fx
  R1 resection → 56-60 Gy at 2 Gy/fx
  R2 resection or unresected disease → 60-66 Gy at 2 Gy/fx
  Nodal Basin
  cN0, no nodal evaluation → 46-50 Gy
  cN0, SLNB negative → no RT (unless potential for false-negative SLNB due to anatomic, operator, or histologic failure)
  cN0, SLNB positive, no formal dissection → 50 Gy
  cN+, no dissection → chemotherapy, then consider 50-60 Gy
  cN+, formal dissection with multiple LNs and/or ECE → 50-56 Gy
- **Target: Primary:** Primary site/scar + 4-cm margin for CTV; when planning electrons, consider penumbra and need to expand edges of field another 7-10 mm to cover the target.
  Lymph nodes: Involved/sentinel nodal basins
- **Technique:** Consider electrons to get adequate dose to the surface for RT to the primary.
  Consider skin collimation and bolus. Photons may be needed for deep primary tumors and for regional RT.

Factors for Adjuvant RT to Primary Site
Positive or close margin
LVSI
Lymph node + OR no lymph node evaluation
Consider for tumors >1 cm
Immunocompromised patient

- **IGRT:** Related to modality used and site of the body. Typically weekly kV for 3D plans.
- **Planning directive:** Standard dose constraints for 2 Gy/fx for ROIs in nearby treatment field (see Appendix).

Surgery

- Primary: Wide local excision with a goal of negative margin when feasible (1- to 2-cm margins). Mohs surgery is an acceptable alternative for smaller lesions. Balance with morbidity of surgery. Avoid complex procedures that would lead to a delay in RT.
- cN0 → sentinel lymph node biopsy. SLNB must be done prior to WLE as to not alter the drainage to the sentinel basin. If SLNB is +, consider completion dissection or RT for cN0.
- cN+ → Nodal basin dissection

Chemotherapy

- Retrospective series fail to show survival benefit. If used, typically given adjuvantly on case-by-case basis; regimen is typically platinum +/– etoposide.
- Metastatic disease: First line is immune checkpoint inhibitor.

Side Effect Management

- Skin care: First-line emollients. Can add Domeboro soaks thereafter. If having further grade 2+ skin toxicity, consider Mepilex. If grade 3 dermatitis, consider Silvadene cream (on weekends or after RT has been completed entirely).

Follow-up

- Complete skin and regional nodal examination every 3-6 months for 2 years. (Most recurrences occur within 2 years.) Can space to every 6-12 months thereafter.
- Can consider imaging in high-risk patients (ie, PET/CT)

Notable Papers

Postoperative RT after WLE

- *Strom et al. Ann Surg Oncol* 2016: Retrospective review of 171 patients treated between 1994 and 2012 at Moffitt Cancer Center. On multivariate analysis, patients receiving XRT had improved 3-year LC (91.2% vs 76.9%, respectively; $P = .01$), LRC (79.5% vs 59.1%; $P = .004$), DFS (57.0% vs 30.2%; $P < .001$), and OS (73% vs 66%; $P = .02$) at 3 years. RT was associated with improved 3-year DSS among node-positive patients (76.2% vs 48.1%; $P = .035$) but not node-negative patients (90.1% vs 80.8%; $P = .79$).

Radiation for stage I-III disease

- *Bishop et al. Head Neck* 2015: Retrospectively analyzed 106 patients treated at MDACC. Majority of patients were post-op. 92% of patients with cN0 disease treated with regional lymph node RT to a median dose of 46 Gy. 5-Year LRC, CSS, and OS were 96%, 76%, and 58%, respectively. Acceptable, 5% long-term grade 3 toxicity noted in this series.

HODGKIN LYMPHOMA

TOMMY SHEU • JILLIAN GUNTHER • BOUTHAINA DABAJA

Background

- **Incidence/prevalence:** 10% of all lymphomas in the United States, 8500 new cases per year
- **Demographics:** Predominantly young adults with slight male predominance, bimodal age distribution (20 and 65)
- **Risk factors:** Delayed/reduced antigen exposure (single family housing, small family size), immunosuppression, EBV virus exposure, autoimmune disease, radiation exposure especially at young age
- **Outcomes:** Stage I/II: 90%-95% OS at 8 years
  Stage III/IV (based on IPS): 0-1, 90%; 2-3, 80%; 4-5, 60% OS at 5 years

IPS, 1 point each: Age ≥ 45, albumin < 4, stage IV, Hgb < 10.5, absolute lymphocyte count < 8%, WBC > 15K, male

Tumor Biology and Characteristics

- **Genetics:** Association with BCL translocations
- **Pathology:** *Classical* (CD15+/CD30+/CD20–, 95% of cases): nodular sclerosing, mixed cellularity, lymphocyte rich, lymphocyte depleted; *NLPHL* (CD15–/CD30–/CD20+/CD45+, 5% of cases)
- **Imaging:** Heterogeneously enhancing mass on CT imaging. PET-avid disease graded utilizing Deauville criteria

Deauville Scale for Treatment Response

(Cheson et al. and Barrington et al. *JCO* 2014)

Score	Description	Interpretation
1	No residual uptake	Negative
2	Uptake < mediastinum	Negative
3	Uptake > mediastinum, but ≤ liver	Negative
4	Uptake > liver	Positive
5	Markedly increased uptake and/or any new lesion	Positive
X	New area of uptake unlikely related to lymphoma	Negative

Workup

- **Laboratory studies:** Core needle or excisional biopsy (FNA is not acceptable), CBC w/ diff, LFTs, LDH, ESR, albumin, bone marrow biopsy (if B symptoms, stage III/IV or BM PET negative), and pregnancy test
- **Imaging:** PET/CT, CT with contrast of the neck, chest, abdomen, and pelvis
- **Other studies:** PFT (for bleomycin) and echocardiogram (for doxorubicin)
- **Referrals:** Oncofertility, cardiology, and endocrinology

Staging and Risk Stratification

Ann Arbor Staging (Lugano Modification)			
I	Single lymph node region or group of adjacent nodes	**IE**	One extra-nodal site
II	≥2 node regions on same side of the diaphragm	**IIE**	≥2 extra-nodal sites on same side of diaphragm
III	Nodes on both sides of the diaphragm or nodes above diaphragm with splenic involvement	**IIISE(1)**	Stage III with splenic involvement
		IIISE(2)	Stage III with localized extra-nodal involvement
		IIISE	Both IIISE(1) and IIISE(2)
IV	Noncontiguous extranodal involvement		

Modifiers			
Bulky (X)	Bulky ≥ 10 cm[a] (removed as of AJCC 8th edition, included here for reference)	**B**	**B symptoms:** unexplained weight loss >10% over 6 months, drenching night sweats, or fever (>38°C)
A	No B symptoms		

[a]Acceptable thresholds for bulky include ≥10 cm on x-ray, 7.5 cm on CT imaging, and >1/2 diaphragm diameter on x-ray.

Nodal regions ("L/R" are considered to be separate)

Supradiaphragmatic regions: Waldeyer ring, L/R cervical/supraclavicular/occipital/preauricular, infraclavicular nodes, L/R axillary/pectoral, mediastinal, L/R hilar, L/R epitrochoidal/brachial

Infradiaphragmatic regions: Spleen, mesenteric, para-aortic, L/R iliac, L/R inguinal/femoral, L/R popliteal

Unfavorable Risk Factors			
Risk Factor	**GHSG**[a]	**EORTC**	**NCCN**
Age		>50	
ESR	>50 if no B symptoms >30 if B symptoms	>50 if A >30 if B	>50 or any B symptoms
Mediastinal mass	MMR > 0.33	MMR > 0.35	MMR > 0.33
Lymph nodal areas	3 or more	4 or more	4 or more
Extranodal lesions	Any		
Bulky			>10 cm

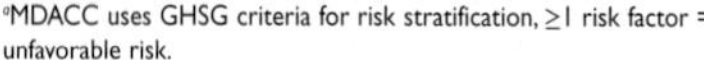

[a]MDACC uses GHSG criteria for risk stratification, ≥1 risk factor = unfavorable risk.

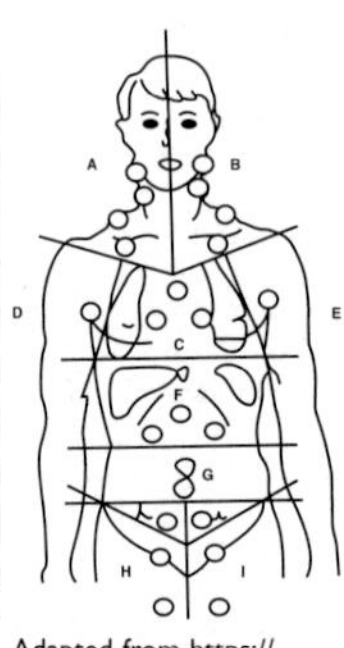

Adapted from https://en.ghsg.org/disease-stages. Reprinted by permission of Dr. Andreas Engert.

Lymph Node Areas (GHSG) for Risk Stratification[a]		
Right	**Midline**	**Left**
A. Cervical/supraclav/infraclav/nuchal	**C.** Hilar/mediastinal	**B.** Cervical/supraclav/infraclav/nuchal
D. Axilla	**F.** Upper abdomen (spleen, liver, celiac)	**E.** Axilla
H. Iliac	**G.** Lower abdomen (spleen, liver, celiac)	**I.** Iliac
K. Inguinal		**L.** Inguinal

[a]Separate lymph node regions are considered for the purpose of Ann Arbor staging and risk stratification.

Treatment Algorithm

Standard of care treatment regimens exist that involve omission of radiation therapy.

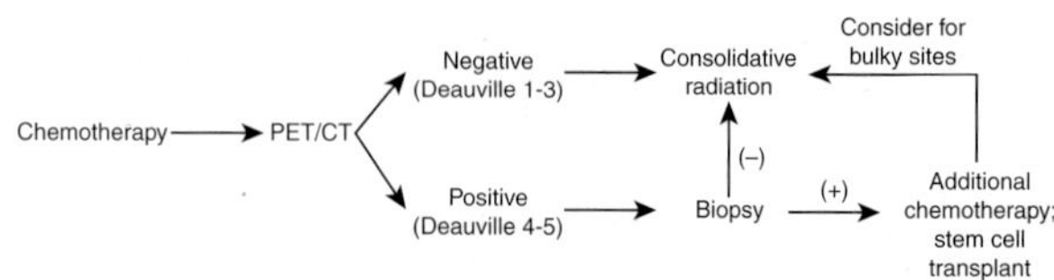

	Stage/Risk	Chemotherapy	Consolidation RT
Classical Hodgkin	Favorable early: Stage I, II nonbulky and no rf	2 cycles of ABVD*	20 Gy/10 fx, ISRT
Classical Hodgkin	Unfavorable early: Stage I, IIA and ≥1 rf or bulky Stage IIB and ≥1 rf (No: MMR, ENE, or bulky)	4 cycles of ABVD*	30.6 Gy/17 fx, ISRT
Classical Hodgkin	Stage IIB bulky	4-6 cycles of ABVD*	30.6 Gy/17 fx, ISRT
Classical Hodgkin	Advanced: Stage III, IV	6 cycles of ABVD*	±30.6-36 Gy/17-20 fx for pre-chemo bulky supradiaphragmatic[§] sites or residual disease after chemo
NLPHL	Stage IA, contiguous IIA	None	30.6 Gy/17 fx ISRT*, 36 Gy/20 fx if bulky
NLPHL	Stage III, IV, or B symptoms	3-6 cycles of R-CHOP	24-30.6 Gy/12-17 fx ISRT, 36 Gy/20 fx if bulky

ISRT, involved site radiation therapy. More generous involved site is permitted.
ABVD refers to potentially holding the last two cycles of bleomycin.

Interim PET/CT imaging should be obtained at the end of planned cycles of chemotherapy for early unfavorable and advanced stage cases. In the event that this is positive (Deauville 4-5), consider additional cycles of ABVD or R-CHOP until a maximum of 6 cycles; if at 6 cycles and PET/CT is positive, consider salvage treatment options including high-dose chemotherapy and stem cell transplant.

Radiation Treatment Technique

Target Location	Technique	Simulation
Neck	IMRT	Supine, thermoplastic mask
Mediastinum	Deep inspiratory breath hold, IMRT with butterfly beam arrangement	Supine, Vac-Lok indexed with Dabaja board (10-15 degrees), thermoplastic mask, hip stopper
Axilla	IMRT or 3DCRT	Supine, arm slightly akimbo or overhead, Vac-Lok
Abdomen	Deep inspiratory breath hold, IMRT	Supine, arms overhead, Vac-Lok, wing board with T-bar

The goal is to reduce low-dose exposure to adjacent OARs. Depending on patient-specific anatomy and tumor location, other techniques and setups may be more optimal.

- **Planning directive**

OAR	Dose Constraint(s)
Heart[a]	Mean < 5 Gy, no higher than 15 Gy
Coronaries and left ventricle	Max < 5 Gy
Total lung	Mean < 13.5 Gy, V20 < 30%, V5 < 55%
Breasts	Mean < 4 Gy or ALARA
Thyroid gland	V5 < 30%, V20 < 33%
Kidneys	V5 < 30%, V20 < 33%
Parotid glands	Mean < 5 Gy or ALARA
Submandibular glands	Mean < 11 Gy
Spleen	Mean < 9 Gy
Liver	Max < 10 Gy

[a]Goal is to keep 5 Gy isodose line off as many critical structures as possible.

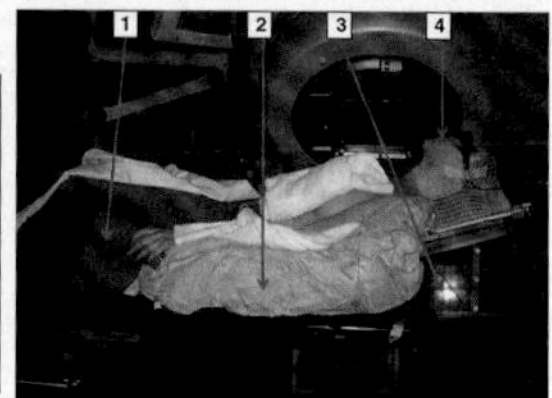

Figure 62.1 Simulation set up for mediastinal HL. (1) Hip stopper, (2) Vac-Lok, (3) Dabaja or incline board at 10-15 degrees, and (4) thermoplastic mask. The patient is wearing goggles that provide real-time visual feedback on the breath cycle.

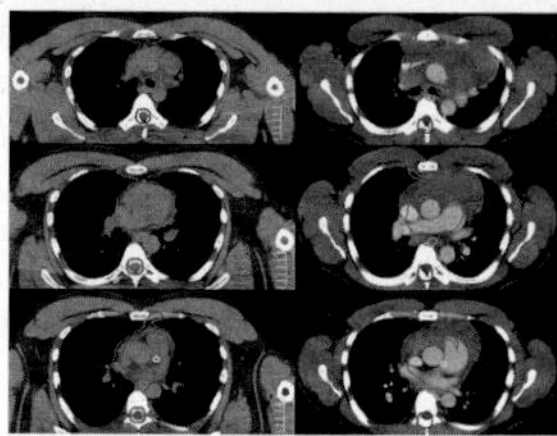

Figure 62.2 Axial view of DIBH (*left* three images) and normal breathing (*right* three images). DIBH can significantly reduce radiation to the coronary arteries, heart, and lungs. Confirm positioning with daily CT on rails or cone beam CT.

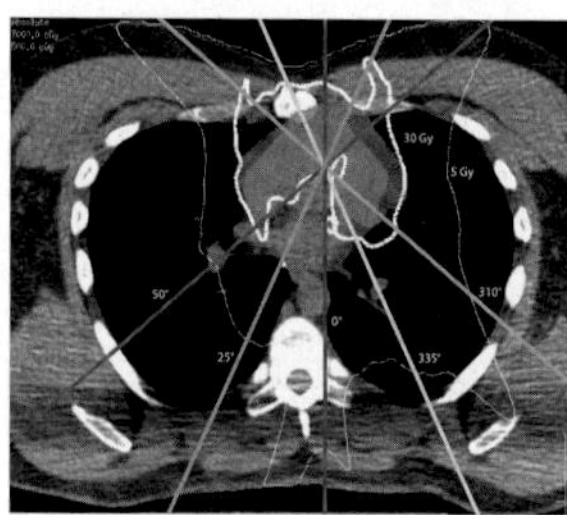

Figure 62.3 Deep inspiratory breath hold with a butterfly technique beam arrangement for anterior mediastinal HL. Anterior beam angles were restricted between 310 and 50 degrees. 30 Gy isodose line is *thick white*; 5 Gy isodose line is *thin white*.

Chemotherapy

- ABVD—doxorubicin (Adriamycin), bleomycin, vinblastine, dacarbazine
  Bleomycin held in the following scenarios: last cycle in early unfavorable, last two cycles in stage IIB bulky if six cycles, and last two cycles of advanced
- BEACOPP—bleomycin, etoposide, doxorubicin (Adriamycin), cyclophosphamide, vincristine (Oncovin), procarbazine, prednisone
  Not routinely used in the United States due to toxicities.

Side Effect Management

- Esophagitis: Xyloxylin (1:1:1 ratio of diphenhydramine, Maalox, viscous lidocaine), 10-15 mL swish/swallow up to 4 times a day
- Pneumonitis (dyspnea or cough): Prednisone 60 mg/day for 4 weeks, taper slowly over 2-3 months

Follow-Up

- Full-body CT with contrast at 6, 12, and 24 months after therapy; PET/CT if previous Deauville 4-5
- Interim H&P 3 months after completion of therapy then Q6 months for first 3 years, then annually
- Late cardiovascular toxicities: Echocardiogram/stress and carotid ultrasound if RT to neck Q10 years
- TSH at least annually if RT to neck to evaluate for potential hypothyroidism, supplement with levothyroxine if detected
- Secondary malignancies: Start annual breast screening the earlier of 8-10 years after therapy or age 40 if chest radiation

Notable Trials

Study	Design	RFS/PFS/DFS	OS	Conclusion
HD10 *Engert NEJM* 2010	Stage I or II no risk factors 2 × 2 randomized: 1. ABVD × 2 vs. ABVD × 4 2. IFRT 30 vs. 20 Gy	**8-y PFS** ABVD × 2 + 20: 87% ABVD × 2 + 30: 85% ABVD × 4 + 20: 90% ABVD × 4 + 30: 88%	**8 y** ABVD × 2 + 20: 95% ABVD × 2 + 30: 94% ABVD × 4 + 20: 95% ABVD × 4 + 30: 94%	Early favorable Hodgkin's lymphoma can be treated with ABVD × 2 and 20 Gy
HD11 *Eich JCO* 2010	Stage IA-IIA and ≥1 risk factors or Stage IIB + ESR ≥30 (no bulky or ENE) 2 × 2 randomized: 1. BEACOPP × 4 vs. ABVD × 4 2. IFRT 20 vs. 30 Gy	**5-y PFS** ABVD + 30: 87% ABVD + 20: 82% BEACOPP + 30: 88% BEACOPP + 20: 87%	**5 y** ABVD + 30: 94% ABVD + 20: 94% BEACOPP + 30: 95% BEACOPP + 20: 95%	Early unfavorable Hodgkin's lymphoma can be treated with AVBD × 4 and 30 Gy
H10 *Andre JCO* 2010	Favorable or unfavorable, stage I or II with **upfront ABVD × 2 → PET** Favorable patients randomized three ways: 1. ABVD × 1 + 30-36 Gy 2a. PET(−):ABVD × 2 2b. PET(+): BEACOPP + 30-36 Gy Unfavorable patients randomization three ways: 1. ABVD × 2 + 30-36 Gy 2a. PET(−):ABVD × 4 2b. PET(+): BEACOPP × 2 + INRT	**5-y PFS** **PET(+)** ABVD + RT: 77% BEACOPP + RT: 91% **Fav, PET(−)** ABVD × 3 + RT: 99% ABVD × 4: 87% **Unfav, PET(−)** ABVD × 4 + RT: 92% ABVD × 6: 90%	**5 y** **PET(+)** ABVD + RT: 89% BEACOPP + RT: 96% **Fav, PET(−)** ABVD × 3 + RT: 100% ABVD × 4: 100% **Unfav, PET(−)** ABVD × 4 + RT: 98% ABVD × 6: 98%	For interim PET(+) patients, radiation therapy improves PFS For interim PET(+) patients, escalation to BEAOPP + RT improves PFS
IIB Bulky *Reddy Clin Lymphoma Myeloma Leuk* 2015	Retrospective, stage IIB bulky treated with chemotherapy and/or radiation	**8 y** All: 77%	**8 y** ABVD: 89% MOPP: 66% >30.1 Gy: 78% <30.1 Gy: 46%	Excellent outcomes treating IIB bulky patients with chemo and RT
Stage III *Phan AJCO* 2011	Retrospective, stage III treated with chemotherapy and/or radiation	**15-y DFS** RT: 65%; No RT: 15% Mediastinal RT associated with improved DFS and OS	**15 y** RT: 80% No RT: 29%	Radiation particularly important for disease above the diaphragm. Less effective in abdomen after 6 cycles of ABVD

Study	Design	RFS/PFS/DFS	OS	Conclusion
RATHL *Johnson NEJM* 2016 *Trotman (Abstract)* 2017	Stage IIB-IV or Stage IIA (bulky or 3+ sites) **upfront ABVD × 2 → PET1** PET1(−) randomization: 1a. ABVD × 4 1b. ABVD × 2 → AVD × 2 PET1(+) additional therapy: **BEACOPP-based therapy → PET2** PET2(+) → radiation PET2(−) → BEACOPP-based therapy	**5-y PFS** ABVD × 6: 83% ABVD × 4 → AVD × 2: 81% PET1(+): 66% 11 of 39 pts with stage II bulky with PET1(+) received RT, 1 progression at median follow-up of 52 months	**5 y** ABVD × 6: 95.3% ABVD × 6: 95.0% PET1(+): 85.1%	Dropping last two cycles of bleomycin for good PET responders does not compromise efficacy RT is efficacious for bulky residual disease
RAPID *Radford NEJM* 2015	Stage IA or IIA PET(−) after ABVD × 3 Randomized: 1. IFRT 2. Observation	**3 y** IFRT: 95% Observation: 91% Noninferiority margin of 7% for PFS not met	**3 y** IFRT: 97% Observation: 99%	For early stage Hodgkin lymphoma, it is not noninferior to omit radiation for good PET responders

DIFFUSE LARGE B-CELL LYMPHOMA

SHANE R. STECKLEIN • CHELSEA C. PINNIX

Background

- **Incidence/prevalence:** Most common form of high-grade non-Hodgkin lymphoma (NHL); accounts for 30%-40% of all NHLs. Approximately 22 000 cases diagnosed in the United States each year.
- **Outcomes:** 5-Year survival across all stages estimated at 60% (SEER data).
- **Demographics:** Typically in middle-aged and elderly adults, median age at diagnosis is 64.
- **Risk factors:** Age, HIV infection, immunosuppression, preexisting B-cell lymphoproliferative disorder (eg, follicular lymphoma, chronic lymphocytic leukemia/small lymphocytic lymphoma [CLL/SLL]).

Tumor Biology and Characteristics

- **Pathology:** Immunophenotype, CD20+, CD45+, and CD3−. Designated as germinal center B cell (GCB) or nongerminal center B cell/activated B cell (non-GCB/ABC) based on gene expression profiling (GEP) studies (*Alizadeh et al. Nature* 2000).
  - **GCB DLBCL:** Arises from centroblasts in the light zone of the lymph node germinal center and may have chromosomal abnormalities affecting *MYC* [t(8;14), *MYC*;IgH/t(2;8), Igκ;*MYC*/t(8;22), *MYC*;Igλ (observed in 10%)] and *BCL2* [t(14;18), IgH:*BCL2* (observed in 40%)] detected by FISH.
  - **Non-GCB/ABC DLBCL:** Arises from postgerminal center lymphocytes that have committed to plasmablastic differentiation and is characterized by NF-κB activation and blockade of terminal differentiation into plasma cells. In general, GCB DLBCL has a better prognosis than non-GCB/ABC DLBCL.

- The Hans algorithm (*Hans et al. Blood* 2004) is a widely used immunohistochemical surrogate for gene expression profiling to discriminate GCB and non-GCB/ABC DLBCL.

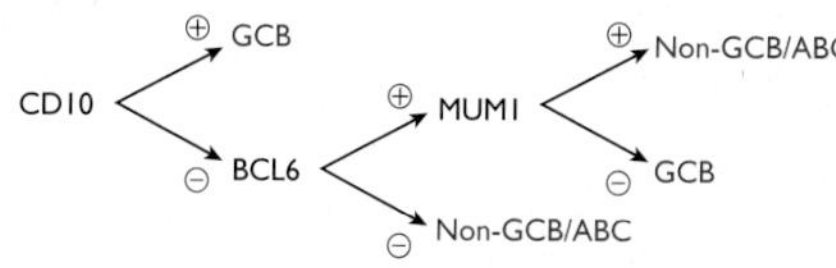

- **Double-hit lymphoma (DHL) and double-protein expression lymphoma:** Aggressive subsets of DLBCL that arise from coexisting genomic rearrangement of *MYC* and *BCL2* or *BCL6* or overexpression of MYC and BCL2 in the absence of simultaneous gene rearrangements (double-protein expression) (*Johnson et al. JCO* 2012). DHL lymphomas are typically GCB DLBCL and have the worst prognosis of all subtypes, while double-protein expression lymphomas are typically non-GCB/ABC DLBCL.
- **Imaging:** ^{18}FDG PET-CT is the most sensitive imaging modality. CT may be used for follow-up. MRI may be useful for imaging the central nervous system (CNS), bulky, or extranodal sites of disease.

Deauville Scale for Treatment Response

(Cheson et al. and Barrington et al. *JCO* 2014)

Score	Description	Interpretation
1	No residual uptake	Negative
2	Uptake < mediastinum	Negative
3	Uptake > mediastinum, but ≤ liver	Negative
4	Uptake > liver	Positive
5	Markedly increased uptake and/or any new lesion	Positive
X	New area of uptake unlikely related to lymphoma	Negative

Workup

- **Laboratory studies:** Core needle or excisional biopsy (FNA is not acceptable), CBC w/diff, ESR, CMP, uric acid, LDH, albumin, bone marrow biopsy (if cytopenic and PET negative)
- **Imaging:** PET/CT, CT with contrast of the neck, chest, abdomen, pelvis
- **Other studies:** Hepatitis B and HIV testing (for rituximab), echocardiogram or MUGA (for doxorubicin). Lumbar puncture is considered for HIV-associated lymphoma, testicular lymphoma, or hit/expression lymphoma.
- **Referrals:** Consider cardiology and infectious diseases.

Ann Arbor Staging System (Lugano Modifications, Cheson et al. *JCO* 2014)

See **"Hodgkin Lymphoma"** chapter.

International Prognostic Index (Ziepert et al. *JCO* 2009)

One Point per Criterion		3-Year Overall Survival	
Age	>60	IPI 0-1	91.4%
ECOG performance status	2, 3, or 4	IPI 2	80.9%
LDH	>Upper limit of normal	IPI 3	65.1%
Extranodal involvement	>1 site	IPI 4-5	59.0%
Ann Arbor stage	III or IV		

Treatment Algorithm for Complete Response to Chemotherapy

Standard-of-care treatment regimens exist that involve omission of radiation therapy.

Stage I/II[a]	Nonbulky **and** IPI 0-1	R-CHOP[a] ×3-4 → 30.6 Gy/17 fx ISRT
	Bulky (≥7.5 cm) **or** IPI > 1	R-CHOP[a] ×6 → 30.6 Gy/17 fx ISRT
Stage III/IV[a]	Bulky or extranodal (especially osseous) sites of disease	R-CHOP[a] × 6 → 30.6-36 Gy/17-20 fx ISRT

[a]For patients with DHL, double-protein expression, or other concerning pathologic features, more aggressive chemotherapy with DA-R-EPOCH can be considered (*Landsburg et al. JCO* 2017).

Treatment Algorithm for Relapsed or Refractory Patients

- The role of radiotherapy for patients with relapsed or refractory DLBCL is individualized and depends on patient- and treatment-related factors, including prior systemic therapy, the extent of disease at diagnosis and relapse, patient performance status, and potential future therapies. Please refer to the International Lymphoma Radiation Oncology Group (ILROG) guidelines for further details and guidance (*Ng et al. IJROBP* 2018).

Radiation Treatment Technique (Not Including Primary CNS or Testicular)

- **SIM:** Highly variable; dependent on area(s) being treated
  - Head and neck: Supine, thermoplastic mask ± bite block, stent as appropriate
  - Axilla: Supine, upper Vac-Lok, arms akimbo
  - Mediastinum: Supine, incline board, upper Vac-Lok, deep inspiration breath hold (DIBH)
  - Abdomen: Supine, upper and/or lower Vac-Lok; consider NPO for 3 hours prior to sim/treatment, may require respiratory motion management
  - Pelvis: Supine, lower Vac-Lok
- **Dose:**

	Response	**Dose**
Consolidation after chemotherapy	Deauville 1-3	30.6 Gy
	Any Deauville 4-5 residual disease after frontline chemotherapy	Salvage chemotherapy and transplant -or- [a]30.6-36 Gy to original sites of disease, integrate boost to 45-50 Gy to Deauville 4-5 areas
Relapsed or refractory	Deauville 1-3 after multiple chemotherapy regimens or peritransplant	30.6-36 Gy to original sites of disease with consideration of integrated boost to 40 Gy to previous sites of persistent disease
	Deauville 4-5 after multiple chemotherapy regimens, including SCT	45-50 Gy to sites of gross disease for salvage (curative intent); consider hypofractionated course (eg, 20 Gy in 5 fractions, 30 Gy in 10 fractions, or 37.5 Gy in 15 fractions) for palliation

[a]For patients with low-volume residual Deauville 4-5 disease, radiation therapy alone can be attempted (in lieu of salvage chemotherapy and autologous stem cell rescue).

- **Targets:**
  - Involved site radiation therapy (ISRT)
    - Prechemotherapy site(s) of disease
    - CTV takes into account changes in size/extent of the tumor, position of nearby normal tissues and organs, and disease pattern and areas of potential subclinical involvement.

- **Technique:** Generally IMRT/VMAT, though 3DCRT may be appropriate for certain geometries. "Butterfly" technique commonly used for mediastinal lymphoma to minimize dose to the heart, lungs, breasts, and spinal cord (*Voong et al. Radiat Oncol* 2014).
- **IGRT:** Dependent on technique and targets; daily kV, CBCT, or CT on rails
- **Dose constraints:**

Organ/Structure	Dose Constraint(s)
Heart[a]	Mean < 5 Gy, no higher than 15 Gy
Coronaries and left ventricle[a]	Max < 5 Gy
Total lung	Mean < 13.5 Gy, V20 < 30%, V5 < 55%
Breasts	Mean < 4Gy
Thyroid gland	V25 < 63.5%
Kidneys	V5 < 30%, V20 < 33%
Parotid glands	Mean < 5 Gy or ALARA
Submandibular glands	Mean < 11 Gy
Spleen	Mean < 9 Gy
Liver	Max < 10 Gy

[a]Goal is to keep 5 Gy isodose line off as many critical structures as possible.

Chemotherapy

- **R-CHOP-21: R**ituximab (375 mg/m² IV on d1), **c**yclophosphamide (750 mg/m² IV on d1), **h**ydroxydaunorubicin (doxorubicin; 50 mg/m² IV on d1), **O**ncovin (vincristine; 1.4 mg/m² [max dose 2 mg] on d1), and **p**rednisone (40 mg/m² po on d1-5) every 21 days.
- **DA-R-EPOCH: R**ituximab (375 mg/m² IV on d1), **e**toposide (50 mg/m²/d IV on d1-4), **p**rednisone (60 mg/m² po bid on d1-5), **O**ncovin (vincristine; 0.4 mg/m²/d IV on d1-4), **c**yclophosphamide (750 mg/m² IV on d5), and **h**ydroxydaunorubicin (doxorubicin; 10 mg/m²/d on d1-4) every 21 days. Subcutaneous Neupogen (filgrastim) is given once daily starting on d6 and continued until WBC count normalizes (can substitute for Neulasta (pegfilgrastim)). Dose-adjusted (DA) protocol increases (etoposide, doxorubicin, cyclophosphamide) or decreases (cyclophosphamide) doses for subsequent cycles based on neutrophil and/or platelet nadirs.

Special Subtypes of DLBCL

- **Primary central nervous system lymphoma (PCNSL)**
  - Classically seen in individuals with primary or acquired immunodeficiency
  - Workup: Slit lamp examination, lumbar puncture, spine MRI (if symptomatic or CSF is positive), HIV test, testicular examination, and testicular ultrasound (especially for men >60 years old)
  - If possible, delay initiation of steroids until biopsy is performed
  - Treatment:
    - R-MPV (rituximab, high-dose methotrexate, procarbazine, vincristine, ± intrathecal chemotherapy).
    - Complete response: High-dose chemotherapy with autologous stem cell transplant or low-dose whole brain radiotherapy (23.4 Gy in 13 fractions at 1.8 Gy/fx; *Morris et al. JCO* 2013).
    - Residual disease: Whole brain radiotherapy (30.6-36 Gy, boost gross disease to 45 Gy) or high-dose chemotherapy with autologous stem cell transplant.
    - Consider omission of radiation in patients with poor functional status or age >60.
- **Primary testicular lymphoma**
  - Generally seen in men >60 years of age.
  - Workup: Lumbar puncture and bilateral testicular ultrasound.
  - R-CHOP or DA-R-EPOCH given per standard DLBCL protocol; intrathecal or high-dose methotrexate for CNS prophylaxis.
  - High risk of contralateral testicular failure after chemotherapy (*Ho et al. Leuk and Lymphoma* 2017). All patients should receive testicle/scrotal/spermatic cord irradiation to 30.6 Gy in 17 fractions (1.8 Gy/fx) after completing chemotherapy (*Vitolo et al. JCO* 2011).
- **Primary mediastinal B-cell lymphoma**
  - Commonly presents in adolescents and young adults (esp. women).
  - Putatively arises from thymic B cells and has significant molecular overlap with nodular sclerosing Hodgkin lymphoma (NSHL). PMBCL cells are typically weakly positive for CD30 and negative for CD15, which helps discriminate PMBCL from NSHL.

- DA-R-EPOCH ×6 without consolidation radiotherapy for patients with Deauville ≤3 metabolic response on [18]FDG PET-CT offers excellent cure rates (*Dunleavy et al. NEJM* 2013).
  - Residual FDG avidity after DA-R-EPOCH should be interpreted cautiously, as not all postchemotherapy metabolic activity denotes active or residual lymphoma and necessitates radiotherapy.
- For patients with low burden residual PET-CT–avid lymphoma after DA-R-EPOCH, salvage radiotherapy to a dose of 45-50 Gy may be considered. Alternate approaches include salvage chemotherapy followed by autologous stem cell transplant with posttransplant consolidative radiotherapy.
- For patients with significant disease progression after DA-R-EPOCH, radiation therapy alone is not desirable (*Filippi et al. Red J* 2016).
- Consolidation radiotherapy to 30.0-36.0 Gy is indicated for patients who receive R-CHOP chemotherapy in lieu of DA-R-EPOCH.

Follow-Up

- No PET-CT for a minimum of 8 weeks after radiotherapy due to chance of false positives.
- H&P and laboratory studies every 3-6 months for 5 years. For stages I and II, repeat imaging only as clinically indicated, and for stages III and IV, CT scan no more often than every 6 months for 2 years and then yearly afterward. TSH at least annually if RT to the neck.
- Secondary malignancies: Start annual breast screening the earlier of 8-10 years after therapy or age 40 if chest radiation.

Notable Trials and Papers

Role of consolidation radiotherapy for early and advanced stage

- DSHNHL-2004-3/UNFOLDER 21/14 (Ongoing; Interim results Held *ICML RT Workshop* 2013). Phase III trial with 2 × 2 randomization of patients with early-stage DLBC IPI = 0-1 with bulky (≥7.5 cm) disease to R-CHOP-21 ×6 vs R-CHOP-21 ×6 → involved field radiotherapy (IFRT) vs R-CHOP-14 ×6 vs R-CHOP-14 ×6 → involved field radiotherapy. Interim analysis terminated no RT arms due to inferior 3-year EFS (81% vs 65%, $P = .004$).
- SWOG 8736 (*Miller et al. NEJM* 1998; *Stephens et al. JCO* 2016). Randomized trial of patients with stage I-IE and nonbulky II-IIE DLBCL to CHOP ×8 vs CHOP ×3 + IFRT to 40 Gy (with boost to 50 Gy for residual disease). CHOP ×3 + IFRT increased PFS (5 years: 77% vs 64%, $p = .03$) and OS (5 years: 82% vs 72%, $p = .02$) compared to CHOP ×8 on initial analysis, but on long-term analysis (median f/u of 17.7 years), the curves overlapped with no significant difference in PFS (median: 12 vs 11.1 years, $p = .73$) or OS (13 vs 13.7 years, $p = .38$) between groups. No significant difference in cumulative incidence of secondary malignancy between groups. Seven patients died from heart failure in CHOP ×8 arm compared to one patient in CHOP ×3 + IFRT arm.
- *Phan et al. JCO* 2010. Retrospective analysis of MDACC patients with stage I-IV DLBCL who received R-CHOP. Approximately 30% received consolidation IFRT to 30-39.6 Gy. Radiotherapy improved PFS and OS for all patients.

Consolidation radiotherapy for bulky and extralymphatic disease

- RICOVER-noRTh (*Held et al. JCO* 2014). Patients >60 years of age with aggressive B-cell lymphoma who received R-CHOP-14+2R + 36 Gy IFRT to bulky (≥7.5 cm) and/or extralymphatic sites of disease (RICOVER-60) were compared to patients treated with same chemotherapy but no radiotherapy on amendment of RICOVER-60 (RICOVER-noRTh). Omission of radiotherapy in patients with bulky or extralymphatic lymphoma was associated with lower EFS (HR = 2.1, $p = .005$) with trends toward lower PFS (HR = 1.8, $p = .058$) and OS (HR = 1.6, $p = .13$).
- German High-Grade NHL Study Group retrospective analysis of patients with skeletal involvement from nine consecutive studies (*Held et al. JCO* 2013). Rituximab failed to improve EFS or OS in patients with skeletal involvement, but consolidation radiotherapy significantly improved EFS.

Consolidation radiotherapy for primary bone DLBCL

- MDACC experience with primary bone DLBCL (*Tao et al. IJROBP* 2015). 72% of patients received rituximab. Receipt of consolidation radiotherapy was associated with improved PFS (5 years: 88% vs 63%, $p = .007$) and OS (5 years: 91% vs 68%, $p = .006$).

MISCELLANEOUS HEMATOLOGIC MALIGNANCIES

ZEINA AYOUB • SARAH MILGROM

FOLLICULAR LYMPHOMA

Background and presentation

- **Incidence/prevalence:** Most common indolent non-Hodgkin lymphoma subtype (70% of indolent lymphomas). Common asymptomatic lymphadenopathy, waxing, and waning for years; rarely with B symptoms. Bone marrow involvement in >70% of patients.
- **Outcomes:** Indolent clinical course with possibility of late relapse; median OS > 10 years.
- **Demographics:** Median age at diagnosis is 60 years.
- **Risk factors:** Age; common association with a history of autoimmune disease, hepatitis, or chronic immunosuppression, exposure to pesticides or chemical plants. Potential for transformation to more aggressive lymphoma can be high (up to 70% in long-time survivors).

Tumor biology and characteristics

- Arises from the germinal center B cells.
  - 85% have the t(14;18), which results in Bcl2 overexpression
  - Morphology shows closely packed follicular nodules
  - Immunophenotype: CD10+, Bcl2, Bcl6
  - Ki-67 significantly lower than DLBCL
- Grade is defined by the number of centroblasts (large cells) per HPF.
  - Grade 1: 0-5 centroblasts/HPF
  - Grade 2: 6-15 centroblasts/HPF
  - Grade 3: >15 centroblasts/HPF
    - 3A: >15 centroblasts, but centrocytes are still present.
    - 3B: Centroblasts form solid sheets with no residual centrocytes.

Workup

- **History and physical:** Physical examination of all node-bearing areas including Waldeyer ring and of size of the spleen and liver. Assessment of performance status and B symptoms (night sweats, weight loss, and fevers).
- **Labs:** CBC, CMP, LDH, ESR, uric acid, β2-microglobulin, hep B/C, HIV, and pregnancy test
- **Procedures/biopsy:** Excisional biopsy is preferred. Bone marrow biopsy (bilateral is encouraged but not mandatory). When chemotherapy is planned, consider MUGA/echo and fertility/sperm banking.
- **Imaging:** CT C/A/P/neck with contrast and/or PET/CT.

Staging *(Lugano modification of Ann Arbor Staging System)*

See "Hodgkin Lymphoma" chapter.

Prognosis

- **FLIPI score** *(Solal-Celigny et al. Blood 2004)*
  - Age > 60
  - Stages III-IV
  - Hemoglobin level < 12 g/dL
  - Number of nodal areas > 4
  - LDH level > ULN

Risk Group (Score)	5-Year OS (%)	10-Year OS (%)
Low (0-1)	90.6	70.7
Intermediate (2)	77.6	50.9
High (≥3)	52.5	35.5

- **FLIPI 2 score** *(Federeico et al. JCO 2009)*
  - Age > 60
  - Hemoglobin level < 12 g/dL
  - Bone marrow involvement
  - β2-microglobulin > upper limit normal
  - Largest diameter of largest involved lymph node > 6 cm

Risk Group (Score)	5-Year OS (%)
Low (0-1)	90.6
Intermediate (2)	77.6
High (≥3)	52.5

Treatment algorithm

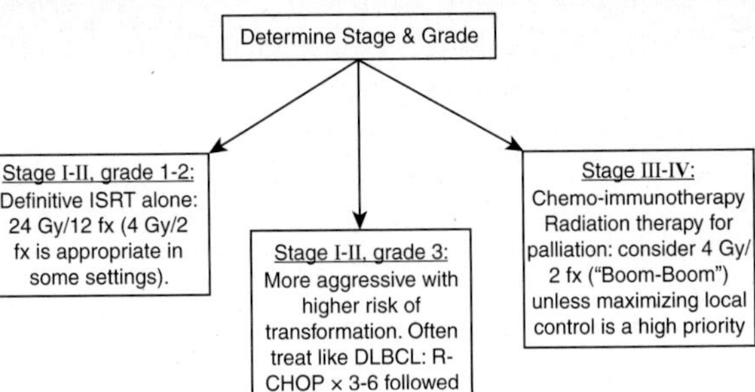

Notable trials

Study	Design	Result	Comment
Lowry et al. 2011	Noninferiority, phase III RCT Inclusion: Any histologic subtype of non-Hodgkin lymphoma randomized to: 1. Indolent lymphomas: 40-45 Gy/20-23 fx vs 24 Gy/12 fx 2. Aggressive lymphomas: 40-45 Gy/20-23 fx vs 30 Gy/15 fx	**1-month overall response** Indolent/40-45 Gy: 93% Indolent/24 Gy: 92% Aggressive/40-45 Gy: 91% Aggressive/30 Gy: 91% No OS or PFS difference, trend for reduced toxicity with lower dose	Established 24 Gy for indolent lymphomas
FORT (Hoskin et al. 2014)	Noninferiority, phase III RCT Inclusion: Follicular or marginal zone lymphoma randomized to: 1. 24 Gy/12 fx 2. 4 Gy/2 fx	**12-week overall response** 24 Gy/12 fx: 91% 4 Gy/2 fx: 81% **12-week complete response** 24 Gy/12 fx: 68% 4Gy/2 fx: 49% Time to progression **not noninferior** for 4 Gy. Higher (3% vs 1%) toxicity in 24 Gy	4 Gy inferior for local progression and time to progression. However, this regime is pragmatic and well tolerated, so it is a good option when durable local control is not critical

Marginal Zone Lymphoma

Background

- **Incidence/prevalence:** 5%-10% non-Hodgkin lymphoma.
- **Outcomes:** Indolent disease. Death due to disease is extremely rare. Gastric site has longer time to progression vs nongastric MALT (8.9 vs 4.9 years). 50% gastric, other sites include orbit, lung, skin, thyroid, salivary gland, etc.
- **Demographics:** Variable age groups depending on the subtype.
- **Risk factors:** Associated with chronic inflammation: autoimmune disease (Sjögren disease), infections (*H. pylori*, *C. psittaci*, *B. burgdorferi*, *C. jejuni*).

Tumor biology and characteristics

- Neoplasm of mature B cells.
- Arise from postgerminal center marginal zone B cells.
- B-cell markers: CD19, CD20, CD22+ (CD5/10/23 –).

- Characterized by proliferation of cells within a lymphoid area where clonal expansion of B cells occurs. Subtypes include:
  - Splenic marginal zone B cells
  - Nodal marginal zone B cells
  - Marginal zone B cells of Peyer patches/extranodal
    - Primary cutaneous
    - Mucosa-associated lymphoid tissue (MALT) lymphoma

Gastric MALT

Presentation

- Majority present with localized stage I/II extranodal disease.
- Most commonly present with abdominal pain and peptic ulcer disease.
- B symptoms are uncommon.
- Outcomes: 5-year OS of 90%-95% and DFS of 75%-80%

Workup

- **History and physical:** Physical examination of all node-bearing areas including Waldeyer ring and of size of the spleen and liver. Assessment of performance status and B symptoms (uncommon for gastric malt).
- **Labs:** CBC, CMP, LDH, ESR, uric acid, β2-microglobulin, hep B/C, HIV, and pregnancy test. Bone marrow biopsy is not routinely done.
- **Procedures/biopsy:** Endoscopic biopsy with *H. pylori* testing by histopathology:
  - If negative → noninvasive testing: Stool antigen test, urea breath test, and blood antibody test
  - PCR or FISH for t(11;18). Translocation associated with lack of response to combination antibiotic therapy
- **Imaging:** CT C/A/P with contrast and/or PET/CT.

Staging *(Lugano Staging for Gastrointestinal Lymphomas; Rohatiner et al. Ann Oncol 1994)*

Stage	Involvement	
Stage I	Tumor confined to GI tract. Single primary or multiple noncontiguous lesions	
Stage II	Tumor extends into the abdomen	
	Stage II1	Local node involvement
	Stage II2	Distant node involvement
	Stage IIE	Tumor penetrates the serosa to invade adjacent organs or tissue
Stage III	No stage III in current system	
Stage IV	Disseminated extranodal involvement or concomitant supradiaphragmatic nodal involvement	

Treatment algorithm

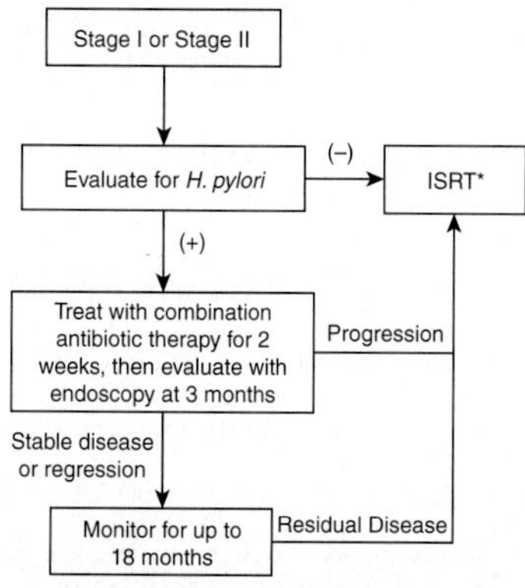

*Can consider ISRT sooner for progression, symptoms or presence of t(11;18).

Radiation treatment technique

Simulation	Supine, upper Vac-Lok cradle, knee wedge, NPO × 4 hours, deep inspiratory breath hold
Target	Entire stomach with a 0.7- to 1.5-cm isometric margin. Cover suspicious perigastric nodes
Dose	24 Gy in 12 fractions or 30 Gy in 15 fractions
Technique	IMRT with daily volumetric imaging. Avoid lateral beams

- Combination antibiotic therapy includes antacid medication and antibiotics (eg, clarithromycin, amoxicillin, and omeprazole).
- Consider chemoimmunotherapy for advanced or relapsed disease.

Orbital MALT

Presentation

- Most common nongastric MALT.
- Can affect the conjunctiva, eyelid, lacrimal gland, and retrobulbar area.
- Associated with *Chlamydia psittaci.*

Treatment approach

- Doxycycline (complete response 65%).
- Consider ISRT if antibiotic therapy failure.

Radiation treatment technique

- 4 Gy in 2 fractions can achieve CR in 90%; for those who do not achieve CR, complete the dose with additional 20 Gy in 10 fractions.

Simulation	Supine. Thermoplastic mask. Skin collimation if indicated
Target	Whole orbit or partial orbit, attempt to avoid lacrimal gland
Dose	MDA practice is 4 Gy/2 fx, if no CR → additional 20 Gy/10 fx
Technique	Wedge pair with photons for whole orbit or electrons for conjunctiva only. Consider IMRT if using 20-24 Gy

Primary Cutaneous B-Cell Lymphomas

Background

- Associated with *B. burgdorferi* infection, preexisting acrodermatitis chronica atrophicans, and vaccination sites
- 20% of all primary cutaneous lymphomas and divided into five subtypes
  - Primary cutaneous marginal zone B-cell lymphoma (PCMZL)
  - Primary cutaneous follicle center lymphoma (PCFCL).
  - Primary cutaneous diffuse large B-cell lymphoma, leg-type (PCLBCL, LT)
  - Primary cutaneous diffuse large B-cell lymphoma, other (PCLBCL, O)
  - Intravascular large B-cell lymphoma (IVLBCL)

Primary Cutaneous Marginal Zone B-cell Lymphoma (PCMZL)

Tumor biology and characteristics

- Pathology shows nodular to diffuse infiltrates of small to medium lymphocytes, with sparing of the epidermis. A reactive germinal center is frequently seen.
- Marginal zone B cells express CD20, CD79, and bcl-2 and are typically negative for CD5, CD10, and bcl 6; translocation t(18;21) is rare.

Presentation

- Multiple painless, nonulcerative, red to violaceous papules, plaques, or nodules occurring mainly on the trunk or the extremities.
- Indolent clinical presentation and spontaneous resolution have been reported.

Treatment approach

- Lesions respond to different treatments (resection, systemic therapy, and radiation). General approach is to treat with least toxic option: ISRT 4 Gy in 2 fractions.
- A noticeable clinical response might not be seen before 4-8 weeks, as effect of radiation may be mostly on the microenvironment rather than on the actual malignant cells.

Outcomes

- The lymphoma-specific survival is close to 100%, while the relapse-free survival for solitary lesions is 77% vs 39% for multifocal lesions.

Primary Cutaneous Follicle Center Lymphoma (PCFCL)

Tumor biology and characteristics

- Pathology demonstrates a monotonous population of large follicle center cells, with nodular or diffuse infiltrates sparing the epidermis.
- Cells that are CD20+, CD79a+, and bcl6+, in a network of CD21+ or CCD35+ follicular dendritic cells.
- Rarely express t(14;18) or bcl2.

Presentation

- Difficult to differentiate from PCMZL, as lesions present as nonulcerative plaques or nodules, most commonly on the scalp, forehead, or trunk.

Treatment approach

- ISRT 4 Gy in 2 fractions.

Outcomes

- Complete remission rates up 100% and a relapse-free survival of 73%-89%; the majority of patients can be salvaged with local radiation.

Primary Cutaneous T-cell Lymphomas

Mycosis Fungoides (MF)

Background

- Represents 2/3 of cutaneous T-cell lymphoma cases
- Indolent disease, may take several years and repeat biopsies
- Incurable disease unless autologous or allogeneic transplant is being considered

Tumor biology and characteristics

- Pathology shows a clonal T-cell population clustered at the basement membrane of the epidermis.
- Characterized by loss of CD7, CD5, and CD2; dim CD3+; and mature clonal CD4+ and CD45RO+.
- Rarely express t(14;18) or bcl2.

Presentation

- Presents with patches, but eventually plaques and tumors with or without erythroderma may develop. Concomitant skin infections are frequent.

Workup

- Inspection and determination of the total body surface area.
- Flow cytometry to determine CD4+/CD8+; if above 4.5, indicates a high level of circulating T-cell lymphoma cells in the blood.
- Imaging and bone marrow biopsy in appropriate cases.
- When limited to the skin, T1 and T2 are patches or plaques involving more than 10% of the skin; T3 is tumor, and T4 is erythroderma.

Treatment approach

- Initial topical therapies: steroids, chemotherapy, bexarotene gel, phototherapy
- Systemic therapies: Retinoids, histone deacetylase inhibitors, denileukin diftitox, monoclonal antibodies, interferon alpha, cytotoxic chemotherapy
- Total skin or local radiation therapy with the goal of avoiding excess skin toxicity

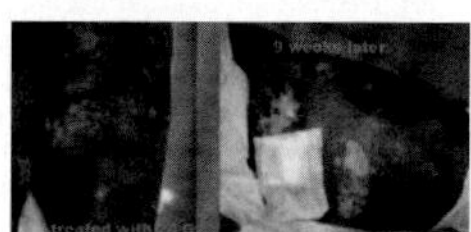

A

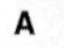

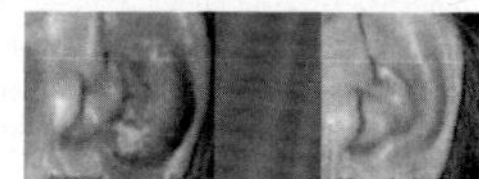

B

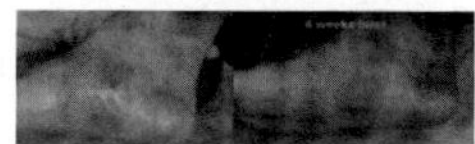

C

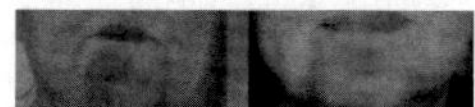

D

Figure 64.1 A–D. Pre- and posttreatment examples of local radiation (4-12 Gy) for the treatment of mycosis fungoides.

- TSEBT reserved for substantial surface involvement and may take up to 8-12 weeks for maximal response
  - Given in 2 Gy fractions twice per week with boosts/supplemental fields for axilla, shoulders, inframammary fold, groins, perineum, perianal area, soles, and skinfolds
  - 10-12 Gy overall response rate of 88% with mild toxicity
  - 30-36 Gy for high disease burden or for pretransplant conditioning
- Local radiation
  - 4-12 Gy to lesion with 1- to 2-cm margin to minimize RT to nonsymptomatic areas. Can retreat with radiation if needed.
  - Electron beam RT in most cases starting at 9 MeV for patch/plaque with higher energy for tumors with bolus to ensure full skin dose.
  - Use simulation CT scan if adjacent to sensitive normal tissue (consider skin collimation also) or unknown tumor depth.

Primary Anaplastic Large Cell Lymphoma (PALCL)

Background

- Second most common type of cutaneous T-cell lymphoma
- Can present along with M
- May take weeks/months for response to radiation and wound healing

Presentation

- Deeper skin involvement and often ulcerative lesions

Treatment approach

- Local radiation
  - Responds to as low as 6 Gy

Plasma Cell Dyscrasias/Solitary Plasmacytomas

Solitary Plasmacytoma

Background

- **Incidence/prevalence:** 10% of plasma cell neoplasms
- **Outcomes:** Localized disease with no evidence of additional lesions, bone marrow involvement, or clinical/laboratory findings consistent with MM (serum calcium > 12, renal dysfunction, Hgb < 10, multiple bone lesions, or >10% plasma cells in bone marrow). Excellent locoregional control with radiation (up to 95%)
  - 80% solitary plasmacytoma of bone (SPB): 55%-80% progress to multiple myeloma
  - 20% extramedullary plasmacytoma (SEP): 35%-50% progress to multiple myeloma
- **Demographics:** Male predominance (2/3 cases); younger median age (55-65) than multiple myeloma
- **Risk factors:** Family prevalence, older age, and male gender

Treatment approach

- Use CT, PET, and MRI (check marrow signal) for target delineation. PTV expansion depending on tumor location. Neither elective vertebral body (superior/inferior) nor elective nodal coverage is necessary if using PET and MRI.
- Typically ISRT to 40-50 Gy
  - If <5 cm, can consider <45 Gy.
  - Lower dose of 30-36 Gy may be sufficient.

Mantle Cell Lymphoma (MCL)

Background

- Usually presents with advanced stage, following an aggressive course
- Male predominance (78%), median age at diagnosis 63 years
- Majority (75%) present in the head and neck
- Age (>60), bulky disease (>5 cm), and stage II → increased treatment failure risk
- Characterized by overexpression of cyclin D and t(11;14) chromosomal translocation

Prognosis

MCL International Prognostic Index (MIPI) (*Lim et al. Oncol Lett* 2010)

Points	Age	ECOG PS	LDH (ULN)	WBC (10^9/L)
0	<50	0-1	<0.67	<6.7
1	50-59	—	0.67-0.99	6.7-9.99
2	60-69	2-4	1.0-1.49	10.0-14.99
3	≥70	—	≥1.5	≥1.5
Risk Group			**Median Survival**	
Low: 0-3 points (44% of patients)			Not reached	
Intermediate: 4-5 points (35% of patients)			51 mo	
High: 6-11 points (21% of patients)			29 mo	

Overall prognosis

- 5-Year freedom from progression, 65% and OS, 76%
- 10-Year freedom from progression, 42% and OS, 64%

Treatment approach

Stage I-II MCL

- Excellent and similar outcomes for chemotherapy, chemoradiation, or radiation alone
- Goal to deintensify therapy to limit treatment-related toxicity. Consider 4 Gy in 2 fractions

Advanced-stage MCL

- RT to palliate bulky nodal or extranodal masses, often after being heavily pretreated.
- 4 Gy in 2 fractions is associated with high response rates, although may take up to 4 weeks to respond.
- Consider additional 24-30 Gy if no response after 4 weeks.

BRAIN METASTASES

BHAVANA S. VANGARA CHAPMAN • JING LI • AMOL JITENDRA GHIA

Background

- **Incidence/prevalence:** Most common intracranial tumor, 20%-40% of all cancer patients will develop intracranial metastases. ~175-200 K diagnosed annually. Incidence increasing due to widespread adoption of MRI, where small lesion detection has improved.
- **Single metastasis**, one intracranial lesion (may have other sites of extracranial disease), vs **solitary metastasis**, one intracranial lesion, which is also the only site of metastatic disease.
- **Outcomes:** Historically, median survival for observation 1 month, steroids 2 months, WBRT 4-6 months, surgical resection for single lesion 6 months, and with adjuvant WBRT 10 months. Outcomes for SRS ± WBRT 6-10 months. Advances in targeted and immunotherapy have resulted in improved outcomes but questionable use due to limitations of the blood-brain barrier.

Tumor Biology and Characteristics

- **Pathology:**
  - Common histologies: Lung, breast, melanoma
  - Less common histologies: GU, GI, H&N, sarcoma, leukemia, lymphoma
  - Hemorrhagic metastases: Melanoma, RCC, choriocarcinoma
- **Imaging:** MRI of the brain ± contrast to visualize abnormal enhancement or ring-enhancing lesions on T1 postcontrast and vasogenic edema on T2 FLAIR; restaging CT CAP and PET-CT to evaluate systemic disease burden

Anatomy

- Most located at gray-white matter junction (watershed areas)
- 80% cerebral hemispheres, 15% cerebellum, 5% brainstem

Workup

- **History and physical:** Common presenting symptoms include headache, nausea, vomiting, seizures, focal neurologic deficits, and vision changes. Assess extent and control of intracranial/extracranial disease, performance status, and neuro exam.
- **Labs:** CBC, CMP (tumor markers to r/o cns primaries vs brain mets)
- **Imaging/procedures/biopsy:** MRI of the brain ± contrast, biopsy or resection if solitary brain lesion or long latency from last known malignancy
- **Initial management:** For symptomatic lesions, steroids 4-16 mg/d in divided doses depending on symptom severity with PPI for gastroprotection, AEDs for seizures (prophylaxis not recommended), radiation oncology, and neurosurgery consults.
- **Prognostic factors:** Age, KPS, cancer type/histology, control of primary disease, extent of metastatic disease, number/size/location of brain metastases, severity of symptoms
  - **Common prognostic scores:** Diagnosis-Specific Graded Prognostic Assessment (DS-GPA) (*Sperduto et al. JCO* 2012), Recursive Partitioning Analysis (RPA) (*Gaspar et al. IJROBP* 1997), Basic Score-Brain Metastasis (BS-BM) (*Lorenzoni et al. IJORBP* 2004), and Score Index for Radiosurgery (SIR) (*Weltman et al. IJROBP* 2000)

RTOG Recursive Partitioning Analysis (RPA) for Brain Metastases

Class	Description	Median Survival
I	KPS ≥ 70 and age > 65 and controlled primary with no extracranial metastases	7.1 mo
II	KPS ≥ 70 and one or more of age ≥ 65, uncontrolled primary, presence of extracranial metastases	4.2 mo
III	KPS < 70	2.3 mo

TREATMENT ALGORITHM

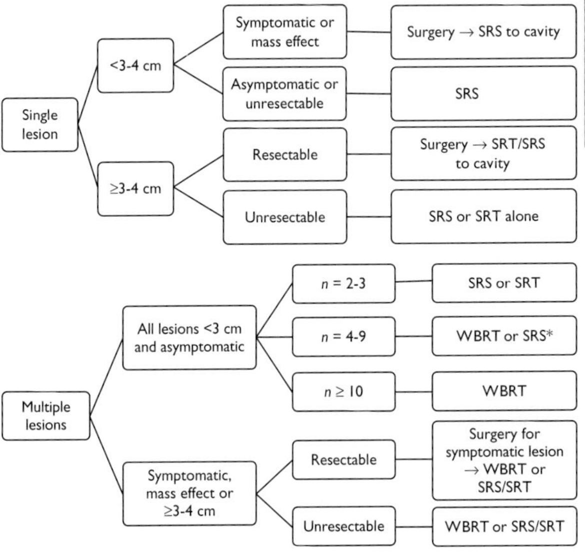

Prognosis ≥3 months

*For 4-9 lesions, standard care remains WBRT due to lack of level I evidence to support the use of SRS in this patient population. We offer SRS only on trials or due to patient refusal.

Prognosis <3 months or KPS < 50

Recommend WBRT or supportive care.

RADIATION TREATMENT TECHNIQUE

SRS: Stereotactic radiosurgery, single fraction SRT: Stereotactic radiotherapy, 2-5 fx WBRT: Whole brain radiation therapy

- **SIM**
  - **WBRT, SRT, and LINAC-based SRS:** Supine, head in neutral position, AquaPlast RT mask, bite block for SRS/SRT
  - **Gamma Knife SRS:** see **SRS** chapter.
- **Dose**
  - **WBRT**
    - Most common: 30 Gy/10 fx
    - For patient with better prognosis and to minimize late toxicity: 37.5 Gy/15 fx or 35 Gy/14 fx
  - **SRT**
    - 21-27 Gy/3 fx or 25-30 Gy/5 fx
  - **SRS** (Based off N107C/CEC•3; *Brown Lancet Oncol* 2017)
    - <4.2 cc — 20-24 Gy
    - 4.2-7.9 cc — 18 Gy
    - ≥8.0 cc, up to 4 cm diameter — 15 Gy
    - Brainstem lesion — 14-18 Gy
- **Target**
  - **WBRT:** Inferior to bottom of C1 or C2, multiple techniques can be utilized to avoid optic lenses (we typically rotate gantry 5 degrees and treat with RAO/LAO technique).

- **SRT or LINAC-based SRS:** GTV +2-mm PTV margin (*PTV margin based on institutional setup uncertainty and IGRT availability).
- **Gamma Knife SRS:** see "SRS" chapter.

- **Technique**
  - **WBRT:** Opposed laterals or IMRT-based hippocampal sparing on trial (*Gondi et al. IJROBP* 2010). Hippocampal sparing is investigational.
  - **SRT or LINAC-based SRS:** IMRT or dynamic conformal arcs
  - **Gamma Knife SRS:** see "SRS" chapter.
- **IGRT:**
  - **WBRT:** Weekly mV imaging
  - **SRT and LINAC-based SRS:** Daily kV imaging, CBCT, ExacTrac
  - **Gamma Knife SRS:** see "SRS" chapter.
- **Planning directive**
  - **SRT**
    - Brainstem* V20 < 1 cc (3 fx), D_{max} < 21 Gy/3 fx, 25 Gy/5 fx
    - Optic nerve D_{max} < 18 Gy/3 fx, 25 Gy/5 fx
  - **SRS**
    - Prescribed to ~80% isodose line for LINAC-based SRS and ~50%-80% isodose line for Gamma Knife SRS depending on size of lesion
    - Brain V12 Gy <5-10 cc; brainstem ≤12 Gy to 1cc*; optic chiasm D_{max} ≤ 10 Gy
    - For additional information, see **SRS** chapter.

  *For targets in the brainstem, normal brainstem defined as brainstem—GTV

Side Effect Management

- **WBRT**
  - **Acute:** Fatigue, alopecia, and ototoxicity. Nausea/vomiting/headaches/vision changes from increased ICP: po dexamethasone + PPI, ondansetron (4 mg q6h prn), or prochlorperazine (10 mg q6h prn)
  - **Long term:** Neurocognitive deficits, leukoencephalopathy, and radiation necrosis (higher for >3 Gy/fx). We recommend prophylactic memantine (based on RTOG 0614) for all WBRT patients, at 10 mg daily for week 1, followed by 10 mg bid for 6 months; consider indefinitely.
- **SRT/SRS**
  - Adverse effects are rare. In one modern SRS series, the 1-year probabilities of symptomatic adverse events are 3% after SRS alone, 4% for SRS preceded by WBRT, and 8% for sequential SRS/WBRT (*Sneed et al. J Neurosurg* 2015).
  - **Acute (rare):** Headache, nausea, vomiting, vestibular dysfunction, seizures; for Gamma Knife SRS, pain at headframe pin sites (OTC analgesic/anti-inflammatory meds; may consider prophylactic dexamethasone, eg, 8-10 mg ×1, when treating large lesions with significant edema seen on recent MRI)
  - **Long term:** Radiation necrosis (PO dexamethasone + PPI, may require surgery or bevacizumab for refractory cases)

Follow-up

- H&P and MRI of the brain in 4-6 weeks → every 3 months for 2 years → then as clinically indicated

Notable Trials

Surgery

- **Patchell II (*Patchell et al. JAMA* 1998):** Two-arm prospective, RCT of patients with a single-brain metastasis, other distant metastases allowed, KPS ≥ 70 with complete resection verified by MRI of the brain randomized to WBRT (50.4 Gy/28 fx) vs observation. WBRT reduced local recurrence (10% vs 46%, P < .001), other intracranial recurrence (18% vs 70%, P < .01), and neurologic death (14% vs 44%, P = .003). There was no difference in OS or time patient remained functionally independent.
- **MD Anderson (*Mahajan et al. Lancet Oncol* 2017):** Two-arm prospective phase III RCT of patients with 1-3 completely resected brain metastases, ≤4-cm cavity, and KPS ≥ 70 randomized to SRS (12-16 Gy) vs observation. Primary end point was time to local recurrence, which was reduced in the SRS arm (42% vs 72%, P =.015). OS was not different between groups.
- **N107C/CEC•3 (*Brown et al. Lancet Oncol* 2017):** Two-arm prospective phase III RCT of patients with a single resected brain metastasis with a cavity ≤5 cm, ≤3 unresected intracranial metastases, and ECOG 0-2 randomized to postoperative SRS

(12/20 Gy) vs WBRT (30 Gy/10 fx or 37.5 Gy/15 fx). On intention-to-treat analyses, OS was not different between groups, but **cognitive-deterioration-free survival** was improved in the SRS arm (median 3.7 vs 3.0 months, *P* < .001).

WBRT vs WBRT + SRS

- **RTOG 9508** **(*Andrews et al. Lancet* 2004)**: Two-arm prospective phase III RCT of patients with 1-3 brain metastases, largest lesion ≤4 cm, additional lesions ≤3 cm, and KPS ≥ 70 randomized to WBRT (30 Gy/10 fx) vs WBRT + SRS (18-24 Gy). Primary end point was OS, which was similar between groups. In patients with a single-brain metastasis, OS improved with the addition of SRS (6.5 vs 4.9 months, *P* = .04). Multivariate analysis also showed patients with RPA I or lung cancer primary had improved OS with an SRS boost. The WBRT + SRS group had improved 1-year local control (82% vs 71%, *P* =.013) and stable or improved KPS at 6 months (43% vs 27%, *P* =.033).
- **JROSG 99-1** **(*Aoyama et al. JAMA* 2006)**: Two-arm prospective, multi-institutional, RCT of patients with 1-4 brain metastases, ≤3 cm, and KPS ≥ 70 randomized to SRS alone (18-25 Gy) vs WBRT (30 Gy/10 fx) + SRS (30% dose reduction). Primary end point was OS, which was not different between groups (SRS alone 8 months; WBRT + SRS 7.5 months, *P* = .42). Intracranial relapse at 1 year and salvage treatment occurred less frequently in the WBRT + SRS arm vs SRS-alone arm (47% vs 76%, *P* < .001).

SRS for multiple brain metastases (2-10)

- **JLGK0901** **(*Yamamoto et al. Lancet Oncol* 2014)**: Prospective observational study of patients with 2-4 vs 5-10 brain metastases, <3 cm, KPS ≥ 70 treated with SRS alone (20-22 Gy). Primary end point was OS with a noninferiority margin of 95% CI with a HR 1.3 on an intention-to-treat analysis. OS was similar between 2-4 vs 5-10 brain metastases groups (median 10.8 months for both). The rate of adverse events was also similar between the arms.

Surgery or SRS → WBRT vs observation

- **EORTC 22952-26001** **(*Kocher et al. JCO* 2011)**: Two-arm prospective phase III RCT of patients with 1-3 brain metastases and WHO PS 0-2 treated with complete surgical resection or SRS (minimum 25 Gy to center and 20 Gy to surface) randomized to WBRT (30 Gy/10 fx) vs observation. Primary end point was time to WHO PS > 2, which was 10 months in the observation arm and 9.5 months in the WBRT arm (not significant). OS was similar between arms. WBRT reduced 2-year local relapse rate (surgery, 59%-27%, *P* < .001; SRS, 31%-19%, *P* = .04) and 2-year relapse at other intracranial sites (surgery, 42%-23%, *P* = .008; SRS, 48%-33%, *P* = .023). Salvage therapies and intracranial progression-related death occurred more frequently in the observation arm.

Neurocognitive function

- **MD Anderson** **(*Chang et al. Lancet Oncol* 2009)**: Two-arm prospective phase III RCT of patients with 1-3 brain metastases, size eligibility for SRS, KPS ≥ 70, RPA class I or 2 randomized to SRS alone (15-24 Gy) vs SRS + WBRT (30 Gy/12 fx) within 3 weeks. Primary end point was neurocognitive function based on HVLT-R recall test at 4 months. SRS + WBRT led to a decline in learning and memory function (52% vs 24%; Bayesian probability *P* = 96% that proportion of SRS + WBRT patients has significant worse neurocognitive function). SRS + WBRT improved local (100% vs 67%, *P* = .012) and distant control (73% vs 27%, *P* = .003). OS was better with SRS (15.2 vs 5.7 months, *P* = .003).
- **RTOG 0614** **(*Brown et al. Neuro-Onc* 2013)**: Two-arm prospective, randomized, double-blind, placebo-controlled trial of patient with brain metastases undergoing WBRT (37.5 Gy/15 fx) randomized to memantine during and after WBRT vs placebo. Primary end point was preserved delayed recall as per the HVLT-R DR at 24 weeks from the start of drug treatment, which trended toward improvement in the memantine arm but was not statistically significant (*P* = .059); a lack of significance was thought to be due to limited statistical power. However, time to cognitive failure improved with memantine (54% vs 65%, *P* = .01).
- **Alliance N0574** **(*Brown et al. JAMA* 2016)**: Two-arm prospective phase III RCT of patients with 1-3 brain metastases <3 cm and ECOG PS randomized to SRS alone (20-24 Gy) vs SRS (18-22 Gy) + WBRT (30 Gy/12 fx) within 2 weeks. Primary end point was cognitive decline >1 SD from baseline on at least 1/7 cognitive tests at 3 months. Cognitive decline was more frequent in the WBRT arm (92% vs 64%, *P* < .001). Although WBRT improved 6 and 12 months local and distant control and decreased salvage rates, there was no difference in OS with the addition of WBRT.

SPINE METASTASES

VINCENT BERNARD • ADNAN ELHAMMALI • AMOL JITENDRA GHIA

Background

- **Incidence/prevalence:** Osseous disease third most common site of metastases. The spine most common site of bone metastases. 70% involve thoracic spine, 20% lumbar, and 10% cervical. Breast, lung, and prostate account for 50%-60% of cases.
- **Radiosensitive histologies:** Breast, prostate, ovarian, and neuroendocrine carcinoma. Patients achieve symptomatic relief and effective local control rates with conventional external beam radiotherapy (cEBRT).
- **Radioresistant histologies:** Sarcoma, melanoma, chordoma, hepatobiliary, and renal cell carcinoma. Do not have good local control rates with conventional radiation. Radiosurgery should be considered.
- **Intermediate resistance histologies:** Lung, colon, and thyroid. Treatment typically dependent on institutional classification and experience.

Workup

- **History and physical:** Characterize pain: Mechanical pain worse with movement and neurologic pain worse when supine. Pain is the most common initial presenting symptom and usually precedes neurologic deficits. Mechanical pain indicates possible need for stabilization. Inquire about neurologic deficits that indicate possible acute cord compression. Does patient have known cancer diagnoses? Ask about prior surgery, prior radiation therapy, concurrent chemotherapy. Assess PFS and ability to tolerate simulation/treatment. Perform complete neurologic examination.
- **Imaging:** MRI T1 with/without contrast of entire spine to delineate disease and identify other sites of involvement. Axial T2 to localize spinal cord. CT myelogram is useful in postoperative SRS above the conus where instrumentation causes increased T2 artifact signal making cord visualization difficult.
- **Surgery consult:** Patient should be evaluated by neurosurgery or spine surgery to determine the need for emergent decompression or spine stabilization prior to radiation therapy.

General Treatment Overview

- **Disease touching the cord (MESCC grade IC or greater)?** If patient is a surgical candidate, we prefer surgery followed by radiation therapy. If not a surgical candidate but otherwise meets clinical indications for SSRS as outlined below, proceed with SSRS respecting spinal cord dose tolerance. Otherwise, cEBRT (see RT Emergencies chapter).
- **Assess the need for surgical stabilization:** Refer patient to neurosurgery or spine surgery for assessment of spine stability and need for stabilization prior to RT based on SINS score (spine instability neoplastic score; *Fisher Radiat Oncol* 2014). **Score 0-6, stable; 7-12, indeterminate; and 13-18, unstable.**
- **Spine radiosurgery:**
  Indications: Reirradiation, radiation-resistant histology, oligometastatic, oligoprogressive
  Contraindications: >3 spinal level involvement, poor PFS, unable to tolerate SRS simulation or treatment (eg, lay flat for an extended period of time)

Component	Score
Location	
Junctional (O-C2; C7-T2; T11-L1; L5-S1)	3
Mobile spine (C3-6; L2-4)	2
Semirigid (T3-10)	1
Rigid (S2-5)	0
Mechanical pain	
Yes	3
No	2
Pain free lesion	1

Component	Score
Bone lesion	
Lytic	2
Mixed (lytic/blastic)	1
Blastic	0
Radiographic spinal alignment	
Subluxation/translation present	4
Deformity (kyphosis/scoliosis)	2
Normal	0
Vertebral body collapse	
>50% collapse	3
<50% collapse	2
No collapse with >50% body involved	1
None of the above	0
Posterolateral involvement	
Bilateral	3
Unilateral	1
None of the above	0

RADIATION TREATMENT TECHNIQUE

Conventional radiotherapy (cEBRT)

- **SIM:** Varies by site and technique. Consider patient pain tolerance.
- **Dose:** Typically 30 Gy in 10 fractions or 20 Gy in 5 fractions; 20 Gy in 8 fractions for lymphoma/multiple myeloma
- **Target:** One vertebral body above and below the site of disease + soft tissue extension + 1-2 cm laterally from the vertebral body
- **Technique:** Depends on level. In general:
  - Cervical (C1-C7): Opposed lateral
  - Thoracic (T1-T12): AP:PA or PA
  - Lumbar (L1-L5): AP:PA or PA
  - Sacrum: Laterals, AP:PA, or 3 field (PA: laterals)

Spine stereotactic surgery

- **SIM:** Supine, full body stereo cradle, head/neck/shoulder Aquaplastic mask for c-spine, body fix device for thoracic/lumbar/sacral spine (Fig. 66.1).

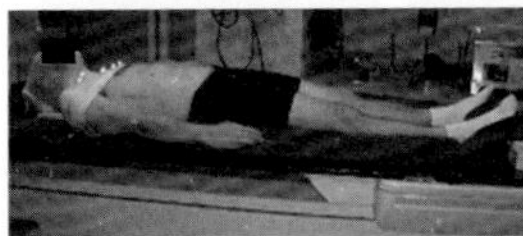

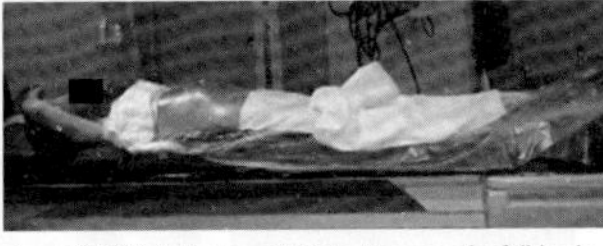

Figure 66.1 Typical set-up for cEBRT (left picture) and SSRS (right picture). Note the use of a full body fix device that covers the entire length of the spine for SSRS treatments, to ensure minimal patient movement and reduce positional error.

- **Dose: *Dosing and target dependent on IGRT availability and physics support.** MDACC SSRS simultaneous integrated boost (SIB) technique:

	Radioresistant (GTV/CTV/fx)	Radiosensitive (GTV/CTV/fx)
No prior RT	24 Gy/16 Gy/1 fx	18 Gy/16 Gy/1 fx
Prior cEBRT	27 Gy/24 Gy/3 fx	27 Gy/21 Gy/3 fx

- **Image fusion:** Axial T1 and/or T1+C for GTV. Identify true cord on axial T2 MRI for intact. CT myelogram preferred for post-op cases as hardware causes T2 artifact.
- **Target (based on SSRS consensus guidelines;** ***Cox et al. IJROBP*** **2012):**
  Intact tumor
  GTV: Visible tumor on CT or MRI

CTV: Contiguous at risk bone as per guidelines (1 echelon beyond; see below) + 5 mm expansion around paraspinal/soft tissue extension of disease
PTV: Depends on institutional setup uncertainty. No expansion at MDACC
Post-op:
GTV: Pre-op disease + residual disease in postoperative imaging
CTV: Same as intact, if bone resected, contour virtual CTV referring to post-op consensus guidelines (Redmond et al. *IJROBP* 2017)
PTV: Same as intact

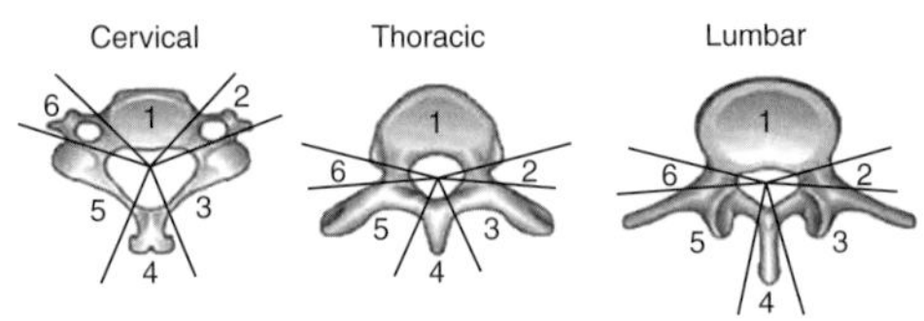

Figure 66.2 Anatomic classification system for consensus target volumes for spine SRS adapted from the international SRS consortium consensus guidelines. *1*, Vertebral body; *2*, left pedicle; *3*, left transverse process and lamina; *4*, spinous process; *5*, right transverse process and lamina; and *6*, right pedicle. (Adapted from Cox BW, Spratt DE, Lovelock M, et al. International Spine Radiosurgery Consortium consensus guidelines for target volume definition in spinal stereotactic radiosurgery. *Int J Radiat Oncol Biol Phys*. 2012;83(5):e597-605. Copyright © 2012 Elsevier. With permission.)

- **Planning directive constraints:** *PRV expansion based on institutional setup uncertainty. No PRV expansion used at MDACC
  Spinal cord:
  Single fraction: V8-10 Gy ≤ 1 cc, D_{max} < 10-12 Gy
  Three fraction (prior cEBRT): 9 Gy ≤ 1 cc, D_{max} ≤ 10 Gy
  Cauda equina:
  Single fraction: V12-14 Gy ≤ 1 cc, D_{max} < 16 Gy
  Three fraction (prior cEBRT): 12 Gy ≤ 1 cc, D_{max} ≤ 18 Gy
  Esophagus:
  Single fraction: V12 Gy ≤ 1 cc, D_{max} < 17 Gy
  Three fraction (prior cEBRT): 12 Gy ≤ 1 cc, D_{max} ≤ 21 Gy
- **Treatment planning:** Step and shoot IMRT with nine coplanar posterior/posterolateral beams. Goal GTV D_{min} > 14 Gy/1 fx or > 21 Gy/3 fx (Bishop *IJROBP* 2015). GTV coverage typically 80%-90%.
- **IGRT:** Daily ExacTrac, CBCT, and orthogonal ports prior to treatment and ExacTrac "snapshot" between each beam. Repeat CBCT if patient moves between beams.

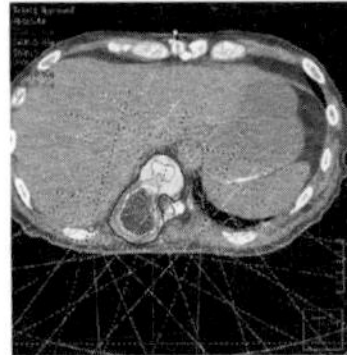
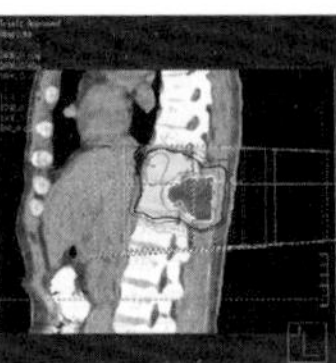
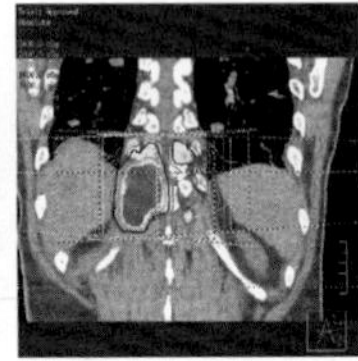

Figure 66.3 Representative treatment plan of a patient undergoing SSRS in axial, sagittal, and coronal (L → R) cross-sectional views. The CTV is highlighted in *yellow color* wash and GTV in *red*. The *blue isodose line* represents 16 Gy and *white isodose line* 24 Gy. This patient was treated with a single fraction. **See color insert**.

SIDE EFFECT MANAGEMENT

Acute
- **Pain flare:** Incidence 20%-63%. Typically self-limiting and salvageable by treating with dexamethasone 4 mg bid over 5-7 days
- **Esophagitis:** Dietary modifications (pureed/bland/soft food, frequent small meals), topical anesthetics (magic mouthwash, etc.), analgesics (acetaminophen, narcotics)

Late
- **Vertebral body fracture:** Rates range from 10% to 40%, although a significant portion is asymptomatic. Risk correlated to dose/fraction, SINS, and preexisting fracture.
- **Myelopathy:** <1%

- **Radiculopathy:** ~10%, risk greatest if disease involves the foramen
- **Esophageal stricture or perforation:** <1%

Follow-up

- Every 3 months with MRI of the entire spine w/contrast for 1-2 years and then every 6 months.
- Local control expected to be >90% at 1 year in radiation-naïve patients regardless of histology and >75% in those receiving reirradiation.

Notable Trials

- **MDACC prospective phase I/II trial** (*Garg Cancer* **2012**)**:** Safety and efficacy using SSRS in 61 patients with 63 tumors receiving 18-24 Gy in a single fraction. 1- and 2-year local control rates were 91% and 88%, respectively, with no significant differences in outcomes with respect to tumor histology. 87% of patients reported complete or partial pain relief. Two patients experienced grade 3 and grade 4 neurologic toxicities.
- **MDACC prospective phase I/II** (*Wang Lancet Oncol* **2012**)**:** Safety and efficacy of SSRS in metastatic spine tumors among 149 patients. Patients who had received prior radiation therapy, treated with 27-30 Gy in 3 fractions, experience 1- and 2-year LC rates of 80.5% and 72.4%, respectively, with 92.9% of patients reporting some degree of pain relief with a significant reduction in opioid use from baseline to 3 (P = .021) and 6 months (P = .011) post SSRS. Rare instances of non-neurologic grade 3 toxicities were reported with no grade 4 toxicities noted.
- **Phase II RTOG 0631 trial** (*Ryu PRO* **2014**)**:** Assessing the feasibility and safety of delivery of an image-guided single 16 Gy SSRS dose for localized spine metastases among 65 institutions. The adopted spinal cord constraints in the study have been reported to be safe with a D_{max} of 10 Gy, ≤0.35 cc or ≤10% of partial spinal cord. There is an ongoing phase III trial comparing single-dose 16 Gy SSRS to single-dose 8 Gy cEBRT for pain control.

NON-SPINE BONE METASTASES

ADNAN ELHAMMALI • QUYNH-NHU NGUYEN

Background

- **Incidence/prevalence:** Approximately 350 000 patients die each year with bone metastases. Pain is the most common presenting symptom.
- **Demographics:** Third most common site of metastatic disease (1st lung, 2nd liver). Axial skeleton more commonly involved (spine > pelvis > ribs > femur > skull)
- **Outcomes:** Highly variable, dependent on histology and extent of disease

Biology and Pathology

- **Pathology:** Most to least common: Prostate > breast > kidney > thyroid > lung. Bone metastases can occur either by direct extension or via hematogenous spread. Alters normal bone remodeling process mediated by osteoblasts and osteoclasts and can present as either lytic (classically RCC, myeloma, melanoma) or blastic (classically prostate and SCLC) lesions

Workup and Evaluation

- **History and physical:** Identify the source of pain, severity, weight-bearing ability, neurologic deficits, pain medication use, performance status, and systemic disease burden.
- **Imaging:** Bone scan (technetium-99) for asymptomatic blastic bone mets. Uptake in bone scan more indicative of osteoblastic activity and may not be as reliable for lytic lesions. For focal assessment of symptomatic lesions, plain films to assess fracture risk, CT, MRI, or PET/CT. For myeloma, get skeletal survey.
- **Biopsy:** Consider if no prior hx of cancer or if site of 1st relapse.
- **Fracture risk:** Determine if surgical stabilization is needed prior to RT. Use Mirels criteria, weight-based scoring system to assess fracture risk (*Mirels et al. Clin Orthop Res* 1989), scoring table shown below

Predictors of pathologic fracture of the femur: >30-mm axial cortical involvement or circumferential cortical involvement >50%, based on analysis of Dutch Bone Metastases Study *(Van der Linden et al. J Bone Joint Surg Br 2004).*

Mirels Score			
Score	1	2	3
Site	Upper extr	Lower extr	Peritrochanteric
Pain	Mild	Mod	Severe
X-ray	Blastic	Mixed	Lytic
% of shaft	0%-33%	33%-66%	67%-100%

Score	Fracture Risk
0-6	0%
7	5%
8	33%
9	57%
10-12	100%

Treatment Principles

- If significant fracture risk (Mirels score ≥ 8, >30 mm femoral cortical involved, >50% femoral circumferential cortical involvement) → surgical fixation followed by radiation therapy.
- Single fraction (SF, 8 Gy) or multifraction (MF, 30 Gy in 10 fractions, 20 Gy in 5 fractions)
  - Equal efficacy of pain relief but higher rates of retreatment in 8 Gy single fraction
  - SF more convenient and cost-effective
  - The United States lags behind SF utilization compared to other countries.
  - Consider PFS, prognosis, risk of cord compression, and tolerance for retreatment.
- Consider radiosurgery for oligometastatic disease (<3 bony sites) or reirradiation. At MDACC, only done on protocol for non-spinal bone metastases.
- Consider radium-223 for diffuse osteoblastic metastatic disease without visceral involvement.
- Reirradiation safe and feasible. Generally 8 Gy in 1 or 20 Gy in 5. Achieves ~50% overall response rate *(Chow et al. Lancet Oncol 2013)*

Radiation Treatment Technique

- **SIM:** Varies by site and technique. Consider patient pain tolerance.
- **Dose:** 8 Gy single fraction, 20 Gy in 5 fractions, or 30 Gy in 10 fractions. Post-op: 30 Gy in 10 fractions.
- **Target (intact):** Contour GTV. PTV = GTV + 1-2 cm (depending on setup reliability and patient's ability to stay still). Add 1.5-2 cm to block edge for dose buildup. Post-op: Cover the entire rod (unless multiple myeloma); split joint space. Leave untreated strip of the skin.
- **Target (post-op):** CT is entire prosthesis and resection area (may require extended SSD technique or may not be able to cover entire prosthesis). PTV = GTV + 1-2 cm (depending on setup reliability and patient's ability to stay still). Add 1.5-2 cm to block edge for dose buildup.
- **Technique:** Depends on location. Generally 2D or 3DCRT, beam arrangement varies by site. Consider IMRT or radiosurgery if retreatment.

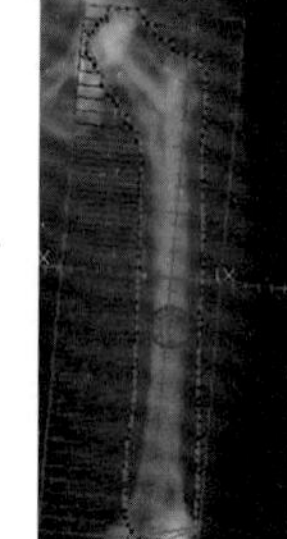

Figure 67.1 Representative postoperative field treating to 20 Gy in 5 fractions.

Surgery

- Done to prevent and/or treat pathologic fractures. For pelvic lesions, orthopedic surgeons typically opt for total hip arthroplasty if the lesion involves the neck and if the patient is able to tolerate. Other options include proximal hip endoprosthesis or stabilization with intramedullary rods (if lesion in the midbone).

Chemotherapy

- RANK-L inhibitors (denosumab): Monoclonal antibody that inhibits the RANK/RANK-L pathway (involved in osteoclast maturation and activity). Has been shown to decrease skeletal-related events in patients with bony mets from advanced cancers when compared to zoledronic acid (*Lipon Eur J Cancer* 2012). Approved for use in metastatic solid tumors. Typically given subcutaneously 120 mg q4wk and continued indefinitely.

- Bisphosphonates (zoledronic acid, pamidronate): Inhibit osteoclast activity, preventing bone resorption. Used in castrate-resistant prostate cancer and breast cancer. Typically given IV q3-4wk (dose adjusted for creatinine clearance). Can also be given q3mo.

Notable Trials

- **RTOG 97-14** ***(Hartsell et al. JNCI* 2005):** 898 breast and prostate points, 1-3 painful bone metastases, randomized to 8 Gy in 1 fraction vs 30 Gy in 10 fractions. Primary outcome was pain relief at 3 months. G2-4 tox greater in 30/10 arm (17% vs 10%, $P = .002$), late tox 4% in both arms. At 3 months, overall response rate to pain was 66%. Complete and partial response rates were 15% and 50%, respectively, in the 8 Gy arm vs 18% and 48% in the 30 Gy arm ($P = .6$). Retreatment was higher in 8 Gy arm vs 30 Gy arm (18% vs 9%, $P < .001$).
- **Norwegian/Swedish Trial** ***(Kaasa et al. Radiother Oncol* 2006):** Phase III RCT, 376 points (planned 1000) with painful bone mets randomized to 8 Gy in 1 vs 30 Gy in 10. Primary end point was pain relief. Trial ended early as initial data showed similar rates of pain control, fatigue, QOL, and survival (8-9 months) between both arms.
- **Chow et al. Meta-analysis** ***(Chow et al. JCO* 2007):** 16 published randomized trials from 1986 onward, SF vs MF (8 Gy in 1 and 30 Gy in 10 most common) regimens compared. Primary outcomes were overall and complete response rate (OR and CR). SF and MF were found to be equivalent in palliation of pain with CR rates of 23% vs 24% for SF and MF, respectively, and OR rates of 58% and 59%. Retreatment rate 2.5× higher with SF (95% CI, 1.76-3.56, $P < .00001$). No difference in pathologic fracture risk.

RADIATION EMERGENCIES

ADNAN ELHAMMALI • MARY FRANCES MCALEER

Cord Compression

- **Definition:** Acute, potentially life-threatening or morbid event caused by cancer for which radiation therapy may be therapeutic and/or offer palliation.
  - Cauda equina syndrome: Lower extremity weakness, saddle anesthesia, bowel/bladder incontinence
- **Incidence/prevalence:** Breast, lung, and prostate account for 50%-60% of cases. 70% involve thoracic spine, 20% lumbar, 10% cervical.
- **Outcomes:** Median OS ~3 months. Pretreatment ambulatory status biggest predictor of functional outcome. If ambulatory medina, OS ~7 months; if nonambulatory, OS ~1.5 months.

Workup

- **History:** Patient must be seen and assessed immediately. Inquire about pain, motor/sensory/bowel/bladder deficits, and duration of symptoms. Also weakness, sensory deficits, bowel/bladder dysfunction. Establish whether patient has known cancer diagnosis with pathology or elevated cancer biomarker (PSA, AFP, CEA, etc.)? Assess performance status. Enquire about prior radiation treatment and last chemotherapy.
- **Examination:** Complete neurologic examination with clinical localization. Check for saddle anesthesia and rectal tone. Back pain most common initial presenting symptom and precedes neurologic deficits, typically worse when lying down.
- **Imaging:** Must image the entire spine as many patients will have epidural disease outside primary symptomatic site. MRI with at least T1 and T2 sequences, preferable with and without contrast. Enhancing mass usually best visualized on T1+C and cord impingement on T2 as CSF is bright (Fig. 68.1). Consider CT myelogram if contraindication to MRI.

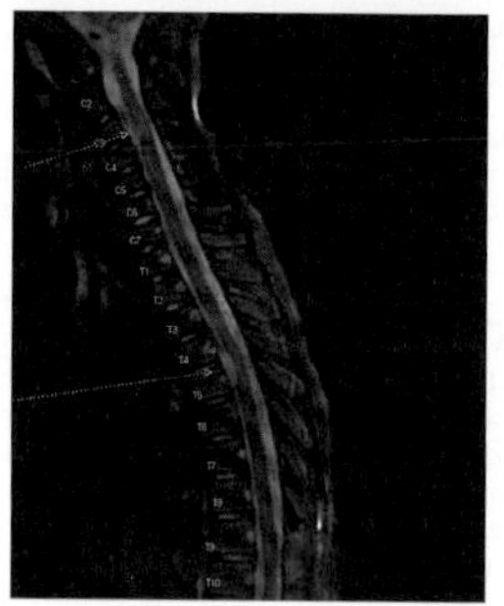

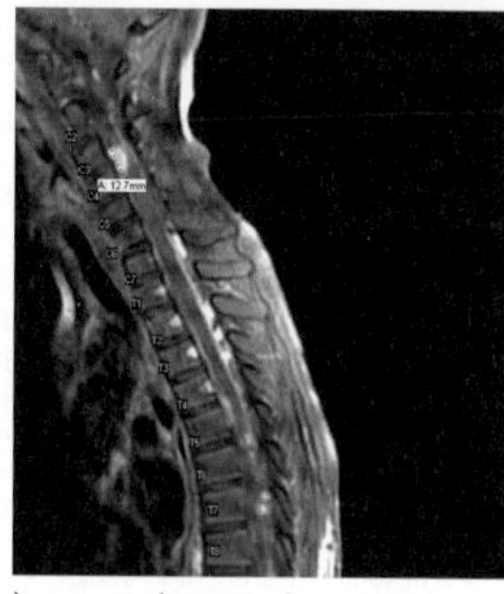

Figure 68.1 MRI T2-FLAIR **(left)** and T1+C **(right)** sequences showing cord compression at C3-C4 and T4-T5 presenting in a 7-year-old male with a new diagnosis of a primitive neuroectodermal tumor (PNET). T2 sequence clearly shows the cord impingement with loss of bright CSF signal in areas where tumor has invaded the spinal canal *(arrows)*.

Treatment principles

- Must establish a cancer diagnosis before radiation therapy, either with tissue or elevated biomarker(s)
- Begin steroids: Dexamethasone 10 mg IV loading dose → 4 mg IV every 6 hours. Start proton pump inhibitor for GI prophylaxis.
- Neurosurgery evaluation to determine if operative candidate. For nonhematologic malignancies, surgery → radiation achieves superior functional outcomes than radiation alone.

Radiation treatment technique

- **SIM:** Varies by site and technique. Consider patient pain tolerance. In emergent cases where CT-based simulation not available (evening, weekends), clinical setup should be used (refer to Clinical Setup chapter for further details).
- **Dose:** Most commonly used regimens: 30 Gy in 10 fractions or 20 Gy in 5 fractions; 20 Gy in 8 fractions for lymphoma/multiple myeloma. Consider radiosurgery post-operatively after decompression for oligometastatic or radioresistant histology (see **Spine Metastases** chapter for more detail).
- **Target:** One vertebral body above and below site of disease + soft tissue extension + 1-2 cm laterally from the vertebral body.
- **Technique:** Depends on level. In general:
  - Cervical (C1-C7): Opposed lateral beams
  - Thoracic (T1-T12): AP:PA or PA
  - Lumbar (L1-L5): AP:PA or PA
  - Sacrum: Opposed laterals, AP:PA, or 3 field (PA:laterals)

Side effect management

- Pain management: NSAIDS, acetaminophen, narcotics. Initiate bowel regimen if narcotics are prescribed.
- Esophagitis: Dietary modification (pureed/bland/soft food, frequent small meals), topical anesthetics (magic mouthwash, glutamine), analgesics (acetaminophen, narcotics).
- Nausea: Antiemetics prior to treatment and PRN. First-line Zofran, add second line if needed.
- Diarrhea: First-line Imodium titrating to a max of 8 pills/day → second line alternating Lomotil and Imodium.
- Cystitis: Rule out UTI, analgesics, cranberry juice, phenazopyridine.

Reirradiation

- If cord compression is identified in a previously irradiated field and patient is not a candidate for surgery or spine stereotactic radiosurgery (SSRS), reirradiation may be offered to select patients.
- Consider life expectancy and extent of neurologic deficit since likelihood of restoring neurologic function is low, but reirradiation may limit progression.

- Based on analysis by *Nieder et al. IJROBP* 2006, risk of myelopathy is <3% if the following conditions are met:
  - Interval between radiation courses ≥6 months
  - Cumulative spinal cord BED ≤ 135 Gy assuming α/β value of 2 for cervical/thoracic cord and 4 for lumbar cord
  - ≤98 Gy BED delivered in any single course

Notable trials

- *Patchell Lancet* 2005: 101 patients with MRI evidence of cord compression with at least 1 symptom (including pain) randomized to surgery + RT vs RT alone (30 Gy in 10 fractions). Excluded: cauda equina–only lesions, paraplegic for >48 hours, radiosensitive histologies, and CNS primary tumors. Primary end point was ambulation at 3 months and was found to be 84% vs 57% (*P* = .001) favoring surgery. Among patients not ambulatory at time of treatment, 62% of surgery patients regained ability to walk vs only 19% of radiation patients (*P* = .01).

Leptomeningeal Disease

Background

- **Definition:** Tumor involvement of the CSF or leptomeninges (pia mater and arachnoid). Note: Involvement of the dura mater does not constitute LMD as CSF is between pia and arachnoid meningeal layers.
- **Incidence/prevalence:** Diagnosed in ~5% of all cancer patients, most commonly in the breast and lung and melanoma.
- **Outcomes:** Prognosis is poor with median survival of 4 months or less.

Workup

- Patients often present with multifocal neurologic symptoms as disease can involve the entire neuroaxis: For example, combination of cranial neuropathy and extremity weakness. Also can present with headache, cerebellar dysfunction, altered mental status, seizure, and cauda equina syndrome.
- Patients suspected of having LMD should have MRI of the complete neuroaxis (brain and cervical, thoracic, lumbar spine) as well as lumbar puncture for CSF cytology analysis. Note: (1) LP should be performed ***after*** spine imaging is completed to prevent false-positive sampling and/or unnecessary procedure if gross evidence of LMD seeding along the spinal cord/cauda nerve roots and (2) sensitivity of CSF cytology 80%-95%, thus repeat LP is warranted in patients with high clinical suspicion or radiographic findings concerning for LMD.

Treatment principles

- Symptomatic patients should receive dexamethasone as outlined in the section on Cord Compression above.
- Primary treatment is intrathecal chemotherapy while radiation therapy reserved for symptomatic sites.
- Note that symptomatic sites may not have radiographic correlate. Localized treatment to suspected site of disease in these patients is reasonable (eg, RT to lumbosacral spine in patient with cauda equina syndrome).
- Use appropriate palliative dosing: 30 Gy in 10 fractions, 20 Gy in 5 fractions, or 8 Gy in 1 fraction for the spine.

SVC Syndrome

- **Definition:** Obstruction of blood flow through the SVC
- **Incidence/prevalence:** 60%-80% caused by malignancy of which 50% NSCLC, 25% SCLC, 10% NHL. Note 20%-40% caused by benign processes (thrombosis from intravascular devices such as catheters or pacemakers, infection). 60% of patients present without prior cancer diagnosis
- **Outcomes:** If SVC syndrome is appropriately managed, survival is comparable to tumor type/stage patients without it.

Workup and treatment

- **History and physical:** Assess respiratory status, signs of airway compromise (stridor, oropharyngeal swelling), and ability of patients to lie down supine. Presenting symptoms include dyspnea, swelling of the face/arm/chest, laryngeal edema causing hoarseness/stridor, cough. Symptoms may be worsened with bending forward or lying down
- **Imaging:** Chest x-ray, CT of the chest with contrast. Consider US if with concern for thrombus.

Treatment principles

- As majority of patients present with undiagnosed cancer, must establish tissue diagnosis prior to initiating treatment unless severe SVC causing airway compromise or, rarely, coma secondary to cerebral edema.
- Consider minimally invasive techniques for rapid diagnoses (sputum/pleural fluid cytology, biopsy of superficial nodes, BM biopsy for lymphoma, cancer biomarkers such as AFP or β-HCG). Alternatively, obtain tissue with CT or bronchoscopic-guided needle techniques.
- For patients with severe symptoms, rapid relief can be achieved with intraluminal stenting to allow time for establishment of a pathologic diagnosis and prior to treatment with chemotherapy/radiation therapy.
- For chemosensitive histologies (SCLC, lymphoma, germ cell tumors), can treat with chemotherapy alone.

Radiation treatment technique

- **SIM:** Generally upper Vac-Lok, arms above head, incline board if unable to lie flat.
- **Dose:** If clinically stable, treat to appropriate dose for the primary histology (eg, 66 Gy in 33 fractions for NSCLC). For palliative intent, 30 Gy in 10 fractions or 20 Gy in 5 fractions. Can consider 3-4 Gy for the first few fractions and then convert to definitive dosing.
- **Target:** Contour GTV. CTV = GTV + 0.5- to 2-cm margin (depending on histology). PTV = CTV + 0.3-1 cm depending on setup and patient's ability to lay still.
- **Technique:** For definitive, consider IMRT, 3DCRT. For palliative or rapid initiation of treatment, 3DCRT or 2D (AP/PA, obliques).

Side effect management

- Esophagitis: Dietary modifications (pureed/bland/soft food, frequent small meals), topical anesthetics (magic mouthwash, glutamine), analgesics (acetaminophen, narcotics).
- Cough: Tessalon Perles, Tussin (dextromethorphan)

AIRWAY COMPROMISE

- **Incidence/prevalence:** Approximately 80 000 cases of malignant airway obstruction occur annually.
- Can lead to cough, dyspnea, and pneumonia and cause significant morbidity and/or mortality.

Treatment principles

- Nonradiation treatment options include therapeutic bronchoscopy with resection or stenting and surgery. These treatment options may provide rapid relief and tissue for diagnostic workup if needed.
- For candidates of definitive radiation therapy, bronchoscopy is preferred to allow for treatment planning and appropriate fractionation.

Radiation treatment technique

- Palliative radiation therapy can be offered, typically external beam for emergent cases. Intraluminal or interstitial brachytherapy can be considered in nonemergent situations.
- Typical external beam doses include 45 Gy in 15 fractions, 30 Gy in 10 fractions (ASTRO guidelines preference), or 20 Gy in 5 fractions. If plan is to convert to definitive therapeutic intent, give 3-4 Gy for the first few fractions and then switch to definitive dosing regimen.

UNCONTROLLED BLEEDING

- **Incidence/prevalence:** Occurs in 6%-10% of cancer patients most typically in the form of hemoptysis, upper/lower GI bleed, epistaxis, hematuria, or vaginal bleeding.

Workup

- Assess patient to confirm he/she is hemodynamically stable, and rule out platelet abnormality, coagulopathy, or iatrogenic (anticoagulants) cause of bleeding.

Treatment principles

- **Nonradiation treatment options**
  - Packing, if accessible, is a least invasive approach and may achieve rapid hemostasis.
  - Endoscopy (EGD, colonoscopy, bronchoscopy, and cystoscopy) can achieve rapid hemostasis and provide tissue for diagnostic workup.

    - IR embolization can achieve rapid hemostasis but requires identification of feeder artery that will not result in significant normal tissue ischemia if embolized.
    - Surgery appropriate for some patients with localized disease.
- **Radiation therapy:** Typically takes days to weeks to achieve hemostasis. If patient is a candidate for definitive treatment, preferable to achieve rapid hemostasis with nonradiation treatment to allow for definitive planning and fractionation.

Radiation treatment technique

- Dosing varies by site, prognosis, severity of bleeding, and desire to convert to definitive treatment.
- Consider 45 Gy in 15 fractions, 30 Gy in 10 fractions, 20 Gy in 5 fractions, 8-10 Gy in 1 fraction, "Quad-shot" for HN cancer *(Corry et al. Radiother Oncol* 2005): 14.8 Gy in 4 fractions bid with >6-hour interfractional interval. If possibly converting to definitive intent, give 3-4 Gy for the first few fractions and then convert to definitive dosing.

BENIGN DISEASE: NON-NEURAL

RACHIT KUMAR • CHRISTOPHER WILKE

Heterotopic Ossification

- Heterotopic ossification (HO) typically appears in the periarticular soft tissues following trauma or surgery. While the estimated frequency varies widely between 10% and 80% of cases, ~10% result in extensive HO, resulting in pain and impairment.
- Highest risk of HO is in patients with previous history of HO, either on the ipsilateral or contralateral side (following second surgery, the risk may be as high as 100%).
- Pain and immobility are the clinical hallmarks of this diagnosis. Typically, clinically relevant osteophytes may be initially seen on plain radiographs of the joint. Brooker, in 1973, described a classification system for HO.

Grade I	Bone islands within soft tissue around the hip
Grade II	Exophytes of the pelvis or proximal femur end with a distance of >1 cm
Grade III	Exophytes of the pelvis or proximal femur end with a distance of <1 cm
Grade IV	Bony ankylosis between proximal femur and pelvis

- Management of HO generally involves surgery and radiotherapy but may also include medical management.
    - Surgery: Remove clinically meaningful ossifications resulting in discomfort.
    - Medical management: NSAIDs (indomethacin) and COX-2 inhibitors have shown promising results in reducing the risk of HO development in the perioperative setting.
    - Radiation: Typically completed 24 hours prior to or within 72 hours after surgery.
- Low-dose radiation has been an effective technique in reducing the risk of HO formation. Both preoperative (24 hours prior to surgery) and postoperative (within 72 hours after surgery) regimens demonstrate efficacy in reducing the risk of HO. Single-fraction doses of 7-8 Gy in the preoperative setting and 7 Gy in the postoperative setting demonstrate excellent efficacy with low toxicity, including no worsening of wound healing. An example field for a patient with heterotopic ossification treated in the postoperative setting is demonstrated in Figure 69.1.

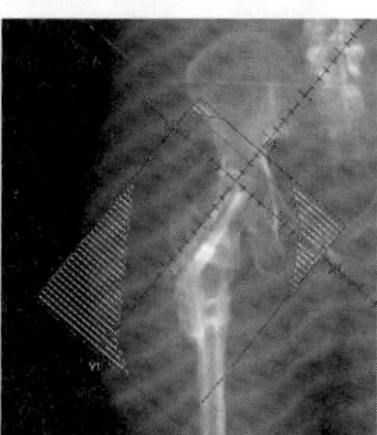

Figure 69.1 Standard AP field for heterotopic ossification.

Keloid

- Keloids are defined as areas of irregular fibrous tissue formed at the site of a scar or injury. Unlike hypertrophic scars, keloids do not regress over time. They may result in local pain and inflammation as a consequence of their infiltrating character. They occur more frequently in areas of high skin tension and are often seen in the upper body, around the joints, and in the earlobes. While the exact cause of keloids remains unknown, a genetic/racial predisposition, particularly in individuals of African descent, has been identified.

- Surgical resection of keloids is the initial treatment, acknowledging that >50% of patients will recur following surgery alone. Nonradiation options following surgery include pressure silicone dressings and steroid injections.
- Radiation helps to reduce the rate of keloid formation after surgery to 20%-25%. Detailed coordination following surgery is required to optimally reduce the rate of keloid formation, with radiation typically completed within 24 hours of operation.
- Typical radiation dose-fractionation schemes vary from single-fraction 7.5-10 Gy to 12-25 Gy in 3 or 4 Gy fractions. Electrons are utilized to optimize dose to the scar with a 1-cm margin, with bolus applied to ensure generous coverage to the postoperative field. Depth of coverage is generally not specified as long as the postoperative field is well treated.

GYNECOMASTIA

- The use of androgen deprivation therapy in men with prostate cancer, particularly in those receiving antiandrogen monotherapy (eg, bicalutamide 150 mg), frequently results in gynecomastia, a benign proliferation of breast tissue, in up to 80% of patients. Prevalence is ~15% in men treated with total androgen blockade (GnRH agonists + antiandrogen).
- This breast enlargement is frequently painful (mastodynia) and is a significant toxicity for many men receiving androgen deprivation therapy.
- Data on the role of radiation therapy in this setting demonstrate that radiation may reduce the incidence of gynecomastia (decreasing from ~80%-50%) but does not decrease mastodynia.
- Classically, radiation has been delivered to a dose of 12-15 Gy in 3 Gy fractions, but single-dose treatment of 9-10 Gy has also been investigated. When used in the prophylactic setting, 10 Gy vs sham radiotherapy successfully reduced the incidence of gynecomastia but did not decrease mastodynia (*Tyrrell IJROBP* 2004).
- A recent *PLoS One* systematic review article compared the results of radiotherapy to tamoxifen, and while both appeared to be effective, tamoxifen was found to be more efficacious (*Fagerlund PLoS One* 2015).
- Based on these results, the utilization of tamoxifen rather than radiotherapy as first-line treatment for gynecomastia should be considered, acknowledging the lack of conclusive trials on the topic and side effect profile of tamoxifen. Prophylactic tamoxifen or radiotherapy should be considered for men treated with long-term antiandrogen therapy.

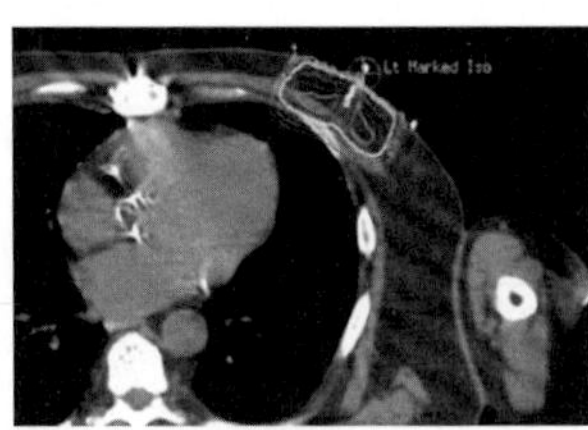

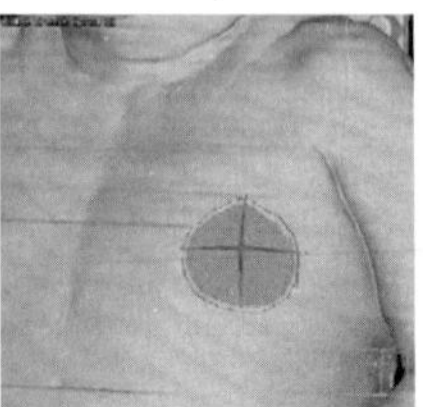

Figure 69.2 Standard electron field for gynecomastia.

DUPUYTREN CONTRACTURE

- Dupuytren contracture, also known as Morbus Dupuytren, is a connective tissue disorder involving the palmar or plantar aponeurosis. This progressive disorder begins with subcutaneous lumps with skin fixation, eventually resulting in periosteal reaction, and connective tissue hardening.
- Eventually, the disorder results in severe flexion contractures of the metacarpophalangeal or proximal interphalangeal joints, limiting the use of the hands or impaired ambulation. The most commonly affected joints are the 4th/5th fingers of the hand and 1st/2nd toes of the foot.

- In more than half of patients, disease progression will occur 5 years after diagnosis. Steroids may be used for small, painful nodules, though the disease will likely progress. Collagenase is effective in patients with limited contractures but with short-term efficacy. If a patient is functionally limited as a consequence of the disorder, surgical intervention is recommended.
- Radiation is typically implemented in the early stages of the disease to limit progression, particularly in patients with asymptomatic lesions or minimal flexion deformities. Doses of 30 Gy in 10 fractions (split course with a 6-week break) or 21 Gy in 3 Gy fractions are used. Targeted disease includes palpable cords and nodules with 1- to 2-cm proximal/distal and 0.5- to 1-cm lateral margins. Orthovoltage (120 kV) or electrons with bolus are used to ensure adequate surface/superficial dose coverage.
- Radiation was able to reduce the risk of progression in a significant number (>70%) of patients with early-stage lesions but rarely resulted in the regression of hallmark lumps and strands. Long-term data demonstrate the most utility for radiation when utilized within the 1st year of diagnosis.

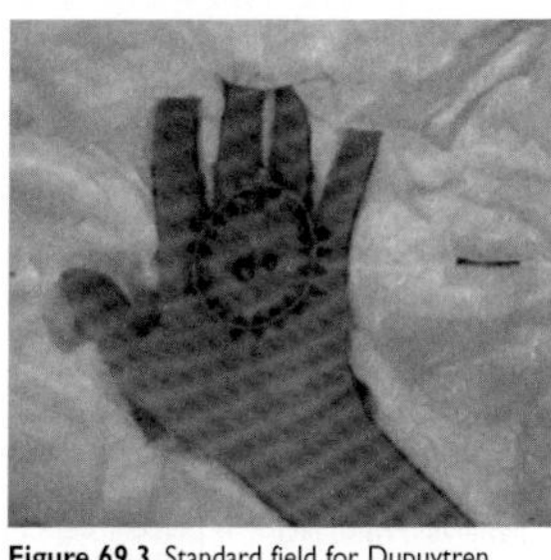

Figure 69.3 Standard field for Dupuytren contracture.

CLINICAL SETUP

CHAD TANG • PETER BALTER

Statements of Calibration

- For each beam, there will be a reference point/geometry for which 1 MU will deliver 1 cGy of dose.
- The most commonly used reference geometries for linear accelerators are source surface distance (SSD) and source axial distance (SAD) (Fig. 70.1):

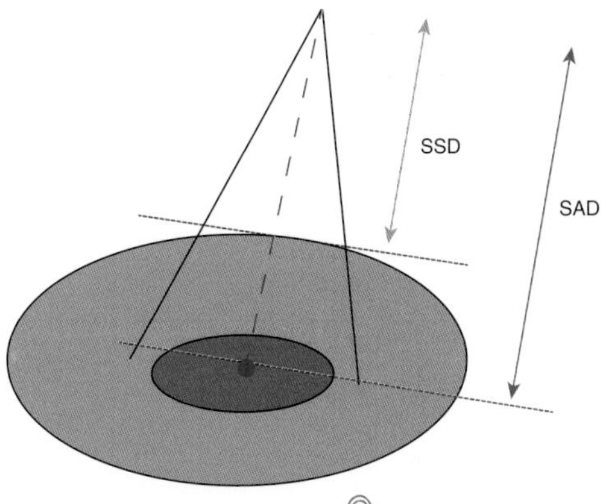

Figure 70.1 Illustration highlighting the difference between SAD and SSD techniques for referencing geometries. Note how the SSD technique maintains constant distance between the source and skin of the patient, whereas the SAD references the isocenter (*maroon spot*).

- SSD: 100 cm to the surface, D_{max} depth for a 10 × 10 cm field 1 MU = 1 cGy (water). Uses constant distance between source and surface/skin. The **patient** is moved for each field.
- SAD: 100 cm to the calculation point, D_{max} depth for a 10 × 10 cm field 1 MU = 1 cGy (water). Uses constant distance between source and the isocenter (100 cm for the modern linear accelerator). The **gantry** is moved for each field.

- If calculations are being done (SSD) and the machine calibration geometry is SSD, PDD tables can be used with no further inverse square corrections.
- If calculations are being done (SAD) and the machine calibration is SAD, the TMR tables can be used with no further inverse square corrections.
- To calculate an SAD setup on a machine with an SSD calibration, multiply the calibration dose rate by the inverse square correction of ((reference SSD + D_{max} Depth)/(reference SSD))^2. This will generally be ((100 + 1.5 cm)/(100 cm))^2 = 1.03 for 6× photons.
- To calculate SSD setup on a machine with an SAD calibration, multiply the calibration dose rate by ((reference SSD)/(reference SSD + D_{max} depth))^2. This will generally be (100 cm)/(10 + 1.5))^2 = 0.971 for 6× photons.

$$MU = \frac{\text{Prescribed Dose per Field}}{\text{Calibration in } \frac{cGy}{MU} \times \text{Depth Factor} \times \text{Field Size Factor} \times \text{Off Axis Factor} \times \text{Beam Attenuation Factor}}$$

- For SSD, depth factor is percent depth dose (%DD)*
- For SAD, depth factors are TMR*
- Field size factors are collimator scatter (Sc) for the jaw setting and phantom scatter (Sp)* for the field size at the reference distance.
- Off-axis factors are presented, but it is not recommended to treat based on hand calculations when using a geometry that requires a significant (>3%) off-axis correction. For nonwedged beams, this is generally true even for significantly off-axis points.
- Beam attenuation factors include wedge factors, tray factors, and other attenuations.

**These factors are usually found in machine-specific tables.*

General Landmarks

- T1: Most prominent posterior process
- T3: Suprasternal notch, root of spine of scapula
- T4: Sternal angle and 2nd rib
- T5: Carina
- T7: Bottom of scapula
- T9: Xiphoid process
- L4: Top of iliac crest
- S2: Posterior superior iliac spine

General Rules

- SAD setup is generally used for photon-based plans to treat deep lesions.
- SSD setup is generally used for electron or orthovoltage-based plans to treat superficial lesions or for single-field treatment.
- Dose falloff: 6 MV ~3.5% per cm; 18 MV ~2.0% per cm
- MU calculations is ~110% of field prescription (eg, prescribe 150 cGy anticipate ~170 MU).
- Agreement between independent calculations must be ±3% (or within 1 MU, whichever is larger).
- If separation <20 cm, consider 6 MV photons.

General Field Setup

First: Decide on setup (SAD vs SSD)
Second: Beam arrangement
Third: Beam energy
Fourth: Treatment depth
Fifth: Field size (X,Y)

- Whole brain: 20 × 20 cm opposed lateral fields covering the entire head, rotate collimator to block face, typical separation 15 ± 2 cm. Expected MUs/field = 166 ± 5 for 300 cGy, 6 MV based on machine calibrated at 100 SSD + D_{max} depth

- Spine: Center field at site of epidural disease or compression, cover 1 vertebral body above and below target vertebral body, expand to cover soft tissue extension, laterally cover 1-2 cm from edge of vertebral body. Review patient records for possible overlap of previous treatment.

General Treatment Plans

	Field(s) Setup	General Doses
Whole brain radiation	L lateral 50%/R lateral 50% prescribed to midplane	30 Gy in 10 fractions
Superior vena cava syndrome	AP 50%/PA 50%	30 Gy in 10 fractions
Painful bone metastasis	AP 50%/PA 50%	30 Gy in 10 fractions or 8 Gy in 1 fractions
Cervical spine	L lateral 50%/R lateral 50%	30 Gy in 10 fractions PA 100% L lateral 50%/R lateral 50% ~50% PA/L lateral ~25%/R lateral ~25%
Thoracic spine	AP ~33%/PA ~67% **OR** PA 100%	
Sacral spine	L lateral 50%/R lateral 50% **OR** AP ~33%/PA ~67% **OR** ~50% PA/L lateral ~25%/R lateral ~25%	
Palpable surface	Electrons	Variable

ABBREVIATIONS

3DCRT	3-D conformal radiation therapy
4DCRT	4-D conformal radiation therapy
4DCT	4D computed tomography
5-FU	fluorouracil
6-MP	mercaptopurine
ABH	lorazepam, diphenhydr-amine, haloperidol
ABMT	autologous bone marrow transplant
ABVD	adriamycin, bleomycin, vinblastine, dacarbazine
AC	adriamycin cyclophosphamide
ACh	acetylcholine
AChE	acetylcholine esterase
ACTH	adrenocorticotropic hormone
ADC	apparent diffusion coefficient
AF	applicator factor
AFP	alpha fetoprotein
AJCC	American Joint Committee on Cancer
ALK	anaplastic lymphoma kinase
ALL	acute lymphoblastic leukemia
ALN	axillary lymph node
ALND	axillary lymph node dissection
AML	acute myelogenous leukemia
AP	anterior-posterior
APBI	accelerated partial breast irradiation
APCs	antigen-presenting cells
APR	abdominoperineal resection
ARR	absolute risk reduction
ASTRO	American Society for Radiation Oncology
ATM	ataxia-telangiectasia mutated
AUA	American Urological Association
AUC	area under curve
AVM	arteriovenous malformation
β-hCG	beta-human chorionic gonadotropin
BCC	basal cell carcinoma
BCL	B-cell lymphoma
BCNU	Carmustine
BCS	breast conserving surgery
BEACOPP	bleomycine, etoposide, doxorubicin (adriamycin), cyclophosphamide, vincristine (oncovin), procarbazine, prednisone
BED	biologically effective dose
BID	two times a day
BI-RADS	breast imaging-reporting and data system
BM	bone marrow
BMBx	bone marrow biopsy
BMI	body mass index
BMT	bone marrow transplant
BOT	base of tongue
BP	blood pressure
BPH	benign prostatic hyperplasia
BSO	bilateral salpingo-oophorectomy
BUN	blood urea nitrogen
Cr	creatinine
C&E	curettage and electrodessication
CAPOX	capecitabine/oxaliplatin
CAR-T	chimeric antigen receptor-T cells
CBC	complete blood count
CBCT	cone beam CT
CCNU	lomustine
CR	clinical response
CCSK	clear cell sarcoma of the kidney
CEA	carcinoembryonic antigen
cEBRT	conventional external beam radiation therapy
CFS	colostomy-free survival
CF-WBI	conventionally fractionated-whole breast irradiation
ChemoRT	chemoradiotherapy
CHF	congestive heart failure
CHT	chemotherapy
CI	conformity index
CIMP	CpG island methylator phenotype
CIN	chromosomal instability
CLL	chronic lymphocytic leukemia
CML	chronic myelogenous leukemia
CMP	comprehensive metabolic panel
CNS	central nervous system
CRM	continual reassessment method
CRPC	castrate resistant prostate cancer
CSF	cerebrospinal fluid
CSI	craniospinal irradiation
CSS	cancer specific survival
CT	computed tomography
CTCL	cutaneous T-cell lymphoma
CTV	clinical target volume
CV	cardiovascular
CW	chest wall
CXR	chest X-ray
DA	dose-adjusted
DAMPs	damage-associated molecu-lar patterns
DCIS	ductal carcinoma in-situ
DD	death dose
ddAC	dose-dense AC
DE-EBRT	dose-escalated external beam radiation therapy
DES	diethylstilbestrol

DEXA	dual-energy X-ray absorptiometry
DFS	disease-free survival
DHL	double-hit lymphoma
DIBH	deep inspiration breath hold
DIPG	diffuse intrinsic pontine gliomas
DLBCL	diffuse large B-cell lymphoma
DM	distant metastasis
DMFS	distant metastasis free survival
DMSO	dimethyl sulfoxide
DNA	deoxyribonucleic acid
DNA-PKcs	DNA-dependent protein kinases
DOI	depth of invasion
DPFS	distant progression free survival
DRE	digital rectal exam
DRR	digitally reconstructed radiography
DSB	double strand break
DS-GPA	diagnosis-specific graded prognostic assessment
DSS	disease specific survival
DTPA	diethylenetriaminepentacetate
DVH	dose-volume histogram
DWI	diffusion-weighted imaging
DX	diagnosis
EBCTCG	Early Breast Cancer Trialists' Collaborative Group
EBRT	external beam radiation therapy
EBUS	endobronchial ultrasound
EBV	Epstein–Barr virus
ECC	epirubicin, cisplatin, capecitabine
ECE	extracapsular extension
ECF	epirubicin, cisplatin, 5-fluorouracil
ECG	electrocardiogram
ECOG	Eastern Cooperative Oncology Group
EFRT	extended field radiation therapy
EFS	event-free survival
EFT	Ewing family of tumors
EGD	esophagogastroduodenoscopy
EGFR	epidermal growth factor receptor
EGFR-MAPK	EGFR-mitogen activated protein kinase
EI-CESS	European Intergroup Cooperative Ewing Sarcoma Studies
ENE	extranodal extension
EOC	epirubicin, oxalipatin, capecitabine
EORTC	European Organisation for Research and Treatment of Cancer
EPID	electronic portal imaging device
EPP	extrapleural pneumonectomy
EQD2	equivalent dose at 2 Gy
ER	estrogen receptor
ERCP	endoscopic retrograde cholangiopancreatography
ESBC	early stage breast cancer
ESMO	European Society of Medical Oncology
ESR	erythrocyte sedimentation rate
ES-SCLC	extensive stage small cell lung cancer
ETV	evaluation target volume
EUA	examination under anesthesia
EUS	endoscopic ultrasound
EWS	Ewing Sarcoma
FA	focal anaplasia
FAC	fluorouracil, adriamycin, and cyclophosphamide
FAP	familial adenomatous polyposis
FAS-L	Fas ligand
FB	free breathing
FDA	Food and Drug Administration
FDG	fludeoxyglucose
FEV1	forced expiratory volume (1 second)
FGFR	fibroblast growth factor receptors
FH	favorable histology
FIGO	International Federation of Gynecology and Obstetrics
FISH	fluorescence in-situ hybridization
FLAIR	fluid-attenuation inversion recovery
FLIPI	Follicular Lymphoma International Prognostic Index
FNA	fine needle aspiration
FOLFIRINOX	folinic acid, fluorouracil, irinotecan, oxaliplatin
FOLFOX	folinic acid, fluorouracil, oxaliplatin
FOV	field-of-view
FSH	follicle-stimulating hormone
GBM	glioblastoma multiforme
GCB	germinal center B-cell
G-CSF	granulocyte-colony-stimulating factor
GCT	germ cell tumor

GEJ	gastroesophageal junction
GEP	gene expression profiling
GERD	gastroesophageal reflux disease
GFAP	glial fibrillary acidic protein
GH	growth hormone
GHSG	German Hodgkin Study Group
GI	gastrointestinal
GIST	gastrointestinal stromal tumor
GM-CSF	granulocyte-macrophage colony-stimulating factor
GnRH	gonadotropin releasing hormone
GOG	Gynecologic Oncology Group
GS	genomically stable
GTR	gross total resection
GTV	gross tumor value
GU	genitourinary
GVHD	graft versus host disease
H&N	head and Neck
H&P	history and physical examination
HA	hinge angle
HAV	hepatitis A virus
HBsAg	hepatitis B surface antigen
HBV	hepatitis B virus
HCC	hepatocellular carcinoma
HDAC	histone deacetylase
HDR	high dose rate
HF-WBI	hypofractionated whole breast irradiation
HGG	high-grade glioma
HIV	human immunodeficiency virus
HL	Hodgkin lymphoma
HLA	human leukocyte antigen
HNC	head and neck cancer
HNPCC	hereditary nonpolyposis colorectal cancer
HNSCC	head and neck squamous cell carcinoma
HO	heterotopic ossification
HPV	human papilloma virus
HPV16	human papilloma virus16
HR	hazard ratio
HR-CTV	high risk clinical target volume
HSCT	hematopoietic stem cell transplantation
HSV-1	herpes simplex virus type 1
HTN	hypertension
HVA	homovanillic acid
HVL	half-value layer
HVLT-R	Hopkins Verbal Learning Test-Revised
IAC	internal auditory canal
IBC	inflammatory breast cancer
IBD	inflammatory bowel disease
IBTR	ipsilateral breast tumor recurrence
ICBT	intracavitary brachytherapy
ICP	intracranial pressure
ICRP	International Commission on Radiological Protection
ICRT	intracavitary radiation therapy
ICRU	International Commission on Radiation Units and Measurements
iCTV	internal clinical target volume
ICV	infraclavicular
IDH	isocitrate dehydrogenase
IDL	isodose line
IFNγ	interferon-gamma
IFRT	involved-field radiotherapy
IGBT	image-guided brachytherapy
IGF-1	insulin growth factor 1
IGRT	image-guided radiation therapy
iGTV	internal gross tumor volume
IHC	immunohistochemistry
IJROBP	International Journal of Radiation Oncology, Biology, Physics
IJV	internal jugular vein
IL	interleukin
IL-2	interleukin 2
ILROG	International Lymphoma Radiation Oncology Group
IM	internal mammary / internal margin
IMA	internal mammary artery
IMC	internal mammary chain
iMLD	ipsilateral mean lung dose
IMN	internal mammary nodes
IMPT	intensity modulated proton therapy
IMRT	intensity-modulated radiation therapy
INR	international normalized ratio
INRT	involved nodal radiation therapy
INSS	International Neuroblastoma Staging System
IPI	International Prognostic Index
IPS	International Prognostic Score
IPSS	International Prostate Symptom Score
IR	interventional radiology
IRB	Institutional Review Board
ISRT	involved site radiation therapy
ISUP	International Society of Urologic Pathologist
ITC	isolated tumor cell
ITV	internal target volume
iTVI	internal tumor vessel interface
IUGR	intrauterine growth restriction
IV	intravenous / irradiated volume

IVF	in vitro fertilization
IVLBCL	intravascular large B-cell lymphoma
JPA	juvenile pilocytic astrocytoma
KPS	Karnofksy Performance Status
KUB	kidney, ureter, and bladder
KV	kilovoltage
LABC	locally advanced breast cancer
LAO	left anterior oblique
LAR	low anterior resection
LC	local control
LDH	lactate dehydrogenase
LDR	low dose rate
LDR-PB	low dose rate prostate brachytherapy
LET	linear energy transfer
LF	local failure
LFTs	liver function tests
LGG	low grade glioma
LH	luteinizing hormone
LHRH	luteinizing hormone-releasing hormone
LINAC	linear accelerator
LMD	leptomeningeal disease
LN	lymph node
LND	lymph node dissection
LOET	late onset efftox model
LOH	loss of heterozygosity
LP	lumbar puncture
LR	local recurrence
LRC	locoregional control
LRF	locoregional failure
LRFS	locoregional failure survival
LRR	local recurrence rate
LSS	limb-sparing surgery
LS-SCLC	limited-stage small cell lung cancer
LUL	left upper lobe
LV	left ventricle
LVI	lymphovascular invasion
LVSI	lymphovascular stromal invasion
MALT	mucosa associated lymphoid tissue
MCC	Merkel cell carcinoma
MCL	mantle cell lymphoma
MCPyV	Merkel cell polyoma virus
mCRC	metastatic colorectal cancer
mCRPC	metastatic castrate resistant prostate cancer
MDACC	MD Anderson Cancer Center
MDP	methylene diphosphonate
MDR	medium dose rate
MDS	myelodysplastic syndrome
MDSC	myeloid-derived suppressor cells
MEC	mucoepidermoid carcinoma
MEN-1	multiple endocrine neoplasia type 1
MEN2	multiple endocrine neoplasia type 2
MESCC	metastatic epidural spinal cord compression
MF	mycosis fungoides
MFO	multi-field optimization
MGMT	O^6-alkylguanine DNA alkyltransferase
MHC	major histocompatibility complex
MIBG	meta-iodobenzylguanidine
MIP	maximum intensity projection
MIPI	MCL International Prognostic Index
MLB	multi-lumen balloon
MLD	metachromatic leukodystrophy
MMC	mitomycin C
MMG	mammogram
MMMT	malignant mixed Müllerian tumor
MMR	mediastinal mass ratio
MMT	mixed malignant tumors
MOPP	mechlorethamine, vincristine, procarbazine, prednisone
MRCP	magnetic resonance cholangiopancreatography
MRI	magnetic resonance imaging
MRM	modified radical mastectomy
mRNA	messenger RNA
MS	multiple sclerosis
MSI	microsatellite instability
MSKCC	Memorial Sloan Kettering Cancer Center
MTD	maximal tolerated dose
MTV	mucosal target volume
MTX	methotrexate
MUGA	multigated acquisition scan
MVA	multivariable analysis
MVAC	methotrexate, vinblastine, adriamycin and cisplatin
MyoD1	myogenic differentiation 1
NAC	neoadjuvant chemotherapy
NASH	nonalcoholic steatohepatitis
NB	neuroblastoma
NCCN	National Comprehensive Cancer Network
NCCTG	North Central Cancer Treatment Group
NCDB	National Cancer Database
NCIC	National Cancer Information Center
NEJM	New England Journal of Medicine
NF	neurofibromatosis
NF1	neurofibromatosis type 1
NGGCT	non-germinomatous GCT
NHEJ	non-homologous end-joining
NHL	non-Hodgkin lymphoma
NK	natural killer
NLPHL	nodular lymphocyte predominant Hodgkin lymphoma
NMSC	non-melanoma skin cancer

NNT	number needed to treat
NPC	nasopharyngeal carcinoma
NPO	nothing by mouth
NPV	negative predictive value
NSABP	National Surgical Adjuvant Breast and Bowel Project
NSAID	non-steroidal anti-inflammatory drug
NSCLC	non-small cell lung cancer
NSHL	nodular sclerosing Hodgkin lymphoma
NTCP	normal tissue complication probability
NTR	near-total resection
NWTS	National Wilms' Tumor Society
OAR	organs at risk
OER	oxygen enhancement ratio
OF	output factor
OPC	oropharyngeal cancer
OR	odds ratio
OS	overall survival
OTC	over the counter
PA	posterior-anterior
PAI	pubic arch interference
PALCL	primary anaplastic large cell lymphoma
PAMPs	pathogen associated molecular patterns
PARP	poly(ADP)ribose polymerase
PBI	partial breast irradiation
PC	posterior commissure
PCA	prostate cancer
PCFCL	primary cutaneous follicle center lymphoma
PCI	prophylactic cranial irradiation
PCLBCL	primary cutaneous diffuse large B-cell lymphoma
PCMZL	primary cutaneous marginal zone B-cell lymphoma
PCNSL	primary central nervous system lymphoma
PCOS	polycystic ovarian syndrome
PCP	primary care physician
PCR	polymerase chain reaction
PCV	procarbazine, lomustine, vincristine
PD	progressive disease
PD-1	programmed cell death protein 1
PDAC	pancreatic ductal adenocarcinoma
PDD	percent depth dose
PDGF	platelet-derived growth factor
PDGFR	platelet-derived growth factor receptor
PD-L1	programmed death-ligand 1
PDR	pulsed dose rate
PE	photoelectric effect
PEG	percutaneous endoscopic gastrostomy
PeIN	penile intraepithelial neoplasia
PET	positron emission tomography
PFS	progression-free survival
PFT	pulmonary function test
PGI	prompt gamma imaging
PLAP	placental alkaline phosphatase
PLT	platelet
PMBCL	primary mediastinal B-cell lymphoma
PMN	polymorphonuclear cell
PMRT	postmastectomy radiation therapy
PNA	pneumonia
PNET	primitive neuroectodermal tumor
PNI	perineural invasion
PNS	peripheral nervous system
PO	by mouth
PORT	post-operative radiation therapy
PP	pair production
PPI	proton pump inhibitor
PPV	positive predictive value
PR	partial response
PR/SD	partial response/stable disease
PRL	prolactin
PRN	as needed
PRV	planning risk volume
PS	performance status
PSA	prostate specific antigen
PSPT	passive scattering proton therapy
pSV	pathologic seminal vesicle specimen
PTC	percutaneous trans-hepatic cholangiography
pts	patients
PTV	planning target volume
QA	quality assurance
QD	every day
QOD	every other day
QOL	quality of life
QUANTEC	quantitative analyses of normal tissue effects in the clinic
RAI	radioactive iodine
RAO	right anterior oblique
RB	retinoblastoma
RBC	red blood cell
RBE	relative biological effectiveness
RCC	renal cell carcinoma
R-CHOP	rituximab-cyclophosphamide, doxorubicin, vincristine, prednisone
RCT	randomized controlled trial
RDL	recommended dose level
RF	radiofrequency
RFA	radiofrequency ablation
RFS	recurrence/relapse-free survival

RHDVRT	reduced high-dose volume radiation therapy
RILD	radiation induced liver disease
R-MPV	rituximab, methotrexate, procarbazine, and vincristine
RMS	rhabdomyosarcoma
RNI	regional nodal irradiation
ROI	region of interest
RP	retroperitoneal
RPA	recursive partitioning analysis
RPLND	retroperitoneal lymph node dissection
RPO	right posterior oblique
RR	risk ratio or relative risk
RT	radiation therapy
RTK	rhabdoid tumor of the kidney
RTOG	Radiation Therapy Oncology Group
RT-PCR	real-time PCR
SABR	stereotactic ablative radiotherapy
SAD	source axial distance
SBC	secondary breast cancer
SBO	small bowel obstruction
SBRT	stereotactic body radiation therapy
SC	short course
SCC	squamous cell carcinoma
SCD	source to calibration distance
SCLC	small-cell lung cancer
SCM	sternocleidomastoid
SCT	stem-cell transplantation
SCV	supraclavicular
SD	stable disease
SEER	surveillance, epidemiology, and end results
SEP	solitary extramedullary plasmacytoma
SERD	selective estrogen receptor degrader
SERM	selective estrogen receptor modulator
SF	single fraction
SFO	single field optimization
SHH	sonic hedgehog
SHIM	sexual health inventory for men
SI	sacroiliac
SIADH	syndrome of inappropriate antidiuretic hormone secretion
SIB	simultaneous integrated boost
SIM	simulation
SINS	spine instability neoplastic score
SIOP	International Society of Paediatric Oncology
SIR	score index for radiosurgery
SLL	small lymphocytic lymphoma
SLN	sentinel lymph node
SLNB	sentinel lymph node biopsy
SLND	sentinel lymph node dissection
SM	setup margin / surgical margin
SMA	superior mesenteric artery
SMN	second malignancy
SMV	superior mesenteric vein
SNEC	small cell neuroendocrine carcinoma
SNL	sentinel lymph node
SNUC	sinonasal undifferentiated carcinoma
SOB	shortness of breath
SOBP	spread-out Bragg peak
SOD	superoxide dismutase
SPB	solitary plasmacytoma of bone
SPD	source to point distance
SRS	stereotactic radiosurgery
SRT	stereotactic radiotherapy
SSBs	single strand breaks
SSD	source surface distance
SSRS	spine stereotactic radiosurgery
STD	sexually transmitted disease
STIR	short T1 inversion recovery
STR	subtotal resection
STS	soft tissue sarcoma
STV	scanning target volume
SUV	standardized uptake value
SV	seminal vesicle
SVC	superior vena cava
SVI	seminal vesicle involvement
TACE	transcatheter arterial chemoembolization
TAH	total abdominal hysterectomy
TAM	tamoxifen
TBI	tolerance by inhibiting
TCGA	The Cancer Genome Atlas
TCHP	paclitaxel, carboplatin, herceptin, pertuzumab
TCR	T-cell receptor
TG	Tamifen, Genox
THP	paclitaxel, herceptin, pertuzumab
TID	three times a day
TIL	tumor infiltrating lymphocyte
TKI	tyrosine kinase inhibitor
TLD	thermoluminescent dosimetry
TLH	total laparoscopic hysterectomy
TLM	transoral laser microsurgery
TME	total mesorectal excision
TMR	tissue maximum ratio
TMZ	temozolamide
TNBC	triple-negative breast cancer

TNF	tumor necrosis factor
TNM	tumor, nodes, metastasis classification system
ToGA	trastuzumab for gastric cancer
TORS	transoral robotic surgery
TPF	docetaxel, cisplatin, fluorouracil
TRUS	transrectal ultrasound
TS	tumor size
TSEBT	total skin electron beam therapy
TSH	thyroid stimulating hormone
TTF	tumor-treating fields
TTP	time to progression
TURBT	transurethral resection of bladder tumor
TURP	transurethral resection of the prostate
TV	treated volume
TVI	tumor vessel interface
TVL	tenth-value layer
UA	urinalysis
UH	unfavorable histology
UPS	undifferentiated pleomorphic sarcoma
URI	upper respiratory infection
US	ultrasound
USPSTF	United States Preventive Services Task Force
UTI	urinary tract infection
UV	ultraviolet
VAA	vincristine/actinomycin D/adriamycin
VAC	vincristine/dactinomycin/cyclophosphamide
VATS	video-assisted thoracic surgery
VBT	vaginal brachytherapy
VCE	vincristine/carboplatin/etoposide
VDC	vincristine/doxorubicin/cyclophosphamide
VDC/IE	vincristine/doxorubicin/cyclophosphamide (VDC) alternating w/ ifosfamide/etoposide (IE)
VEGF	vascular endothelial growth factor
vGTV	virtual gross tumor volume
VIP	VP-16/ifosfamide/cisplatin
VMA	vanillylmandelic acid
VMAT	volumetric-modulated arc therapy
VOD	veno-occlusive disease
VTE	venous thromboembolism
WA	wedge angle
WAGR	WT, aniridia, GU malformations, retardation
WAI	whole abdomen irradiation
WART	whole pelvic radiation therapy
WBC	white blood cell count
WBI	whole breast irradiation
WBRT	whole brain radiation therapy
WF	weighting factor
WHO	World Health Organization
WLE	wide local excision
WPRT	whole-pelvis RT
WT	Wilms tumor
WV-PTV	whole ventricular planning target volume
WVRT	whole ventricle RT
XRT	radiation therapy

INDEX

Page numbers followed by a "f" denote figures; those followed by a "t" denote tables.

E

M

N

P

R

X

Z

BT 2-2

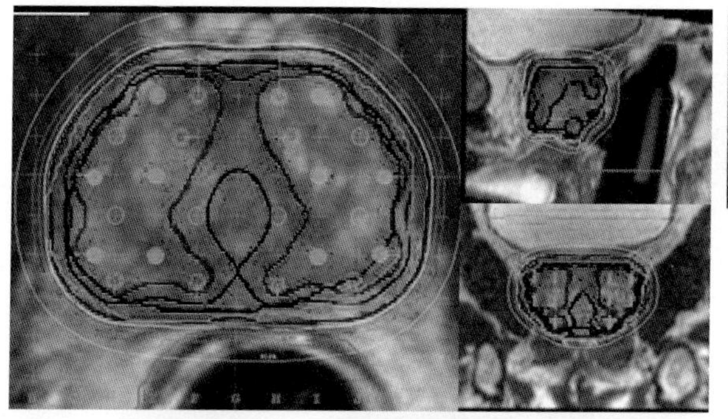

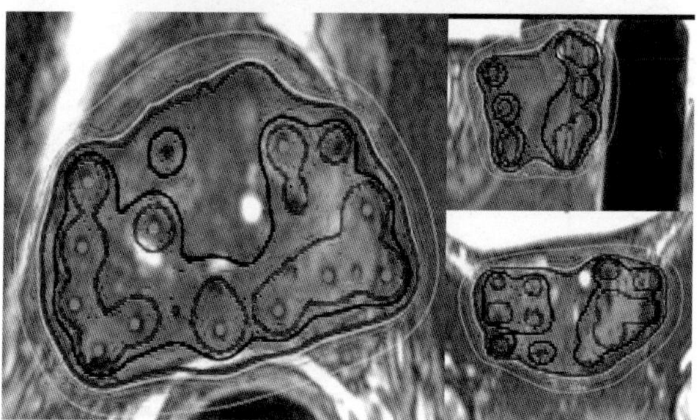

Figure 6.1: example MRI LDR Preplan (left side) and D0 plan for 144 Gy I-125 brachytherapy monotherapy implant to treat intermediate risk prostate cancer. Showing the 100%, 150% and 200% isodose lines.

PT 2-7

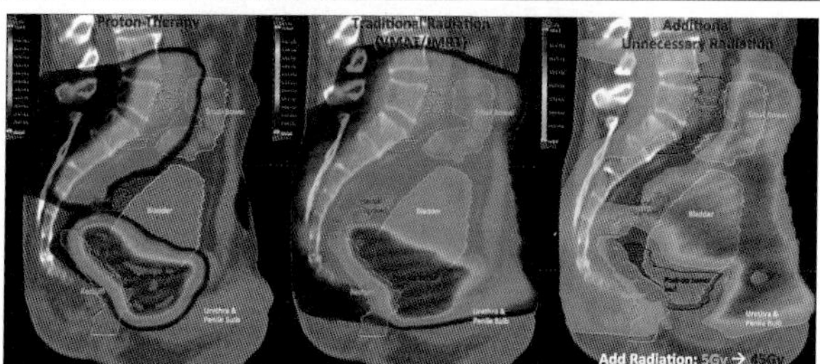

Figure 7.2: Comparitive plan showing intensity modulated proton therapy (left) versus a VMAT/IMRT plan (middle). Excess radiation dose (right) is calculated by subtracting the proton therapy plan from the VMAT/IMRT plan.

HGG 3-6

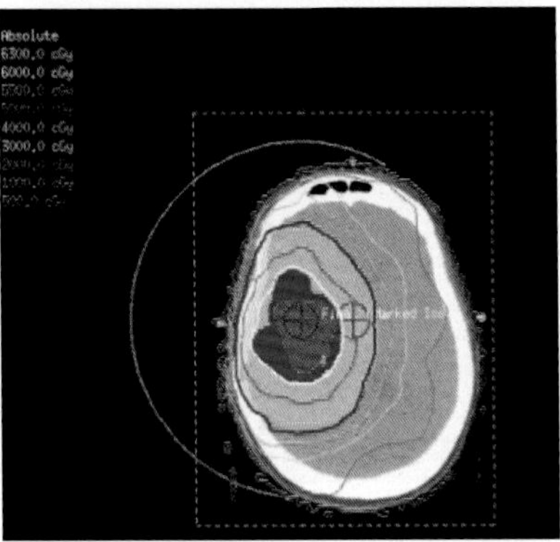

Figure 12.2: Representative plan for a patient with a grade IV glioblastoma. The 60 Gy isodose line (white) can be seen surrounding the red GTV/resection cavity (red colorwash). The 50 Gy isodose line (blue) covers GTV+2cm (tan colorwash) which is expanded to include hyperintense signal on T2Flair sequence.

OC 5-2

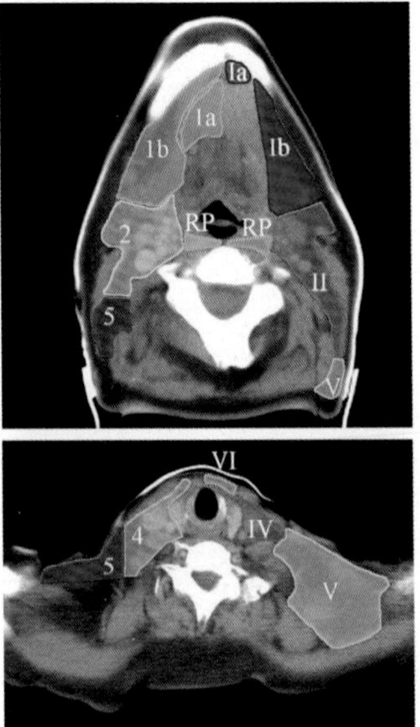

Figure 25.2: Axial CT images showing LN levels at the lower edge of the mandible (upper pane) and low neck (lower pane). Images adapted from Gregoire et al. *Radiother and Onc* 2003.

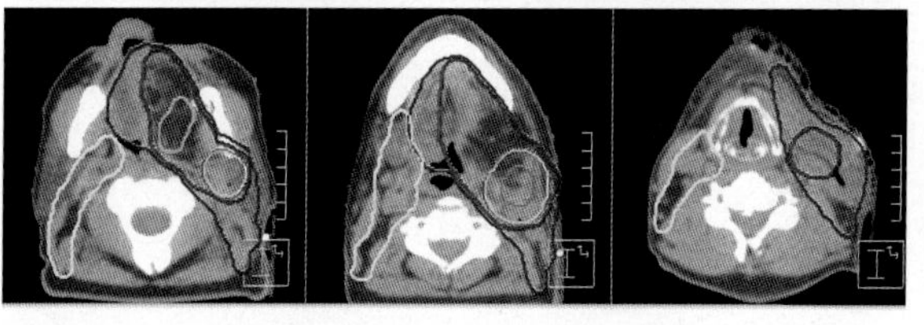

Figure 25.3: 64yo with a resected pT2N2a (4.5cm LN with ECE) SCC of the oral tongue reconstructed with a pectoralis flap treated with chemoRT. GTV (green), GTV-N (forest green), CTV63 (aqua), CTV60 (red), CTV57 (blue), CTV54 (yellow) in 30 fractions

THYROID 5-28

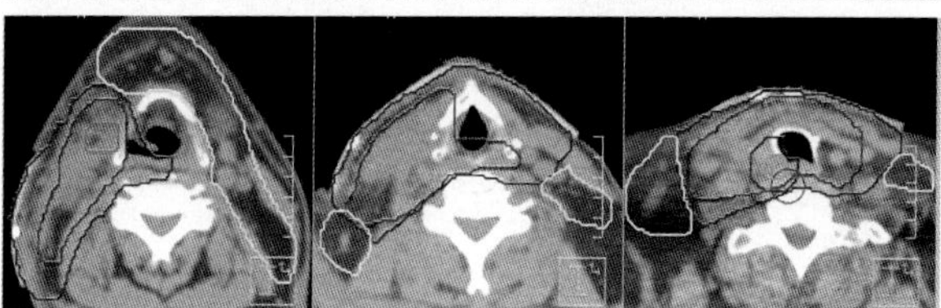

Figure 30.1: 74yo with 4 previous resections for papillary thyroid cancer. Following surgery, he was found to have a 3cm right level II node with ECE, 2/10 level right level III nodes up to 2cm as well as a right tracheal sidewall mass resected with SM+. Contours shown are GTV-LN (green), CTV63 (purple), CTV60 (red), CTV57 (blue), CTV54 (yellow). Treatment was delivered utilizing simultaneous integrated boost in 30 fractions

UHNP 5-31

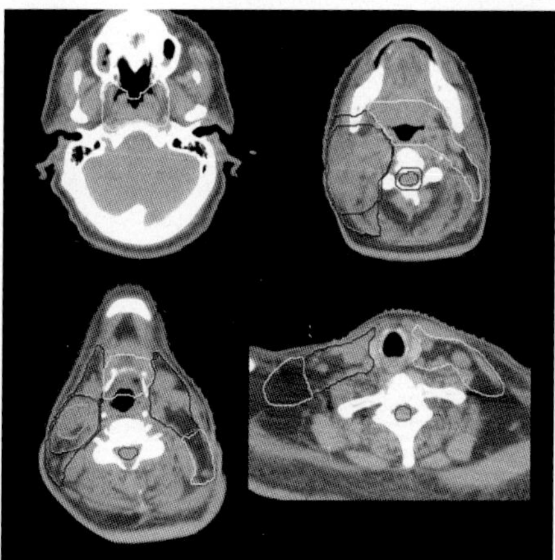

Figure 31.1: Target volumes for CUP with metastasis to left LN level II-III, showing CTV_{HD} (red), CTV_{ID}(blue) and CTV_{ED} (yellow).

SCLC 6-10

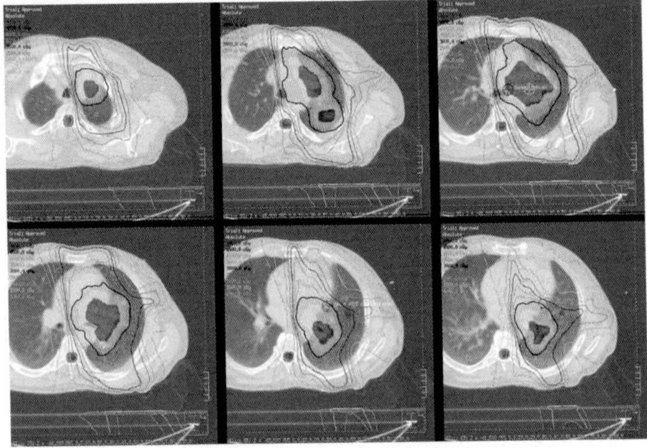

Figure 34.3: Limited Stage SCLC IMRT Plan. 45 Gy isodose line showed in blue surrounding PTV (sky blue colorwash), CTV (tan), and GTV (red). Note sparing of contralateral lung.

ESOPHAGEAL 6-23

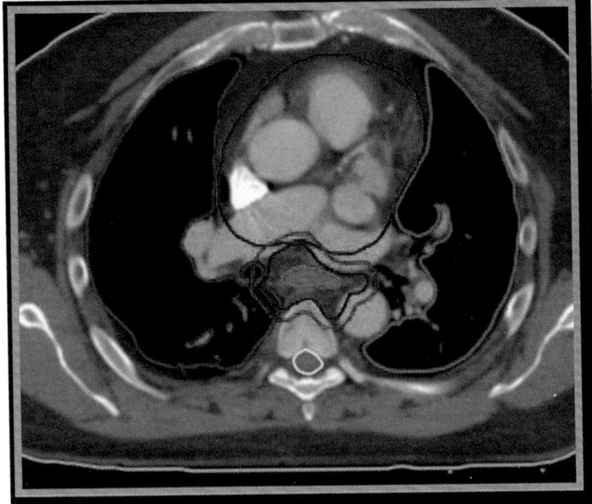

Figure 37.2: Representative cross-sectional image illustrating typical contours for an esophageal adenocarcinoma patient. GTV, CTV, and PTV contours showed in orange, red, and pink, respectively.

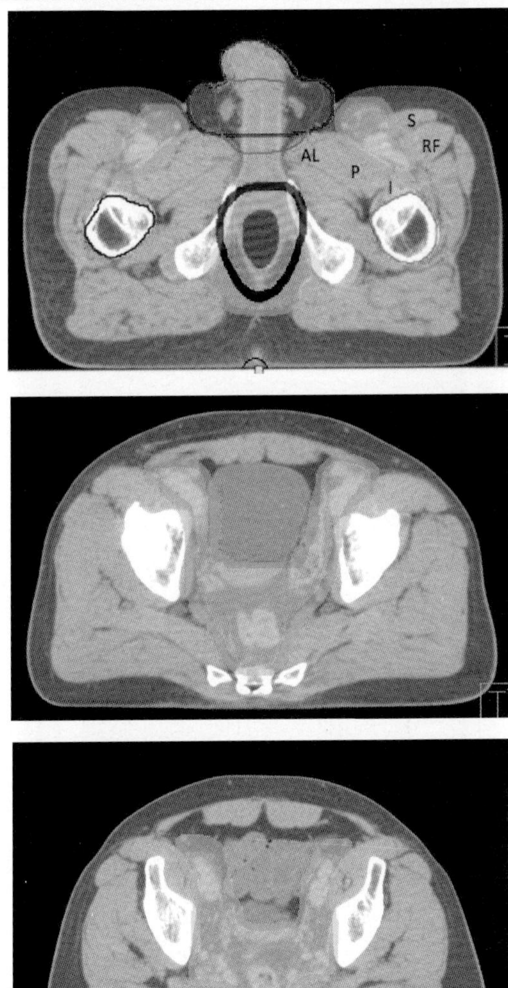

Figure 39.1: RTOG Atlas (used for RTOG 0529) https://www.rtog.org/CoreLab/ContouringAtlases/Anorectal.aspx (Australasian GI Trials Group Atlas: Ng et al, Int J *Radiat Oncol Biol Phys*, 2012.; Inguinal Nodal Atlas: Kim et al, *Pract Rad Onc*, 2012.)

PC 7-11

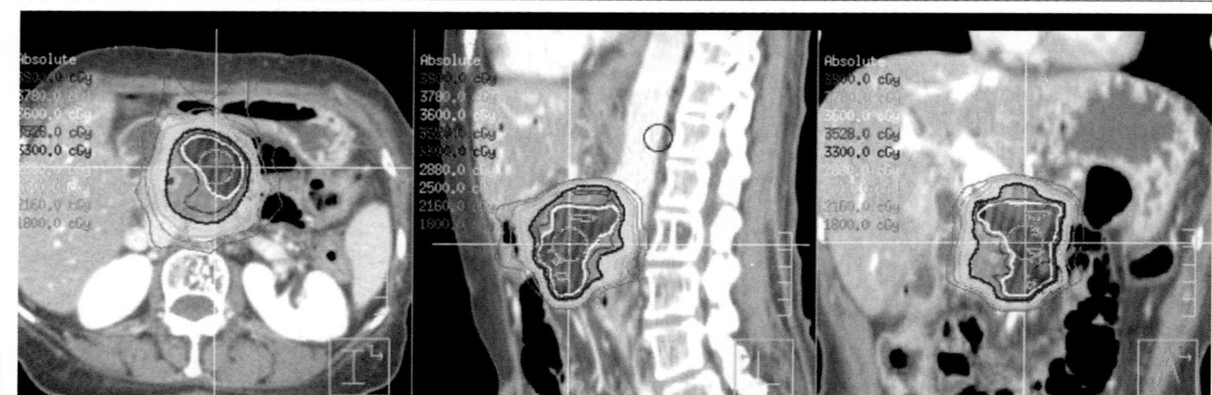

Figure 40.1: Representative cross sectional axial, sagittal and coronal images (L→R) from a SBRT treatment plan for locally advanced pancreatic cancer. The white isodose line represents 36 Gy encompassing the red colorwash which delineates PTV3 (tumor vessel interface minus PRV). The sky blue isodose line represents 25 Gy which is encompassing the yellow contour that represents PTV1 (gross tumor + TVI + 3 mm). This patient had fiducials placed which was used daily for image guidance along with CBCT.

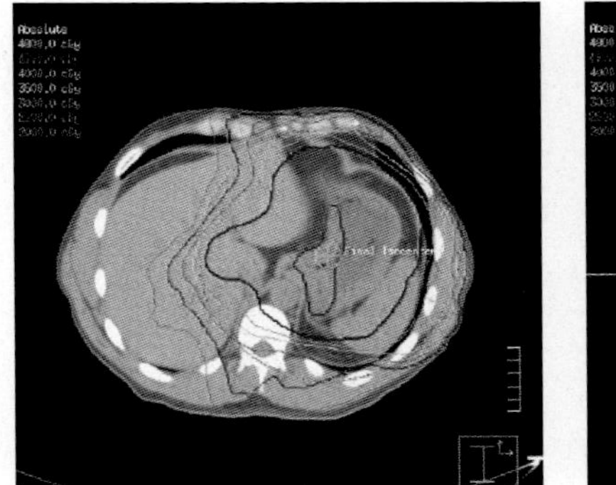

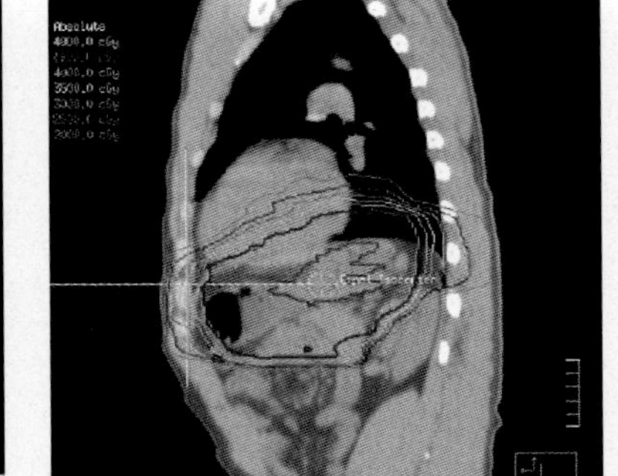

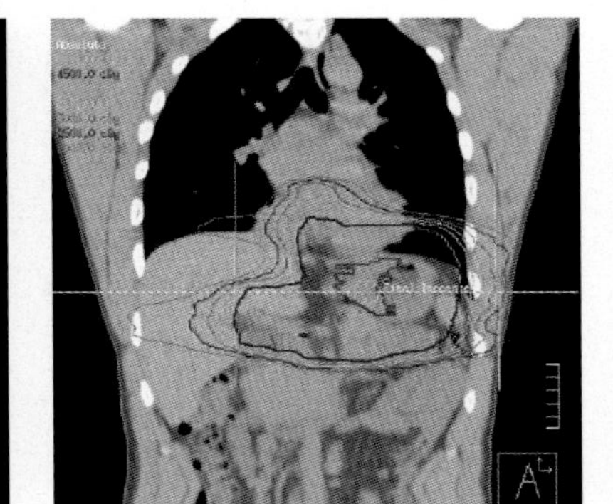

Figure 41.2: Representative axial, sagittal, and coronal cross-sectional images (L→R) illustrating a typically IMRT treatment plan for pre-operative radiation for gastric adenocarcinoma. The 45 Gy isodose line is shown in blue which encompasses the MTV (red line), involved and elective nodes, with a 1 cm expansion. This patient's primary tumor was located at the GEJ extending 4 cm into the cardia.

LABC 8-11

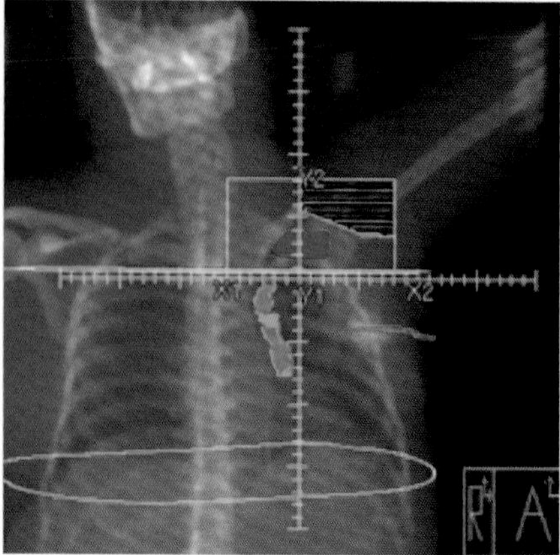

Figure 46.1: Supraclavicular/Infraclavicular Field Design: DRR matched to non-divergent tangent fields. Contours: Blue, Level III axilla on DRR; Green, IM nodes in 1st 3 interspaces; Orange, Mastectomy scar. Lines: Yellow, Superior and inferior borders of tangent fields. Blocks: Purple, Humeral head block

LABC 8-11

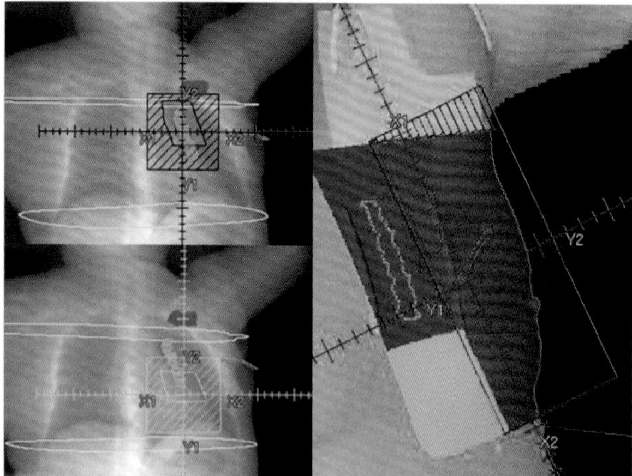

Figure 46.2: IMC Field Design: DRRs and skin rendering matched to non-divergent tangent fields and SCV field. Contours: Blue, Level III axilla on DRR; Green, IM nodes in 1st 3 interspaces; Orange, Mastectomy scar. Lines: Yellow, Superior and inferior borders of tangent fields. Fields: Yellow, AP oblique SCV field; Purple/Aqua, appositional upper and lower IMC fields; Red, Medial tangent field

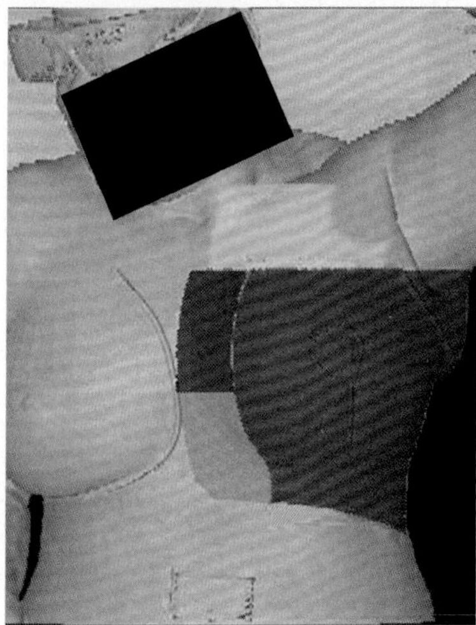

Figure 46.2: Composite Skin Rendering of Comprehensive Treatment Fields (w/o Boost). Fields: Yellow, AP oblique SCV field; Purple/Orange, appositional upper and lower IMC fields; Red/Aqua, Medial and lateral tangent fields

PC 9-8

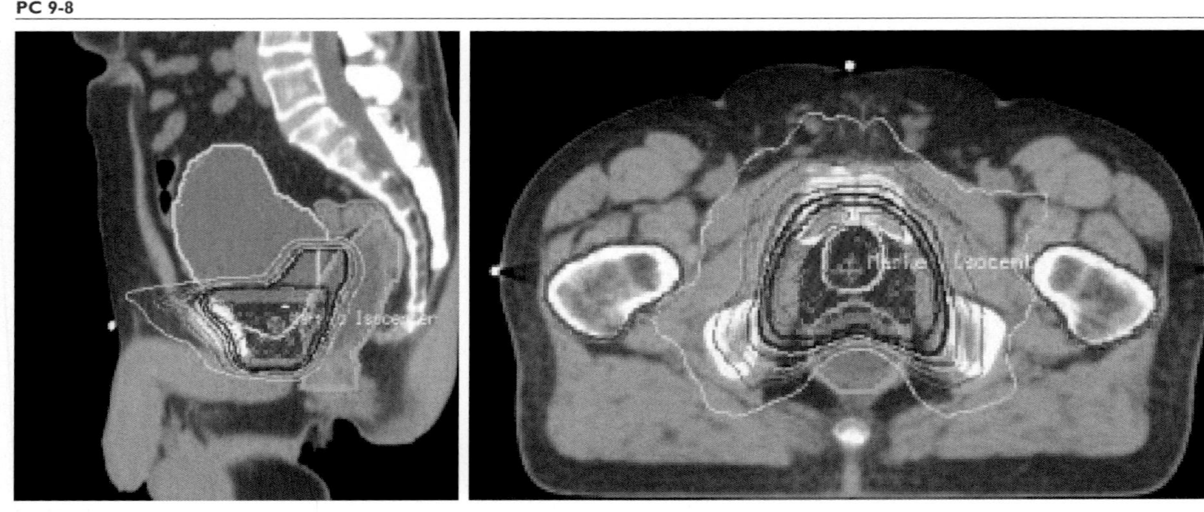

Figure 49.1: Sagittal and axial views showing an RT plan treating the prostate fossa to 70 Gy (blue colorwash) and SV fossa (yellow colorwash) to 63 Gy.

BC 9-11

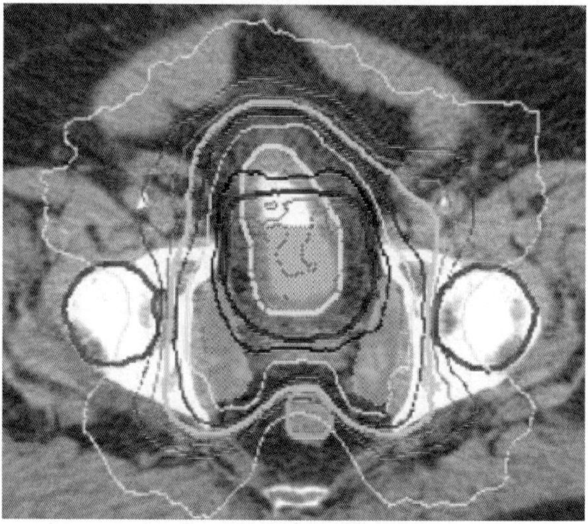

Figure 50.2: IMRT bladder conservation radiation plan treating to 45 Gy (blue isodose line) in 25 fractions to LNs and whole bladder followed by a sequential boost to the bladder resection cavity to 64.8 Gy (red isodose line) in 26 fractions.

CC 10-3

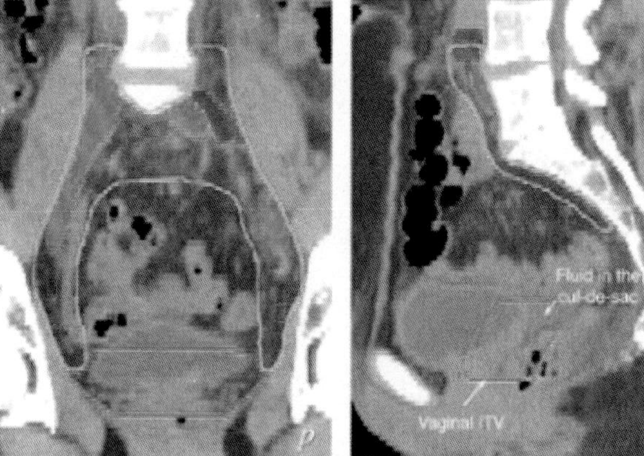

Figure 53.2: Aqua blue contour line in coronal (left) and sagittal (right) planes representing target lymph nodes in a post-operative cervical cancer case that was treated with IMRT. Note the vaginal ITV in turquoise. *Adopted from Eifel and Klopp, Gynecologic Radiation Oncology, a practical guide.*

EC 10-7

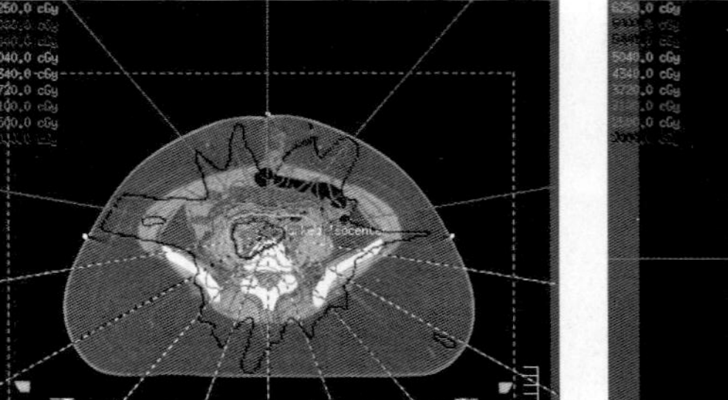

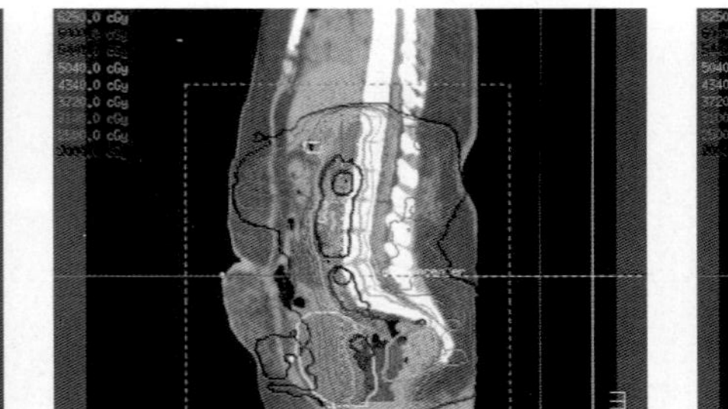

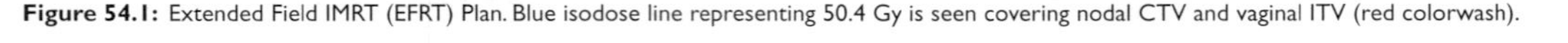

Figure 54.1: Extended Field IMRT (EFRT) Plan. Blue isodose line representing 50.4 Gy is seen covering nodal CTV and vaginal ITV (red colorwash).

VC 10-13

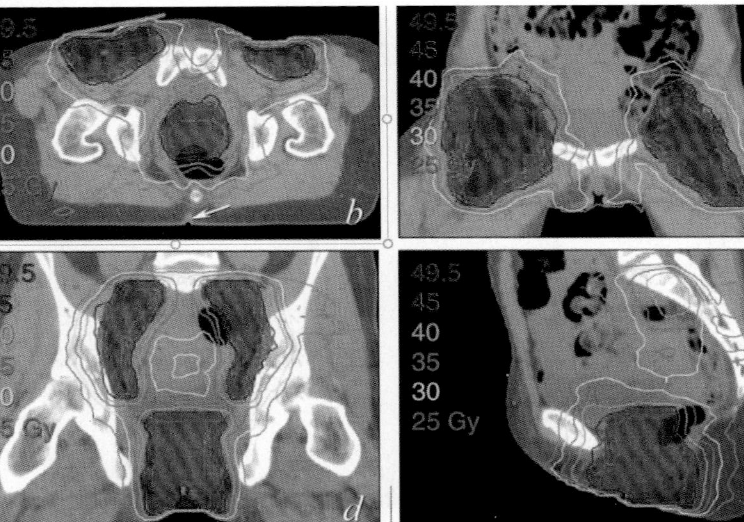

Figure 56.1: Representative treatment plan illustrating coverage of classical CTV (red colorwash) and PTV (purple colorwash) volumes for a vulvar cancer patient undergoing IMRT. *Adopted from Eifel and Klopp, Gynecologic Radiation Oncology, a practical guide.*

STS 11-2

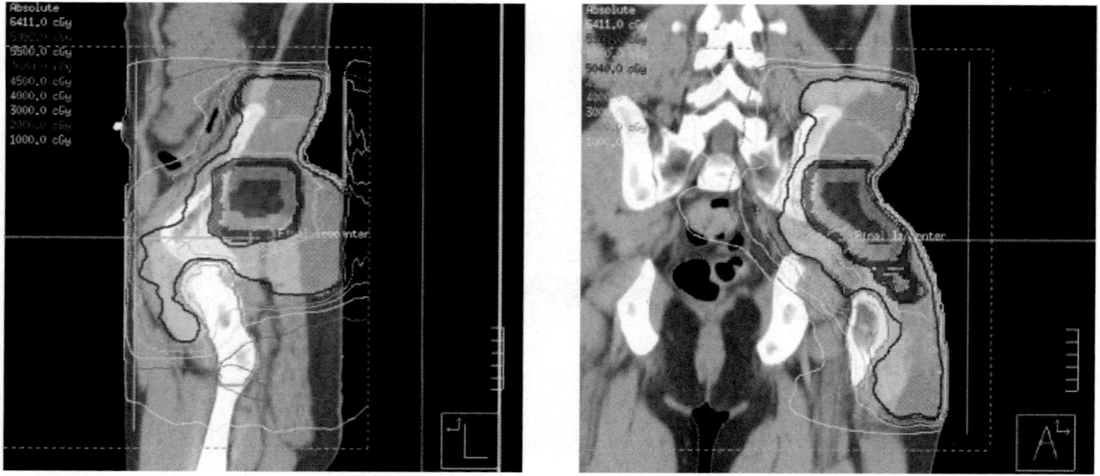

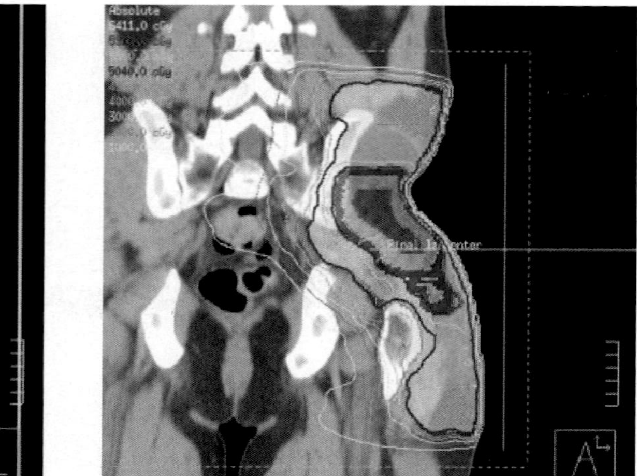

Figure 58.1: Representative sagittal and coronal (L→R) images of an IMRT treatment plan for a 40 y/o male being treated with adjuvant RT following R0 resection of a grade III PNET of the left lower extremity. Using IMRT in this case allowed for reduced dose to the left femoral head/proximal femur. The red isodose line represents 59.92 Gy (covering GTV) and blue represents 50.40 Gy (covering CTV).

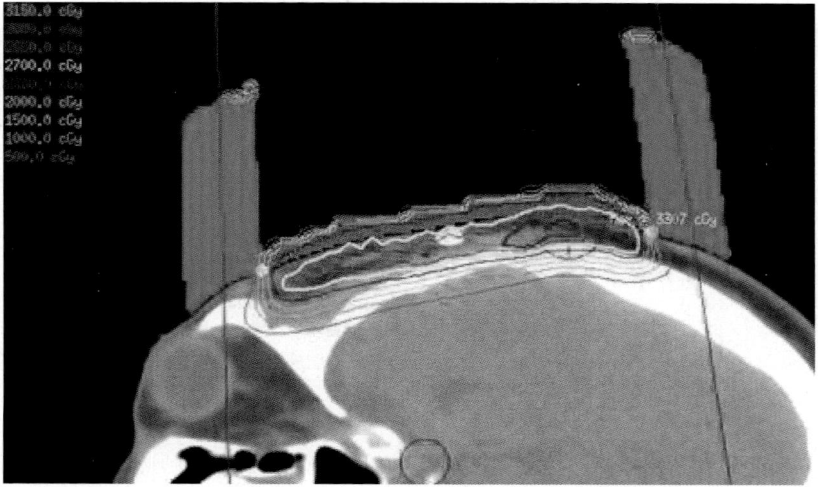

Figure 59.1: Sample RT treatment plan for a patient with a melanoma of the scalp. This patient was treated post-operatively with electrons to the tumor bed to a total dose of 30 Gy in 5 fractions. Note the 27 Gy isodose line in yellow which is used to evaluate target coverage. 30 Gy hotspots are seen in red.

SM 13-7

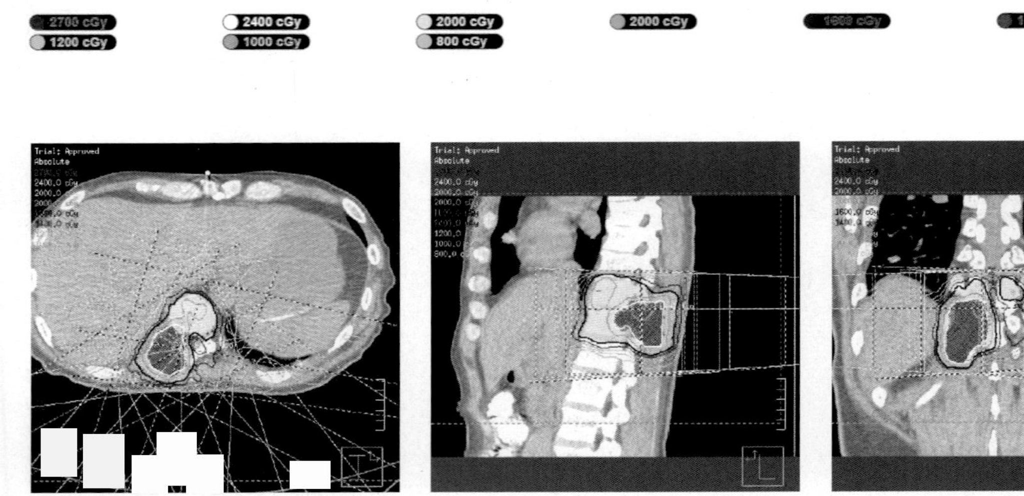

Figure 66.3: Representative treatment plan of a patient undergoing SSRS in axial, sagittal, and coronal (L→R) cross-sectional views. The CTV is highlighted in yellow color-wash and GTV in red. The blue isodose line represents 16 Gy, and white isodose line, 24 Gy. This patient was treated with a single fraction.

CCS0220